Penguin Education

# Health Economics

Edited by M. H. Cooper
and A. J. Culyer

Penguin Modern Economics Readings

*General Editor*

B. J. McCormick

*Advisory Board*

K. J. W. Alexander
R. W. Clower
G. Fisher
P. Robson
J. Spraos
H. Townsend

# Health Economics

**Selected Readings**

Edited by M. H. Cooper and A. J. Culyer

Penguin Books

Penguin Books Ltd, Harmondsworth,
Middlesex, England
Penguin Books Inc., 7110 Ambassador Road,
Baltimore, Md 21207, USA
Penguin Books Australia Ltd,
Ringwood, Victoria, Australia

First published 1973
This selection copyright © M. H. Cooper and A. J. Culyer, 1973
Introduction and notes copyright © M. H. Cooper and A. J. Culyer, 1973
Copyright acknowledgement for items in this volume
will be found on page 383

Made and printed in Great Britain by
Richard Clay (The Chaucer Press) Ltd,
Bungay, Suffolk
Set in Monotype Times

# Contents

# Introduction

As a subject for specialized economic study, health, or ill-health, is as yet only in its adolescence. An obvious indication of this lies in the fact that not one of the readings selected for reprinting in this volume belongs to a period earlier than the 1960s. Another is that major problem areas remain unresearched. Indeed, it may generally be said that there are currently many more questions than satisfactory answers.

Not all of this is due merely to the youth of the subject, for the nature of the area poses important problems of scruple, of analysis and of application. A person's health is an emotional and very personal matter. It is also of concern to other persons. The production and distribution of motor vehicles may appear to be 'obviously' in the economist's province, but the production and distribution of health care is less 'obviously' an economic matter. Health is 'special'. The doctor–patient relationship is not the same as the motor car manufacturer–customer relationship. Patients consult. Clients instruct. Customers order. A mystique surrounds the medical practitioner. He is accorded a special status in the community. In any case, is it not often said that economics is about prices whilst, at least under the British NHS, one pays scarcely any price for medical care?

One purpose of this selection is to show how economists have approached health service problems and have begun to carve out for themselves certain areas which at least partly, if not largely, demand the use of the economic box of tools. Indeed, the study of health problems has produced some new additions to the box. It is too early to pronounce definitively upon the usefulness of economic contributions or to assess the direction which professional economic interest is taking. One thing, however, does appear to be clear, and this is that the earlier preoccupation with rather rarified discussions of the best ways of organizing whole systems of health care – the so-called 'market versus the state' debate – is now in the past. The current trend is towards the study of the specific problems thrown up under various systems. The trend is towards empiricism, applying theory to solve real-world problems rather than engaging in abstract speculation.

The selection in this book reflects, we believe, this trend. Part One contains some of the major theoretical contributions in the field. Parts Two, Three and Four present a variety of different applications of economic analysis. The sorts of question which demand economic analysis in the health sector are: how much should a country spend on health services? How should its expenditure be financed? Is health expenditure an investment or is it consumption? What is the output of health care institutions? What is the most efficient combination of doctors, nurses, hospitals etc. in producing a given output? How many doctors, nurses, hospitals, etc. ought we to have today, next year, at the end of the century? What effects do the methods of payment of doctors, nurses, etc. have on their behaviour and attitudes? What is the demand for health care and what determines it? Is demand different from need? What effect does a change in one part of the health sector have upon the inputs and outputs of the rest? What contribution does better health make to the growth of GNP?

The answers to some of these questions are still very unsatisfactory and the answers to others barely exist, as is to be expected in a young subject. The reprinted papers will, however, give the reader the flavour of the economic approach and an idea of its strengths and weaknesses. One of its strengths is its lack of sentimentality. Economics takes it as axiomatic that not all can or will be done to give persons the full potential benefit of modern medical science. To do so would mean giving up too many other good things: housing, education, food and 'luxuries' that are not really luxuries any more. But in any case, better health, whether physical, mental or emotional, requires housing, education, food and 'luxuries'. Choices have therefore to be made and economics is the science of choice. Many people could benefit from a greater availability of kidney machines. We would all benefit from greater emphasis on preventive medicine. Many people are sicker, and die sooner than they need if more were done to help them. But do we 'need' more? Are these 'shortages' *really* shortages. We are, after all, also short of fillet steaks, holidays, clean air . . . in the same sense that we would like to have more. But would we like more regardless of the cost? In this sense, while fillet steaks and transplanted kidneys may rank differently in social and humanitarian priorities, the basic problem of choosing how much to make available and for whom is the same.

The economics of health derives entirely from this dilemma confronting society and economists believe they can help society arrive at better resolutions of the dilemma than might otherwise arise. For *operationality*, however, – to be *practically* useful – four general questions require answers. These four questions are not unique to the economic approach, for *any* method of making choices that is not entirely arbitrary requires answers to this quartet. They are:

1. What is the output of health services and how is it affected by other things?
2. How does society rank these outputs in its priority list?
3. What is required in the way of 'inputs' to produce any of the outputs?
4. What must society lose in providing the outputs?

In the case of health possibly more than any other economic good, the answers are very difficult. The problem of the 'output' – the most fundamental problem of all – has yet to be resolved satisfactorily. Is the output the numbers of patients treated? Patients treated successfully? (What is a 'successful' treatment?). Is it 'health'? (What *is* health?) Is it more working hours available? Can the knowledge that *people care* be part of the output? No single answer has yet been obtained. Even if there existed a measure of output – whether it is the output of your local kidney dialysis centre or of the entire national complex of health services – how is it to be valued? In a *narrow* economic sense there are certain obvious monetary gains from improved health. But in a wider (but equally economic) sense, what of the social and humanitarian value of a reduction in pain and suffering, of a mother restored fit and healthy to her children, of a dangerous psychotic successfully treated, of the love and sympathy so readily provided by the majority of the men and women who provide medical care? Even if the output were known and the social and humanitarian value can be assessed, how is it to be produced? There is no unique medical technology prescribing the inputs required in the treatment of each condition. Even the form of treatment itself may be in dispute by the medical experts. Finally, the social and humanitarian costs of providing the output present the same set of problems as the assessment of its social and humanitarian benefits. If one patient occupies a hospital bed and necessarily excludes another, what cost, in addition to the social costs of the inputs, has been incurred?

This volume is divided into four parts. In Part One some of the fundamental characteristics of medical care viewed as an economic good are surveyed. In a sense, Part One can be viewed as containing justifications for adopting the method of economics in an area where it has traditionally not been applied. The respects in which medical care is unique and different from other economic goods are identified and the implications of these special characteristics are explored. The rest of the book is more down to earth in that all the remaining contributions can be seen clearly as contributing towards a solution, or a method of solution, for some real policy problems. Part Two presents a selection of studies of particular problems: health as an investment in human capital akin to education and manpower training; the effects of good health on national output; the meaning and means of curing shortages of manpower; the interrelationships in a macro system of health services; the choice of least cost technique for treating patients with kidney disease. Part Three concentrates exclusively on the problems of hospitals. In particular, the readings selected here investigate the problems involved in developing a behavioural model of a hospital and of interpreting and using cost data. Part Four is devoted exclusively to a discussion of the value of human life, including the value of preventing births. Conceptually, it is probably the hardest part of the discussion to come to emotional terms with, for the economic view that life is not of infinite 'value' appears to assert something contrary to that which we all believe in our hearts.

Finally, in a book such as this, much has had to be omitted. The reader will find little extended discussion here of the health problems of the poor countries. There is little on the problems of health insurance firms. There is nothing from the health indicators literature. Most of the readings deal with personal health services rather than public health services. There is no descriptive material at all nor is there anything on the relationship between health spending and the social accounts or on comparative international expenditure on health. In our choice of readings we have been guided by a number of criteria. The most general one is that we have tried to reflect in our choice the emphasis that has been chiefly placed upon topics by the writers in the field. We have also, however, tried to present 'results' or conclusions as far as possible. Areas which have been no more than tentatively explored to date have been excluded. Thus, if the book appears patchy in its coverage, we believe that it is due to the patchy development of our adolescent subject. We hope, however, that the reader will agree that the marginal value of the items *included* exceeds that of those *excluded*. If this is true, then the volume will have served its purpose.

# Part One
# Economic Efficiency

The initial interest in health problems shown by
English-speaking economists concentrated very much on the
theoretical expectations that could be derived from an abstract
consideration of various ways in which it has been, and could
be, organized. There were probably two reasons for this: one
methodological and the other practical. The former derives
from a proper inclination, shared by most economists, to sort
out the appropriate theoretical framework in a general way
before applying it to specific problems. Facts have never
spoken for themselves. To give them meaning and to draw
inferences about them requires a theoretical or conceptual
framework. In health, this step has been thought of as
particularly important since many regard it as being a very
special case in which the economists' traditional 'box of tools'
was not readily applicable without special developments. The
second set of reasons derived from the impressions that
economists had of the way that health services operated in
their own countries. Some felt, for example, that the British
NHS left a great deal to be desired in terms of efficiency and
fairness. It was certainly characterized right from its inception
in 1948 with a concern – initially very optimistic but
subsequently pessimistic – about its costliness. On the other
side of the Atlantic many felt that the US system was wasteful
and unfair, denying proper care to many and beset by a
variety of oppressive restrictive practices by insurance
companies, hospitals and the medical profession.

Reading 1 in this selection is a classic by Kenneth Arrow,
who examined the actual US health care system in relation to a
hypothetically ideal market and found that some of the
characteristics of medical care that distinguish it from other
economic goods cause the actual resource allocation to fall
substantially short of the ideal. The conceptual framework

conceived by Arrow has proved of great value to economists working in the area though many of the specific inferences he drew from his analysis have been hotly disputed. The controversies that existed before Arrow's contribution as well as the sharpening up of the differences that existed among economists resulting from the contribution are surveyed and assessed in Reading 2 by Anthony Culyer. His general conclusion is that the whole of the debate on 'the market versus the state' which preoccupied so many in the early sixties cannot be resolved in *a priori* terms but that the conceptual framework of welfare economics can be useful in specific applications, by identifying the appropriate factors that make for good decision-making and improved resource allocation. In addition, this article claims that health care, though evidently not the same thing as other economic goods, is nevertheless capable of being treated by the traditional analytical apparatus, a view that has frequently been challenged in the past.

Reading 3 in Part One is a recent paper by Cotton Lindsay in which a new theoretical approach to the National Health Service is presented. In this paper, Lindsay faces up to an important feeling, frequently ignored by economists but evidently of prime significance in society, that everyone ought to have an equal right to life. By an exceedingly ingenious and simple change in the utility functions of individuals, Lindsay incorporates this aspect of the ethics of medical care into the mainstream of economic analysis, and shows that it has important implications for the form of organization chosen for producing and distributing health care to the community.

The most recent trend in health economics has been a healthy one (in our view) away from the purely *a priori* approach towards an integration of theory and specific real life problems. To those who regard the essential form of organization currently existing in any given country as being unlikely to be substantially changed, at least in the near future, this more empirical and specific interest is clearly the more useful if policy decisions are to be informed and affected by economists.

# 1 Kenneth J. Arrow

## The Welfare Economics of Medical Care[1]

Excerpt from Kenneth J. Arrow, 'Uncertainty and the welfare economics of medical care', *American Economic Review*, vol. 53, 1963, pp. 941–73.

### I Introduction: scope and method

This paper is an exploratory and tentative study of the specific differentia of medical care as the object of normative economics. It is contended here, on the basis of comparison of obvious characteristics of the medical-care industry with the norms of welfare economics, that the special economic problems of medical care can be explained as adaptations to the existence of uncertainty in the incidence of disease and in the efficacy of treatment.

It should be noted that the subject is the *medical-care industry*, not *health*. The causal factors in health are many, and the provision of medical care is only one. Particularly at low levels of income, other commodities such as nutrition, shelter, clothing, and sanitation may be much more significant. It is the complex of services that center about the physician, private and group practice, hospitals, and public health, which I propose to discuss.

The focus of discussion will be on the way the operation of the medical-care industry and the efficacy with which it satisfies the needs of society differ from a norm, if at all. The 'norm' that the economist usually uses for the purposes of such comparisons is the operation of a competitive model, that is, the flows of services that would be offered and purchased and the prices that would be paid for them if each individual in the market offered or purchased services at the going prices as if his decisions had no influence over them, and the going prices were such that the amounts of services which were available equalled the total amounts which other individuals were willing to purchase, with no imposed restrictions on supply or demand.

1. The author is Professor of Economics at Stanford University. He wishes to express his thanks for useful comments to F. Bator, R. Dorfman, V. Fuchs, Dr S. Gilson, R. Kessel, S. Mushkin, and C. R. Rorem. This paper was prepared under the sponsorship of the Ford Foundation as part of a series of papers on the economics of health, education, and welfare.

The interest in the competitive model stems partly from its presumed descriptive power and partly from its implications for economic efficiency. In particular, we can state the following well-known proposition (First Optimality Theorem). If a competitive equilibrium exists at all, and if all commodities relevant to costs or utilities are in fact priced in the market, then the equilibrium is necessarily *optimal* in the following precise sense (due to V. Pareto): There is no other allocation of resources to services which will make all participants in the market better off.

Both the conditions of this optimality theorem and the definition of optimality call for comment. A definition is just a definition, but when the *definiendum* is a word already in common use with highly favorable connotations, it is clear that we are really trying to be persuasive; we are implicitly recommending the achievement of optimal states (Little, 1950, pp. 71–4; Stevenson, 1945, pp. 210–17). It is reasonable enough to assert that a change in allocation which makes all participants better off is one that certainly should be made; this is a value judgment, not a descriptive proposition, but it is a very weak one. From this it follows that it is not desirable to put up with a non-optimal allocation. But it does not follow that if we are at an allocation which is optimal in the Pareto sense, we should not change to any other. We cannot indeed make a change that does not hurt someone; but we can still desire to change to another allocation if the change makes enough participants better off and by so much that we feel that the injury to others is not enough to offset the benefits. Such interpersonal comparisons are, of course, value judgments. The change, however, by the previous argument ought to be an optimal state; of course there are many possible states, each of which is optimal in the sense here used.

However, a value judgment on the desirability of each possible new distribution of benefits and costs corresponding to each possible reallocation of resources is not, in general, necessary. Judgments about the distribution can be made separately, in one sense, from those about allocation if certain conditions are fulfilled. Before stating the relevant proposition, it is necessary to remark that the competitive equilibrium achieved depends in good measure on the initial distribution of purchasing power, which consists of ownership of assets and skills that command a price on the market. A transfer of assets among individuals will, in general, change the final supplies of goods and services and the prices paid for them. Thus, a transfer of purchasing power from the well to the ill will increase the demand for medical services. This will manifest itself in the short run in an increase in the price of medical services and in the long run in an increase in the amount supplied.

With this in mind, the following statement can be made (Second Optimality Theorem): If there are no increasing returns in production, and if certain other minor conditions are satisfied, then every optimal state is a competitive equilibrium corresponding to some initial distribution of purchasing power. Operationally, the significance of this proposition is that if the conditions of the two optimality theorems are satisfied, and if the allocation mechanism in the real world satisfies the conditions for a competitive model, then social policy can confine itself to steps taken to alter the distribution of purchasing power. For any given distribution of purchasing power, the market will, under the assumptions made, achieve a competitive equilibrium which is necessarily optimal; and any optimal state is a competitive equilibrium corresponding to some distribution of purchasing power, so that any desired optimal state can be achieved.

The redistribution of purchasing power among individuals most simply takes the form of money: taxes and subsidies. The implications of such a transfer for individual satisfactions are, in general, not known in advance. But we can assume that society can *ex post* judge the distribution of satisfactions and, if deemed unsatisfactory, take steps to correct it by subsequent transfers. Thus, by successive approximations, a most preferred social state can be achieved, with resource allocation being handled by the market and public policy confined to the redistribution of money income.[2]

If, on the contrary, the actual market differs significantly from the competitive model, or if the assumptions of the two optimality theorems are not fulfilled, the separation of allocative and distributional procedures becomes, in most cases, impossible.[3]

2. The separation between allocation and distribution even under the above assumptions has glossed over problems in the execution of any desired redistribution policy; in practice, it is virtually impossible to find a set of taxes and subsidies that will not have an adverse effect on the achievement of an optimal state. But this discussion would take us even further afield than we have already gone.

3. The basic theorems of welfare economics alluded to so briefly above have been the subject of voluminous literature, but no thoroughly satisfactory statement covering both the theorems themselves and the significance of exceptions to them exists. The positive assertions of welfare

The first step then in the analysis of the medical-care market is the comparison between the actual market and the competitive model. The methodology of this comparison has been a recurrent subject of controversy in economics for over a century. Recently, Friedman (1953, pp. 3–43) has vigorously argued that the competitive or any other model should be tested solely by its ability to predict. In the context of competition, he comes close to arguing that prices and quantities are the only relevant data. This point of view is valuable in stressing that a certain amount of lack of realism in the assumptions of a model is no argument against its value. But the price–quantity implications of the competitive model for pricing are not easy to derive without major – and, in many cases, impossible – econometric efforts.

In this paper, the institutional organization and the observable mores of the medical profession are included among the data to be used in assessing the competitiveness of the medical-care market. I shall also examine the presence or absence of the preconditions for the equivalence of competitive equilibria and optimal states. The major competitive preconditions, in the sense used here, are three: the *existence* of competitive equilibrium, the *marketability* of all goods and services relevant to costs and utilities, and *non-increasing returns*. The first two, as we have seen, insure that competitive equilibrium is necessarily optimal; the third insures that every optimal state is the competitive equilibrium corresponding to some distribution of income (Koopmans, 1957, pp. 50–55). The first and third conditions are interrelated; indeed, non-increasing returns plus some additional conditions not restrictive in a modern economy imply the existence of a competitive equilibrium, i.e., imply that there will be some set of prices which will clear all markets (Koopmans, pp. 56–60; Debreu, 1959, ch. 5).

The concept of marketability is somewhat broader than the traditional divergence between private and social costs and benefits. The latter concept refers to cases in which the organization of the market does not require an individual to pay for costs that he imposes on others as the result of his actions or does not permit him to receive compensation for benefits he confers. In the medical field, the obvious example is the spread of communicable diseases. An individual who fails to be immunized not only risks

economics and their relation to the theory of competitive equilibrium are admirably covered in Koopmans (1957). The best summary of the various ways in which the theorems can fail to hold is probably Bator's (1958).

his own health, a disutility which presumably he has weighed against the utility of avoiding the procedure, but also that of others. In an ideal price system, there would be a price which he would have to pay to anyone whose health is endangered, a price sufficiently high so that the others would feel compensated; or, alternatively, there would be a price which would be paid to him by others to induce him to undergo the immunization procedure. Either system would lead to an optimal state, though the distributional implications would be different. It is, of course, not hard to see that such price systems could not, in fact, be practical; to approximate an optimal state it would be necessary to have collective intervention in the form of subsidy or tax or compulsion.

By the absence of marketability for an action which is identifiable, technologically possible, and capable of influencing some individual's welfare, for better or for worse, is meant here the failure of the existing market to provide a means whereby the services can be both offered and demanded upon payment of a price. Non-marketability may be due to intrinsic technological characteristics of the product which prevent a suitable price from being enforced, as in the case of communicable diseases, or it may be due to social or historical controls, such as those prohibiting an individual from selling himself into slavery. This distinction is, in fact, difficult to make precise, though it is obviously of importance for policy; for the present purposes, it will be sufficient to identify non-marketability with the observed absence of markets.

The instance of non-marketability with which we shall be most concerned is that of risk-bearing. The relevance of risk-bearing to medical care seems obvious; illness is to a considerable extent an unpredictable phenomenon. The ability to shift the risks of illness to others is worth a price which many are willing to pay. Because of pooling and of superior willingness and ability, others are willing to bear the risks. Nevertheless, as we shall see in greater detail, a great many risks are not covered, and indeed the markets for the services of risk-coverage are poorly developed or nonexistent. Why this should be so is explained in more detail in section IV *C* below; briefly, it is impossible to draw up insurance policies which will sufficiently distinguish among risks, particularly since observation of the results will be incapable of distinguishing between avoidable and unavoidable risks, so that incentives to avoid losses are diluted.

The optimality theorems discussed above are usually presented in the literature as referring only to conditions of certainty, but there is no difficulty in extending them to the case of risks, provided the additional services of risk-bearing are included with other commodities (see Allais, 1953; Arrow, 1953; Baudier, 1959; Debreu, 1959, 1960).

However, the variety of possible risks in the world is really staggering. The relevant commodities include, in effect, bets on all possible occurrences in the world which impinge upon utilities. In fact, many of these 'commodities', i.e., desired protection against many risks, are simply not available. Thus, a wide class of commodities is non-marketable, and a basic competitive precondition is not satisfied.[4]

There is a still more subtle consequence of the introduction of risk-bearing considerations. When there is uncertainty, information or knowledge becomes a commodity. Like other commodities, it has a cost of production and a cost of transmission, and so it is naturally not spread out over the entire population but concentrated among those who can profit most from it. (These costs may be measured in time or disutility as well as money.) But the demand for information is difficult to discuss in the rational terms usually employed. The value of information is frequently not known in any meaningful sense to the buyer; if, indeed, he knew enough to measure the value of information, he would know the information itself. But information, in the form of skilled care, is precisely what is being bought from most physicians, and, indeed, from most professionals. The elusive character of information as a commodity suggests that it departs considerably from the usual marketability assumptions about commodities.[5]

That risk and uncertainty are, in fact, significant elements in

4. It should also be remarked that in the presence of uncertainty, indivisibilities that are sufficiently small to create little difficulty for the existence and viability of competitive equilibrium may nevertheless give rise to a considerable range of increasing returns because of the operation of the law of large numbers. Since most objects of insurance (lives, fire hazards, etc.) have some element of indivisibility, insurance companies have to be above a certain size. But it is not clear that this effect is sufficiently great to create serious obstacles to the existence and viability of competitive equilibrium in practice.

5. One form of production of information is research. Not only does the product have unconventional aspects as a commodity, but it is also subject to increasing returns in use, since new ideas, once developed, can be used over and over without being consumed, and to difficulties of market control, since the cost of reproduction is usually much less than that of production. Hence, it is not surprising that a free enterprise economy will tend to underinvest in research; see Nelson (1959) and Arrow (1962).

medical care hardly needs argument. I will hold that virtually all the special features of this industry, in fact, stem from the prevalence of uncertainty.

The non-existence of markets for the bearing of some risks in the first instance reduces welfare for those who wish to transfer those risks to others for a certain price, as well as those who would find it profitable to take on the risk at such prices. But it also reduces the desire to render or consume services which have risky consequences; in technical language, these commodities are complementary to risk-bearing. Conversely, the production and consumption of commodities and services with little risk attached act as substitutes for risk-bearing and are encouraged by market failure there with respect to risk-bearing. Thus the observed commodity pattern will be affected by the non-existence of other markets.

The failure of one or more of the competitive preconditions has as its most immediate and obvious consequence a reduction in welfare below that obtainable from existing resources and technology, in the sense of a failure to reach an optimal state in the sense of Pareto. But more can be said. I propose here the view that, when the market fails to achieve an optimal state, society will, to some extent at least, recognize the gap, and non-market social institutions will arise attempting to bridge it.[6] Certainly this process is not necessarily conscious; nor is it uniformly successful in approaching more closely to optimality when the entire range of consequences is considered. It has always been a favorite activity of economists to point out that actions which on their face achieve a desirable goal may have less obvious consequences, particularly over time, which more than offset the original gains.

But it is contended here that the special structural characteristics of the medical-care market are largely attempts to overcome the lack of optimality due to the non-marketability of the bearing of suitable risks and the imperfect marketability of information. These compensatory institutional changes, with some reinforcement from usual profit motives, largely explain the observed non-competitive behavior of the medical-care market, behavior

6. An important current situation in which normal market relations have had to be greatly modified in the presence of great risks is the production and procurement of modern weapons; see Peck and Scherer (1962, pp. 581–2) (I am indebted for this reference to V. Fuchs) and Alchian *et al.* 1958, pp. 71–5).

which, in itself, interferes with optimality. The social adjustment towards optimality thus puts obstacles in its own path.

The doctrine that society will seek to achieve optimality by non-market means if it cannot achieve them in the market is not novel. Certainly, the government, at least in its economic activities, is usually implicitly or explicitly held to function as the agency which substitutes for the market's failure (Baumol, 1952). I am arguing here that in some circumstances other social institutions will step into the optimality gap, and that the medical-care industry, with its variety of special institutions, some ancient, some modern, exemplifies this tendency.

It may be useful to remark here that a good part of the preference for redistribution expressed in government taxation and expenditure policies and private charity can be reinterpreted as desire for insurance. It is noteworthy that virtually nowhere is there a system of subsidies that has as its aim simply an equalization of income. The subsidies or other governmental help go to those who are disadvantaged in life by events the incidence of which is popularly regarded as unpredictable: the blind, dependent children, the medically indigent. Thus, optimality, in a context which includes risk-bearing, includes much that appears to be motivated by distributional value judgments when looked at in a narrower context.[7]

This methodological background gives rise to the following plan for this paper. Section II is a catalogue of stylized generalizations about the medical-care market which differentiate it from the usual commodity markets. In Section III the behavior of the market is compared with that of the competitive model which disregards the fact of uncertainty. In Section IV, the medical-care market is compared, both as to behavior and as to preconditions, with the ideal competitive market that takes account of uncertainty; an attempt will be made to demonstrate that the characteristics outlined in Section II can be explained either as the result of deviations from the competitive preconditions or as attempts to compensate by other institutions for these failures. The discussion is not designed to be definitive, but provocative. In particular, I have been chary about drawing policy inferences; to a considerable extent, they depend on further research, for which the present paper is intended to provide a framework.

7. Since writing the above, I find that Buchanan and Tullock (1962, ch. 13) have argued that all redistribution can be interpreted as 'income insurance'.

## II A survey of the special characteristics of the medical-care market[8]

This section will list selectively some characteristics of medical care which distinguish it from the usual commodity of economics textbooks. The list is not exhaustive, and it is not claimed that the characteristics listed are individually unique to this market. But, taken together, they do establish a special place for medical care in economic analysis.

### A The nature of demand

The most obvious distinguishing characteristics of an individual's demand for medical services is that it is not steady in origin as, for example, for food or clothing, but irregular and unpredictable. Medical services, apart from preventive services, afford satisfaction only in the event of illness, a departure from the normal state of affairs. It is hard, indeed, to think of another commodity of significance in the average budget of which this is true. A portion of legal services, devoted to defense in criminal trials or to lawsuits, might fall in this category but the incidence is surely very much lower (and, of course, there are, in fact, strong institutional similarities between the legal and medical-care markets).[9]

In addition, the demand for medical services is associated, with a considerable probability, with an assault on personal integrity. There is some risk of death and a more considerable risk of impairment of full functioning. In particular, there is a major potential for loss or reduction of earning ability. The risks are not by themselves unique; food is also a necessity, but avoidance of deprivation of food can be guaranteed with sufficient income, where the same cannot be said of avoidance of illness. Illness is, thus, not only risky but a costly risk in itself, apart from the cost of medical care.

### B Expected behavior of the physician

It is clear from everyday observation that the behavior expected of sellers of medical care is different from that of business men in general. These expectations are relevant because medical care

8. For an illuminating survey to which I am much indebted, see S. Mushkin (1958).

9. In governmental demand, military power is an example of a service used only irregularly and unpredictably. Here too, special institutional and professional relations have emerged, though the precise social structure is different for reasons that are not hard to analyse.

belongs to the category of commodities for which the product and the activity of production are identical. In all such cases, the customer cannot test the product before consuming it, and there is an element of trust in the relation.[10] But the ethically understood restrictions on the activities of a physician are much more severe than on those of, say, a barber. His behavior is supposed to be governed by a concern for the customer's welfare which would not be expected of a salesman. In Parsons's terms, there is a 'collectivity-orientation', which distinguishes medicine and other professions from business, where self-interest on the part of participants is the accepted norm (Parsons, 1951, p. 463).

A few illustrations will indicate the degree of difference between the behavior expected of physicians and that expected of the typical businessman.[11] (1) Advertising and overt price competition are virtually eliminated among physicians. (2) Advice given by physicians as to further treatment by himself or others is supposed to be completely divorced from self-interest. (3) It is at least claimed that treatment is dictated by the objective needs of the case and not limited by financial considerations.[12] While the ethical compulsion is surely not as absolute in fact as it is in theory, we can hardly suppose that it has no influence over resource allocation in this area. Charity treatment in one form or another does exist because of this tradition about human rights to adequate medical care.[13] (4) The physician is relied on as an expert in certifying to the existence of illnesses and injuries for

10. Even with material commodities, testing is never so adequate that all elements of implicit trust can be eliminated. Of course, over the long run, experience with the quality of product of a given seller provides a check on the possibility of trust.

11. I am indebted to Herbert Klarman of Johns Hopkins University for some of the points discussed in this and the following paragraph.

12. The belief that the ethics of medicine demands treatment independent of the patient's ability to pay is strongly ingrained. Such a perceptive observer as René Dubos has made the remark that the high cost of anticoagulants restricts their use and may contradict classical medical ethics, as though this were an unprecedented phenomenon. (Dubos, 1959, p. 419). 'A time *may come* when medical ethics will have to be considered in the harsh light of economics' (emphasis added). Of course, this expectation amounts to ignoring the scarcity of medical resources; one has only to have been poor to realize the error. We may confidently assume that price and income do have some consequences for medical expenditures.

13. A needed piece of research is a study of the exact nature of the variations of medical care received and medical care paid for as income rises. (The relevant income concept also needs study.) For this purpose, some disaggregation is needed; differences in hospital care which are essentially

various legal and other purposes. It is socially expected that his concern for the correct conveying of information will, when appropriate, outweigh his desire to please his customers (Field, 1957, ch. 9).

Departure from the profit motive is strikingly manifested by the overwhelming predominance of non-profit over proprietary hospitals.[14] The hospital *per se* offers services not too different from those of a hotel, and it is certainly not obvious that the profit motive will not lead to a more efficient supply. The explanation may lie either on the supply side or on that of demand. The simplest explanation is that public and private subsidies decrease the cost to the patient in non-profit hospitals. A second possibility is that the association of profit-making with the supply of medical services arouses suspicion and antagonism on the part of patients and referring physicians, so they do prefer non-profit institutions. Either explanation implies a preference on the part of some group, whether donors or patients, against the profit motive in the supply of hospital services.[15]

Conformity to collectivity-oriented behavior is especially important since it is a commonplace that the physician–patient relation affects the quality of the medical care product. A pure cash nexus would be inadequate; if nothing else, the patient expects that the same physician will normally treat him on successive occasions. This expectation is strong enough to persist even in the Soviet Union, where medical care is nominally removed from the market place (Field, 1957, pp. 194–6). That purely psychic interactions between physician and patient have effects which are objectively indistinguishable in kind from the effects of medication is evidenced by the use of the placebo as a control in medical experimentation; see Shapiro (1960).

---

matters of comfort should, in the above view, be much more responsive to income than, e.g., drugs.

14. About 3 per cent of beds were in proprietary hospitals in 1958, against 30 per cent in voluntary non-profit, and the remainder in federal, state, and local hospitals; see (Somers and Somers, 1961, p. 60).

15. C. R. Rorem has pointed out to me some further factors in this analysis. (1) Given the social intention of helping all patients without regard to immediate ability to pay, economies of scale would dictate a predominance of community-sponsored hospitals. (2) Some proprietary hospitals will tend to control total costs to the patient more closely, including the fees of physicians, who will therefore tend to prefer community-sponsored hospitals.

## C Product uncertainty

Uncertainty as to the quality of the product is perhaps more intense here than in any other important commodity. Recovery from disease is as unpredictable as is its incidence. In most commodities, the possibility of learning from one's own experience or that of others is strong because there is an adequate number of trials. In the case of severe illness, that is, in general, not true; the uncertainty due to inexperience is added to the intrinsic difficulty of prediction. Further, the amount of uncertainty, measured in terms of utility variability, is certainly much greater for medical care in severe cases than for, say, houses or automobiles, even though these are also expenditures sufficiently infrequent so that there may be considerable residual uncertainty.

Further, there is a special quality to the uncertainty; it is very different on the two sides of the transaction. Because medical knowledge is so complicated, the information possessed by the physician as to the consequences and possibilities of treatment is necessarily very much greater than that of the patient, or at least so it is believed by both parties.[16] Further, both parties are aware of this informational inequality, and their relation is colored by this knowledge.

To avoid misunderstanding, observe that the difference in information relevant here is a difference in information as to the consequence of a purchase of medical care. There is always an inequality of information as to production methods between the producer and the purchaser of any commodity, but in most cases the customer may well have as good or nearly as good an understanding of the utility of the product as the producer.

## D Supply conditions

In competitive theory, the supply of a commodity is governed by the net return from its production compared with the return derivable from the use of the same resources elsewhere. There are several significant departures from this theory in the case of medical care.

Most obviously, entry to the profession is restricted by licensing. Licensing, of course, restricts supply and therefore increases

16. Without trying to assess the present situation, it is clear in retrospect that at some point in the past the actual differential knowledge possessed by physicians may not have been much. But from the economic point of view, it is the subjective belief of both parties, as manifested in their market behavior, that is relevant.

the cost of medical care. It is defended as guaranteeing a minimum of quality. Restriction of entry by licensing occurs in most professions, including barbering and undertaking.

A second feature is perhaps even more remarkable. The cost of medical education today is high and, according to the usual figures, is borne only to a minor extent by the student. Thus, the private benefits to the entering student considerably exceed the costs. (It is, however, possible that research costs, not properly chargeable to education, swell the apparent difference.) This subsidy should, in principle, cause a fall in the price of medical services, which, however, is offset by rationing through limited entry to schools and through elimination of students during the medical-school career. These restrictions basically render superfluous the licensing, except in regard to graduates of foreign schools.

The special role of educational institutions in simultaneously subsidizing and rationing entry is common to all professions requiring advanced training.[17] It is a striking and insufficiently remarked phenomenon that such an important part of resource allocation should be performed by non-profit-oriented agencies.

Since this last phenomenon goes well beyond the purely medical aspect, we will not dwell on it longer here except to note that the anomaly is most striking in the medical field. Educational costs tend to be far higher there than in any other branch of professional training. While tuition is the same, or only slightly higher, so that the subsidy is much greater, at the same time the earnings of physicians rank highest among professional groups, so there would not at first blush seem to be any necessity for special inducements to enter the profession. Even if we grant that, for reasons unexamined here, there is a social interest in subsidized professional education, it is not clear why the rate of subsidization should differ among professions. One might expect that the tuition costs of medical students would be higher than that of other students.

The high cost of medical education in the United States is itself a reflection of the quality standards imposed by the American Medical Association since the Flexner Report, and it is, I believe, only since then that the subsidy element in medical education has become significant. Previously, many medical schools paid their way or even yielded a profit.

17. The degree of subsidy in different branches of professional education is worthy of a major research effort.

Another interesting feature of limitation on entry to subsidized education is the extent of individual preferences concerning the social welfare, as manifested by contributions to private universities. But whether support is public or private, the important point is that both the quality and the quantity of the supply of medical care are being strongly influenced by social non-market forces.[18]

One striking consequence of the control of quality is the restriction on the range offered. If many qualities of a commodity are possible, it would usually happen in a competitive market that many qualities will be offered on the market, at suitably varying prices, to appeal to different tastes and incomes. Both the licensing laws and the standards of medical-school training have limited the possibilities of alternative qualities of medical care. The declining ratio of physicians to total employees in the medical-care industry shows that substitution of less trained personnel, technicians, and the like, is not prevented completely, but the central role of the highly trained physician is not affected at all.[19]

### E Pricing practices

The unusual pricing practices and attitudes of the medical profession are well known: extensive price discrimination by income (with an extreme of zero prices for sufficiently indigent patients) and, formerly, a strong insistence on fee for services as against such alternatives as prepayment.

The opposition to prepayment is closely related to an even stronger opposition to closed-panel practice (contractual arrangements which bind the patient to a particular group of physicians). Again these attitudes seem to differentiate professions from business. Prepayment and closed-panel plans are virtually non-

18. Strictly speaking, there are four variables in the market for physicians: price, quality of entering students, quality of education and quantity. The basic market forces, demand for medical services and supply of entering students, determine two relations among the four variables. Hence, if the non-market forces determine the last two, market forces will determine price and quality of entrants. The supply of PhD's is similarly governed, but there are other conditions in the market which are much different, especially on the demand side.

19. Today only the Soviet Union offers an alternative lower level of medical personnel, the feldshers, who practice primarily in the rural districts (the institution dates back to the eighteenth century). According to Field (1957, pp. 98–100, 132–3), there is clear evidence of strain in the relations between physicians and feldshers, but it is not certain that the feldshers will gradually disappear as physicians grow in numbers.

existent in the legal profession. In ordinary business, on the other hand, there exists a wide variety of exclusive service contracts involving sharing of risks; it is assumed that competition will select those which satisfy needs best.[20]

The problems of implicit and explicit price-fixing should also be mentioned. Price competition is frowned on. Arrangements of this type are not uncommon in service industries, and they have not been subjected to antitrust action. How important this is is hard to assess. It has been pointed out many times that the apparent rigidity of so-called administered prices considerably understates the actual flexibility. Here, too, if physicians find themselves with unoccupied time, rates are likely to go down, openly or covertly; if there is insufficient time for the demand, rates will surely rise. The 'ethics' of price competition may decrease the flexibility of price responses, but probably that is all.

## III Comparisons with the competitive model under certainty
### A Non-marketable commodities

As already noted, the diffusion of communicable diseases provides an obvious example of non-market interactions. But from a theoretical viewpoint, the issues are well understood, and there is little point in expanding on this theme. (This should not be interpreted as minimizing the contribution of public health to welfare; there is every reason to suppose that it is considerably more important than all other aspects of medical care.)

Beyond this special area there is a more general interdependence, the concern of individuals for the health of others. The economic manifestations of this taste are to be found in individual donations to hospitals and to medical education, as well as in the widely accepted responsibilities of government in this area. The taste for improving the health of others appears to be stronger than for improving other aspects of their welfare.[21]

In interdependencies generated by concern for the welfare of others there is always a theoretical case for collective action if each participant derives satisfaction from the contributions of all.

20. The law does impose some limits on risk-shifting in contracts, for example, its general refusal to honor exculpatory clauses.

21. There may be an identification problem in this observation. If the failure of the market system is, or appears to be, greater in medical care than in, say, food an individual otherwise equally concerned about the two aspects of others' welfare may prefer to help in the first.

## B Increasing returns

Problems associated with increasing returns play some role in allocation of resources in the medical field, particularly in areas of low density or low income. Hospitals show increasing returns up to a point; specialists and some medical equipment constitute significant indivisibilities. In many parts of the world the individual physician may be a large unit relative to demand. In such cases it can be socially desirable to subsidize the appropriate medical-care unit. The appropriate mode of analysis is much the same as for water-resource projects. Increasing returns are hardly apt to be a significant problem in general practice in large cities in the United States, and improved transportation to some extent reduces their importance elsewhere.

## C Entry

The most striking departure from competitive behavior is restriction on entry to the field, as discussed in II $D$ above. Friedman and Kuznets (1945, pp. 118–37), in a detailed examination of the pre-Second World War data, have argued that the higher income of physicians could be attributed to this restriction (see Noyes in Friedman and Kuznets, pp. 407–10).

There is some evidence that the demand for admission to medical school has dropped (as indicated by the number of applicants per place and the quality of those admitted), so that the number of medical-school places is not as significant a barrier to entry as in the early 1950s (US Department of Health, Education and Welfare, 1959, pp. 14–15). But it certainly has operated over the past and it is still operating to a considerable extent today. It has, of course, constituted a direct and unsubtle restriction on the supply of medical care.

There are several considerations that must be added to help evaluate the importance of entry restrictions: (1) Additional entrants would be, in general, of lower quality; hence, the addition to the supply of medical care, properly adjusted for quality, is less than purely quantitative calculations would show.[22] (2) To achieve genuinely competitive conditions, it would be necessary not only

22. It might be argued that the existence of racial discrimination in entrance has meant that some of the rejected applicants are superior to some accepted. However, there is no necessary connection between an increase in the number of entrants and a reduction in racial discrimination; so long as there is excess demand for entry, discrimination can continue unabated and new entrants will be inferior to those previously accepted.

to remove numerical restrictions on entry but also to remove the subsidy in medical education. Like any other producer, the physician should bear all the costs of production, including, in this case, education.[23] It is not so clear that this change would not keep even unrestricted entry down below the present level. (3) To some extent, the effect of making tuition carry the full cost of education will be to create too few entrants, rather than too many. Given the imperfections of the capital market, loans for this purpose to those who do not have the cash are difficult to obtain. The lender really has no security. The obvious answer is some form of insured loans, as has frequently been argued; not too much ingenuity would be needed to create a credit system for medical (and other branches of higher) education. Under these conditions the cost would still constitute a deterrent, but one to be compared with the high future incomes to be obtained.

If entry were governed by ideal competitive conditions, it may be that the quantity on balance would be increased, though this conclusion is not obvious. The average quality would probably fall, even under an ideal credit system, since subsidy plus selected entry draw some highly qualified individuals who would otherwise get into other fields. The decline in quality is not an overall social loss, since it is accompanied by increase in quality in other fields of endeavor; indeed, if demands accurately reflected utilities, there would be a net social gain through a switch to competitive entry.[24]

There is a second aspect of entry in which the contrast with competitive behavior is, in many respects, even sharper. It is the exclusion of many imperfect substitutes for physicians. The licensing laws, though they do not effectively limit the number of physicians, do exclude all others from engaging in any one of the activities known as medical practice. As a result, costly physician time may be employed at specific tasks for which only a small fraction of their training is needed, and which could be performed by others less well trained and therefore less expensive. One might expect immunization centers, privately operated, but not necessarily requiring the services of doctors.

In the competitive model without uncertainty, consumers are

23. One problem here is that the tax laws do not permit depreciation of professional education, so that there is a discrimination against this form of investment.

24. To anticipate later discussion, this condition is not necessarily fulfilled. When it comes to quality choices, the market may be inaccurate.

presumed to be able to distinguish qualities of the commodities they buy. Under this hypothesis, licensing would be, at best, superfluous and exclude those from whom consumers would not buy anyway; but it might exclude too many.

## D Pricing

The pricing practices of the medical industry (see II E above) depart sharply from the competitive norm. As Kessel (1958) has pointed out with great vigor, not only is price discrimination incompatible with the competitive model, but its preservation in the face of the large number of physicians is equivalent to a collective monopoly. In the past, the opposition to prepayment plans has taken distinctly coercive forms, certainly transcending market pressures, to say the least.

Kessel has argued that price discrimination is designed to maximize profits along the classic lines of discriminating monopoly and that organized medical opposition to prepayment was motivated by the desire to protect these profits. In principle, prepayment schemes are compatible with discrimination, but in practice they do not usually discriminate. I do not believe the evidence that the actual scale of discrimination is profit-maximizing is convincing. In particular, note that for any monopoly, discriminating or otherwise, the elasticity of demand in each market at the point of maximum profits is greater than one. But it is almost surely true for medical care that the price elasticity of demand for all income levels is less than one. That price discrimination by income is not completely profit-maximizing is obvious in the extreme case of charity; Kessel argues that this represents an appeasement of public opinion. But this already shows the incompleteness of the model and suggests the relevance and importance of social and ethical factors.

Certainly one important part of the opposition to prepayment was its close relation to closed-panel plans. Prepayment is a form of insurance, and naturally the individual physician did not wish to assume the risks. Pooling was intrinsically involved, and this strongly motivates, as we shall discuss further in section IV below, control over prices and benefits. The simplest administrative form is the closed panel; physicians involved are, in effect, the insuring agent. From this point of view, Blue Cross solved the prepayment problem by universalizing the closed panel.

The case that price discrimination by income is a form of profit maximization which was zealously defended by opposition to fees for service seems far from proven. But it remains true that this price discrimination, for whatever cause, is a source of non-optimality. Hypothetically, it means everyone would be better off if prices were made equal for all, and the rich compensated the poor for the changes in the relative positions. The importance of this welfare loss depends on the actual amount of discrimination and on the elasticities of demand for medical services by the different income groups. If the discussion is simplified by considering only two income levels, rich and poor, and if the elasticity of demand by either one is zero, then no reallocation of medical services will take place and the initial situation is optimal. The only effect of a change in price will be the redistribution of income as between the medical profession and the group with the zero elasticity of demand. With low elasticities of demand, the gain will be small. To illustrate, suppose the price of medical care to the rich is double that to the poor, the medical expenditures by the rich are 20 per cent of those by the poor, and the elasticity of demand for both classes is 0·5; then the net social gain due to the abolition of discrimination is slightly over 1 per cent of previous medical expenditures.[25]

25. It is assumed that there are two classes, rich and poor; the price of medical services to the rich is twice that to the poor, medical expenditures by the rich are 20 per cent of those by the poor, and the elasticity of demand for medical services is 0·5 for both classes. Let us choose our quantity and monetary units so that the quantity of medical services consumed by the poor and the price they pay are both one. Then the rich purchase 0·1 unit of medical services at a price of two. Given the assumption about the elasticities of demand, the demand function of the rich is $D_R(p) = 0.14\,p^{-0.5}$ and that of the poor is $D_P(p) = p^{-0.5}$. The supply of medical services is assumed fixed and therefore must equal 1·1. If price discrimination were abolished, the equilibrium price, $\bar{p}$, must satisfy the relation

$$D_R(\bar{p}) + D_P(\bar{p}) = 1.1$$

and therefore $\bar{p} = 1.07$. The quantities of medical care purchased by the rich and poor, respectively, would be $D_R(\bar{p}) = 0.135$ and $D_P(\bar{p}) = 0.965$.

The inverse demand functions, the price to be paid corresponding to any given quantity, are $d_R(q) = 0.02/q^2$, and $d_P(q) = 1/q^2$. Therefore, the consumers' surplus to the rich generated by the change is

$$\int_{0.1}^{0.135} (0.02/q^2)dq - \bar{p}(0.135 - 0.1) \qquad\qquad 1$$

and similarly the loss in consumers' surplus by the poor is:

$$\int_{0.965}^{1} (1/q^2)dq - \bar{p}(1 - 0.965) \qquad\qquad 2$$

If 2 is subtracted from 1, the second terms cancel, and the aggregate increase in consumers' surplus is 0·0156, or a little over 1 per cent of the initial expenditures.

The issues involved in the opposition to prepayment, the other major anomaly in medical pricing, are not meaningful in the world of certainty and will be discussed below.

## IV Comparison with the ideal competitive model under uncertainty
### A Introduction

In this section we will compare the operations of the actual medical-care market with those of an ideal system in which not only the usual commodities and services but also insurance policies against all conceivable risks are available.[26] Departures consist for the most part of insurance policies that might conceivably be written, but are in fact not. Whether these potential commodities are non-marketable, or, merely because of some imperfection in the market, are not actually marketed, is a somewhat fine point.

To recall what has already been said in section I, there are two kinds of risks involved in medical care: the risk of becoming ill, and the risk of total or incomplete or delayed recovery. The loss due to illness is only partially the cost of medical care. It also consists of discomfort and loss of productive time during illness, and, in more serious cases, death or prolonged deprivation of normal function. From the point of view of the welfare economics of uncertainty, both losses are risks against which individuals would like to insure. The non-existence of suitable insurance policies for either risk implies a loss of welfare.

### B The theory of ideal insurance

In this section, the basic principles of an optimal regime for risk-bearing will be presented. For illustration, reference will usually be made to the case of insurance against cost in medical care. The principles are equally applicable to any of the risks. There is no single source to which the reader can be easily referred, though I think the principles are at least reasonably well understood.

As a basis for the analysis, the assumption is made that each individual acts so as to maximize the expected value of a utility function. If we think of utility as attached to income, then the

26. A striking illustration of the desire for security in medical care is provided by the expressed preferences of *émigrés* from the Soviet Union as between Soviet medical practice and German or American practice; see Field (1957, ch. 12). Those in Germany preferred the German system to the Soviet, but those in the United States preferred (in a ratio of 3 to 1) the Soviet system. The reasons given boil down to the certainty of medical care, independent of income or health fluctuations.

costs of medical care act as a random deduction from this income, and it is the expected value of the utility of income after medical costs that we are concerned with. (Income after medical costs is the ability to spend money on other objects which give satisfaction. We presuppose that illness is not a source of satisfaction in itself; to the extent that it is a source of dissatisfaction, the illness should enter into the utility function as a separate variable.) The expected-utility hypothesis, due originally to Daniel Bernoulli (1738), is plausible and is the most analytically manageable of all hypotheses that have been proposed to explain behavior under uncertainty. In any case, the results to follow probably would not be significantly affected by moving to another mode of analysis.

It is further assumed that individuals are normally risk-averters. In utility terms, this means that they have a diminishing marginal utility of income. This assumption may reasonably be taken to hold for most of the significant affairs of life for a majority of people, but the presence of gambling provides some difficulty in the full application of this view. It follows from the assumption of risk aversion that if an individual is given a choice between a probability distribution of income, with a given mean $m$, and the certainty of the income $m$, he would prefer the latter. Suppose, therefore, an agency, a large insurance company plan, or the government, stands ready to offer insurance against medical costs on an actuarially fair basis; that is, if the costs of medical care are a random variable with mean $m$, the company will charge a premium $m$, and agree to indemnify the individual for all medical costs. Under these circumstances, the individual will certainly prefer to take out a policy and will have a welfare gain thereby.

Will this be a social gain? Obviously yes, if the insurance agent is suffering no social loss. Under the assumption that medical risks on different individuals are basically independent, the pooling of them reduces the risk involved to the insurer to relatively small proportions. In the limit, the welfare loss, even assuming risk aversion on the part of the insurer, would vanish and there is a net social gain which may be of quite substantial magnitude. In fact, of course, the pooling of risks does not go to the limit; there is only a finite number of them and there may be some interdependence among the risks due to epidemics and the like. But then a premium, perhaps slightly above the actuarial level, would be sufficient to offset this welfare loss. From the point of view of the individual, since he has a strict preference for the actuarially fair policy over assuming the risks himself, he will still have a preference for an actuarially unfair policy, provided, of course, that it is not too unfair.

In addition to a residual degree of risk aversion by insurers, there are other reasons for the loading of the premium (i.e., an excess of premium over the actuarial value). Insurance involves administrative costs. Also, because of the irregularity of payments there is likely to be a cost of capital tied up. Suppose, to take a simple case, the insurance company is not willing to sell any insurance policy that a consumer wants but will charge a fixed-percentage loading above the actuarial value for its premium. Then it can be shown that the most preferred policy from the point of view of an individual is a coverage with a deductible amount; that is, the insurance policy provides 100 per cent coverage for all medical costs in excess of some fixed-dollar limit. If, however, the insurance company has some degree of risk aversion, its loading may also depend on the degree of uncertainty of the risk. In that case, the Pareto optimal policy will involve some element of co-insurance, i.e., the coverage for costs over the minimum limit will be some fraction less than 100 per cent (for proofs of these statements, see Appendix).

These results can also be applied to the hypothetical concept of insurance against failure to recover from illness. For simplicity, let us assume that the cost of failure to recover is regarded purely as a money cost, either simply productive opportunities foregone or, more generally, the money equivalent of all dissatisfactions. Suppose further that, given that a person is ill, the expected value of medical care is greater than its cost; that is, the expected money value attributable to recovery with medical help is greater than resources devoted to medical help. However, the recovery, though on the average beneficial, is uncertain; in the absence of insurance a risk-averter may well prefer not to take a chance on further impoverishment by buying medical care. A suitable insurance policy would, however, mean that he paid nothing if he doesn't benefit; since the expected value is greater than the cost, there would be a net social gain.[27]

### C Problems of insurance

*1. The moral hazard.* The welfare case for insurance policies of all sorts is overwhelming. It follows that the government should undertake insurance in those cases where this market, for what-

27. It is a popular belief that the Chinese, at one time, paid their physicians when well but not when sick.

ever reason, has failed to emerge. Nevertheless, there are a number of significant practical limitations on the use of insurance. It is important to understand them, though I do not believe that they alter the case for the creation of a much wider class of insurance policies than now exists.

One of the limits which has been much stressed in insurance literature is the effect of insurance on incentives. What is desired in the case of insurance is that the event against which insurance is taken be out of the control of the individual. Unfortunately, in real life this separation can never be made perfectly. The outbreak of fire in one's house or business may be largely uncontrollable by the individual, but the probability of fire is somewhat influenced by carelessness, and of course arson is a possibility, if an extreme one. Similarly, in medical policies the cost of medical care is not completely determined by the illness suffered by the individual but depends on the choice of a doctor and his willingness to use medical services. It is frequently observed that widespread medical insurance increases the demand for medical care. Co-insurance provisions have been introduced into many major medical policies to meet this contingency as well as the risk aversion of the insurance companies.

To some extent the professional relationship between physician and patient limits the normal hazard in various forms of medical insurance. By certifying to the necessity of given treatment or the lack thereof, the physician acts as a controlling agent on behalf of the insurance companies. Needless to say, it is a far from perfect check; the physicians themselves are not under any control and it may be convenient for them or pleasing to their patients to prescribe more expensive medication, private nurses, more frequent treatments, and other marginal variations of care. It is probably true that hospitalization and surgery are more under the casual inspection of others than is general practice and therefore less subject to moral hazard; this may be one reason why insurance policies in those fields have been more widespread.

2. *Alternative methods of insurance payment.* It is interesting that no less than three different methods of coverage of the costs of medical care have arisen: prepayment, indemnities according to a fixed schedule, and insurance against costs, whatever they may be. In prepayment plans, insurance in effect is paid in kind – that is, directly in medical services. The other two forms both involve cash payments to the beneficiary, but in the one case the amounts

to be paid involving a medical contingency are fixed in advance, while in the other the insurance carrier pays all the costs, whatever they may be, subject, of course, to provisions like deductibles and co-insurance.

In hypothetically perfect markets these three forms of insurance would be equivalent. The indemnities stipulated would, in fact, equal the market price of the services, so that value to the insured would be the same if he were to be paid the fixed sum or the market price or were given the services free. In fact, of course, insurance against full costs and prepayment plans both offer insurance against uncertainty as to the price of medical services, in addition to uncertainty about their needs. Further, by their mode of compensation to the physician, prepayment plans are inevitably bound up with closed panels so that the freedom of choice of the physician by the patient is less than it would be under a scheme more strictly confined to the provision of insurance. These remarks are tentative, and the question of coexistence of the different schemes should be a fruitful subject for investigation.

*3. Third-party control over payments.* The moral hazard in physicians' control noted in paragraph one above shows itself in those insurance schemes where the physician has the greatest control, namely, major medical insurance. Here there has been a marked rise in expenditures over time. In prepayment plans, where the insurance and medical services are supplied by the same group, the incentive to keep medical costs to a minimum is strongest. In the plans of the Blue Cross group, there has developed a conflict of interest between the insurance carrier and the medical-service supplier, in this case particularly the hospital.

The need for third-party control is reinforced by another aspect of the moral hazard. Insurance removes the incentive on the part of individuals, patients and physicians to shop around for better prices for hospitalization and surgical care. The market forces, therefore, tend to be replaced by direct institutional control.

*4. Administrative costs.* The pure theory of insurance sketched in section *B* above omits one very important consideration: the costs of operating an insurance company. There are several types of operating costs, but one of the most important categories includes commissions and acquisition costs, selling costs in usual economic terminology. Not only does this mean that insurance policies must be sold for considerably more than their actuarial value, but it also means there is a great differential among different types of insurance. It is very striking to observe that among health insurance policies of insurance companies in 1958, expenses of one sort or another constitute 51·6 per cent of total premium income for individual policies, and only 9·5 per cent for group policies (Somers and Somers, 1961, Table 14-1, p. 272). This striking differential would seem to imply enormous economies of scale in the provision of insurance, quite apart from the coverage of the risks themselves. Obviously, this provides a very strong argument for widespread plans, including, in particular, compulsory ones.

*5. Predictability and insurance.* Clearly, from the risk-aversion point of view, insurance is more valuable, the greater the uncertainty in the risk being insured against. This is usually used as an argument for putting greater emphasis on insurance against hospitalization and surgery than other forms of medical care. The empirical assumption has been challenged by Anderson and others (1957, pp. 53–4), who asserted that out-of-hospital expenses were equally as unpredictable as in-hospital costs. What was in fact shown was that the probability of costs exceeding $200 is about the same for the two categories, but this is not, of course, a correct measure of predictability, and a quick glance at the supporting evidence shows that in relation to the average cost the variability is much lower for ordinary medical expenses. Thus, for the city of Birmingham, the mean expenditure on surgery was $7, as opposed to $20 for other medical expenses, but of those who paid something for surgery the average bill was $99, as against $36 for those with some ordinary medical cost. Eighty-two per cent of those interviewed had no surgery, and only 20 per cent had no ordinary medical expenses (1957, Tables A-13, A-18, and A-19 on pp. 72, 77, and 79, respectively).

The issue of predictability also has bearing on the merits of insurance against chronic illness or maternity. On a lifetime insurance basis, insurance against chronic illness makes sense, since this is both highly unpredictable and highly significant in costs. Among people who already have chronic illness, or symptoms which reliably indicate it, insurance in the strict sense is probably pointless.

*6. Pooling of unequal risks.* Hypothetically, insurance requires for its full social benefit a maximum possible discrimination of risks. Those in groups of higher incidences of illness should pay higher premiums. In fact, however, there is a tendency to equalize, rather than to differentiate, premiums, especially in the Blue Cross and similar widespread schemes. This constitutes, in effect, a redistribution of income from those with a low propensity to illness to those with a high propensity. The equalization, of course, could not in fact be carried through if the market were genuinely competitive. Under those circumstances, insurance plans could arise which charged lower premiums to preferred risks and draw them off, leaving the plan which does not discriminate among risks with only an adverse selection of them.

As we have already seen in the case of income redistribution, some of this may be thought of as insurance with a longer time perspective. If a plan guarantees to everybody a premium that corresponds to total experience but not to experience as it might be segregated by smaller subgroups, everybody is, in effect, insured against a change in his basic state of health which would lead to a reclassification. This corresponds precisely to the use of a level premium in life insurance instead of a premium varying by age, as would be the case for term insurance.

7. *Gaps and coverage.* We may briefly note that, at any rate to date, insurances against the cost of medical care are far from universal. Certain groups – the unemployed, the institutionalized, and the aged – are almost completely uncovered. Of total expenditures, between one fifth and one fourth are covered by insurance. It should be noted, however, that over half of all hospital expenses and about 35 per cent of the medical payments of those with bills of $1000 a year and over, are included (Somers and Somers, 1961, p. 376). Thus, the coverage on the more variable parts of medical expenditure is somewhat better than the overall figures would indicate, but it must be assumed that the insurance mechanism is still very far from achieving the full coverage of which it is capable.

### D Uncertainty of effects of treatment

1. There are really two major aspects of uncertainty for an individual already suffering from an illness. He is uncertain about the effectiveness of medical treatment, and his uncertainty may be quite different from that of his physician, based on the presumably quite different medical knowledges.

2. Ideal insurance. This will necessarily involve insurance against a failure to benefit from medical care, whether through recovery, relief of pain, or arrest of further deterioration. One

form would be a system in which the payment to the physician is made in accordance with the degree of benefit. Since this would involve transferring the risks from the patient to the physician, who might certainly have an aversion to bearing them, there is room for insurance carriers to pool the risks, either by contract with physicians or by contract with the potential patients. Under ideal insurance, medical care will always be undertaken in any case in which the expected utility, taking account of the probabilities, exceeds the expected medical cost. This prescription would lead to an economic optimum. If we think of the failure to recover mainly in terms of lost working time, then this policy would, in fact, maximize economic welfare as ordinarily measured.

3. The concepts of trust and delegation. In the absence of ideal insurance, there arise institutions which offer some sort of substitute guarantees. Under ideal insurance the patient would actually have no concern with the informational inequality between himself and the physician, since he would only be paying by results anyway, and his utility position would in fact be thoroughly guaranteed. In its absence he wants to have some guarantee that at least the physician is using his knowledge to the best advantage. This leads to the setting up of a relationship of trust and confidence, one which the physician has a social obligation to live up to. Since the patient does not, at least in his belief, know as much as the physician, he cannot completely enforce standards of care. In part, he replaces direct observation by generalized belief in the ability of the physician.[28] To put it another way, the social obligation for best practice is part of the commodity the physician sells, even though it is a part that is not subject to thorough inspection by the buyer.

One consequence of such trust relations is that the physician cannot act, or at least appear to act, as if he is maximizing his income at every moment of time. As a signal to the buyer of his intentions to act as thoroughly on the buyer's behalf as possible, the physician avoids the obvious stigmata of profit-maximizing. Purely arms-length bargaining behavior would be incompatible, not logically, but surely psychologically, with the trust relations. From these special relations come the various forms of ethical behavior discussed above, and so also, I suggest, the relative unimportance of profit-making in hospitals. The very word, 'profit', is a signal that denies the trust relations.

28. Francis Bator points out to me that some protection can be achieved, at a price, by securing additional opinions.

Price discrimination and its extreme, free treatment for the indigent, also follow. If the obligation of the physician is understood to be first of all to the welfare of the patient, then in particular it takes precedence over financial difficulties.

As a second consequence of informational inequality between physician and patient and the lack of insurance of a suitable type, the patient must delegate to the physician much of his freedom of choice. He does not have the knowledge to make decisions on treatment, referral, or hospitalization. To justify this delegation, the physician finds himself somewhat limited, just as any agent would in similar circumstances. The safest course to take to avoid not being a true agent is to give the socially prescribed 'best' treatment of the day. Compromise in quality, even for the purpose of saving the patient money, is to risk an imputation of failure to live up to the social bond.

The special trust relation of physicians (and allied occupations, such as priests) extends to third parties so that the certifications of physicians as to illness and injury are accepted as especially reliable (see section II $B$ above). The social value to all concerned of such presumptively reliable sources of information is obvious.

Notice the general principle here. Because there are barriers to the information flow and because there is no market in which the risks involved can be insured, co-ordination of purchase and sales must take place through convergent expectations, but these are greatly assisted by having clear and prominent signals, and these, in turn, force patterns of behavior which are not in themselves logical necessities for optimality.[29]

4. Licensing and educational standards. Delegation and trust are the social institutions designed to obviate the problem of informational inequality. The general uncertainty about the prospects of medical treatment is socially handled by rigid entry requirements. These are designed to reduce the uncertainty in the mind of the consumer as to the quality of product insofar as this is possible.[30] I think this explanation, which is perhaps the naive one, is much more tenable than any idea of a monopoly seeking to increase

29. The situation is very reminiscent of the crucial role of the focal point in Schelling's theory of tacit games, in which two parties have to find a common course of action without being able to communicate (Schelling, 1960, esp. pp. 225 ff).

30. How well they achieve this end is another matter. R. Kessel points out to me that they merely guarantee training, not continued good performance as medical technology changes.

incomes. No doubt restriction on entry is desirable from the point of view of the existing physicians, but the public pressure needed to achieve the restriction must come from deeper causes.

The social demand for guaranteed quality can be met in more than one way, however. At least three attitudes can be taken by the state or other social institutions toward entry into an occupation or toward the production of commodities in general; examples of all three types exist. (1) The occupation can be licensed, nonqualified entrants being simply excluded. The licensing may be more complex than it is in medicine; individuals could be licensed for some, but not all, medical activities, for example. Indeed, the present all-or-none approach could be criticized as being insufficient with regard to complicated specialist treatment, as well as excessive with regard to minor medical skills. Graded licensing may, however, be much harder to enforce. Controls could be exercised analogous to those for foods; they can be excluded as being dangerous, or they can be permitted for animals but not for humans. (2) The state or other agency can certify or label, without compulsory exclusion. The category of Certified Psychologist is now under active discussion; canned goods are graded. Certification can be done by non-governmental agencies, as in the medical-board examinations for specialists. (3) Nothing at all may be done; consumers make their own choices.

The choice among these alternatives in any given case depends on the degree of difficulty consumers have in making the choice unaided, and on the consequences of errors of judgment. It is the general social consensus, clearly, that the *laissez faire* solution for medicine is intolerable. The certification proposal never seems to have been discussed seriously. It is beyond the scope of this paper to discuss these proposals in detail. I wish simply to point out that they should be judged in terms of the ability to relieve the uncertainty of the patient in regard to the quality of the commodity he is purchasing, and that entry restrictions are the consequences of an apparent inability to devise a system in which the risks of gaps in medical knowledge and skill are borne primarily by the patient, not the physician.

## Postscript

I wish to repeat here what has been suggested above in several places: that the failure of the market to insure against uncertainties has created many social institutions in which the usual assumptions of the market are to some extent contradicted. The medical profession is only one example, though in many respects an extreme one. All professions share some of the same properties. The economic importance of personal and especially family relationships, though declining, is by no means trivial in the most advanced economies; it is based on non-market relations that create guarantees of behavior which would otherwise be afflicted with excessive uncertainty. Many other examples can be given. The logic and limitations of ideal competitive behavior under uncertainty force us to recognize the incomplete description of reality supplied by the impersonal price system.

## Appendix
### On optimal insurance policies

The two propositions about the nature of optimal insurance policies asserted in section IV B above will be proved here.

*Proposition 1.* If an insurance company is willing to offer any insurance policy against loss desired by the buyer at a premium which depends only on the policy's actuarial value, then the policy chosen by a risk-averting buyer will take the form of 100 per cent coverage above a deductible minimum.

Note: The premium will, in general, exceed the actuarial value; it is only required that two policies with the same actuarial value will be offered by the company for the same premium.

*Proof:* Let $W$ be the initial wealth of the individual, $X$ his loss, a random variable, $I(X)$ the amount of insurance paid if loss $X$ occurs, $P$ the premium, and $Y(X)$ the wealth of the individual after paying the premium, incurring the loss, and receiving the insurance benefit.

$$Y(X) = W - P - X + I(X). \qquad 1$$

The individual values alternative policies by the expected utility of his final wealth position, $Y(X)$. Let $U(y)$ be the utility of final wealth, $y$; then his aim is to maximize,

$$E\{U[Y(X)]\}, \qquad 2$$

where the symbol, $E$, denotes mathematical expectation.

An insurance payment is necessarily non-negative, so the insurance policy must satisfy the condition,

$$I(X) \geqslant 0 \quad \text{for all } X. \qquad 3$$

If a policy is optimal, it must in particular be better in the sense of the criterion (2), than any other policy with the same actuarial expectation, $E[I(X)]$. Consider a policy that pays some positive amount of insurance at one level of loss, say $X_1$, but which permits the final wealth at some other loss level, say $X_2$, to be lower than that corresponding to $X_1$. Then, it is intuitively obvious that a risk-averter would prefer an alternative policy with the same actuarial value which would offer slightly less protection for losses in the neighborhood of $X_1$ and slightly higher protection for those in the neighborhood of $X_2$, since risk aversion implies that the marginal utility of $Y(X)$ is greater when $Y(X)$ is smaller: hence, the original policy cannot be optimal.

To prove this formally, let $I_1(X)$ be the original policy, with $I_1(X) > 0$ and $Y_1(X_1) > Y_2(X_2)$, where $Y_1(X)$ is defined in terms of $I_1(X)$ by $(I)$. Choose $\delta$ sufficiently small so that,

$$I_1(X) > 0 \quad \text{for} \quad X_1 \leqslant X \leqslant X_1 + \delta, \qquad\qquad 4$$
$$Y_1(X') < Y_1(X) \text{ for } X_2 \leqslant X' \leqslant X_2 + \delta, \ X_1 \leqslant X \leqslant X_1 + \delta. \quad 5$$

(This choice of $\delta$ is possible if the functions $I_1(X)$, $Y_1(X)$ are continuous; this can be proved to be true for the optimal policy, and therefore we need only consider this case.)

Let $\pi_1$ be the probability that the loss, $X$, lies in the interval $\langle X_1, X_1 + \delta \rangle$, $\pi_2$ the probability that $X$ lies in the interval $\langle X_2, X_2 + \delta \rangle$. From 4 and 5 we can choose $\varepsilon > 0$ and sufficiently small so that

$$I_1(X) - \pi_2 \varepsilon \geqslant 0 \quad \text{for} \quad X_1 \leqslant X \leqslant X_1 + \delta, \qquad\qquad 6$$
$$Y_1(X') + \pi_1 \varepsilon < Y_1(X) - \pi_2 \varepsilon$$
$$\text{for} \quad X_2 \leqslant X' \leqslant X_2 + \delta, \ X_1 \leqslant X \leqslant X_1 + \delta. \qquad\qquad 7$$

Now define a new insurance policy, $I_2(X)$, which is the same as $I_1(X)$ except that it is smaller by $\pi_2 \varepsilon$ in the interval from $X_1$ to $X_1 + \delta$ and larger by $\pi_1 \varepsilon$ in the interval from $X_2$ to $X_2 + \delta$. From (6), $I_2(X) \geqslant 0$ everywhere, so that (3) is satisfied. We will show that $E[I_1(X)] = E[I_2(X)]$ and that $I_2(X)$ yields the higher expected utility, so that $I_1(X)$ is not optimal.

Note that $I_2(X) - I_1(X)$ equals $-\pi_2 \varepsilon$ for $X_1 \leqslant X \leqslant X_1 + \delta$, $\pi_1 \varepsilon$ for $X_2 \leqslant X \leqslant X_2 + \delta$, and 0 elsewhere. Let $\varphi(X)$ be the density of the random variable $X$. Then,

$$E[I_2(X) - I_1(X)] = \int_{X_1}^{X_1 + \delta} [I_2(X) - I_1(X)] \varphi(X) dX$$
$$+ \int_{X_2}^{X_2 + \delta} [I_2(X) - I_1(X)] dX$$
$$= (-\pi_2 \varepsilon) \int_{X_1}^{X_1 + \delta} \varphi(X) dX + (\pi_1 \varepsilon) \int_{X_2}^{X_2 + \delta} \varphi(X) dX$$
$$= -(\pi_2 \varepsilon) \pi_1 + (\pi_1 \varepsilon) \pi_2 = 0,$$

so that the two policies have the same actuarial value and, by assumption, the same premium.

Define $Y_2(X)$ in terms of $I_2(X)$ by (1). Then $Y_2(X) - Y_1(X) = I_2(X) - I_1(X)$. From (7)

$$Y_1(X') < Y_2(X') < Y_2(X) < Y_1(X)$$
for $\quad X_2 \leqslant X' \leqslant X_2 + \delta, \quad X_1 \leqslant X \leqslant X_1 + \delta.$ \qquad **8**

Since $Y_1(X) - Y_2(X) = 0$ outside the intervals $\langle X_1, X_1 + \delta \rangle$, $\langle X_2, X_2 + \delta \rangle$, we can write

$$E\{U[Y_2(X)] - U[Y_1(X)]\}$$
$$= \int_{X_1}^{X_1+\delta} \{U[Y_2(X)] - U[Y_1(X)]\}\varphi(X)dX$$
$$+ \int_{X_2}^{X_2+\delta} \{U[Y_2(X)] - U[Y_1(X)]\}\varphi(X)dX. \qquad \textbf{9}$$

By the Mean Value Theorem, for any given value of $X$,

$$U[Y_2(X)] - U[Y_1(X)] = U'[Y(X)][Y_2(X) - Y_1(X)]$$
$$= U'[Y(X)][I_2(X) - I_1(X)], \qquad \textbf{10}$$

where $Y(X)$ lies between $Y_1(X)$ and $Y_2(X)$. From (8)

$$Y(X') < Y(X) \quad \text{for} \quad X_2 \leqslant X' \leqslant X_2 + \delta, \quad X_1 \leqslant X \leqslant X_1 + \delta,$$

and, since $U'(y)$ is a diminishing function of $y$ for a risk-averter,

$$U'[Y(X')] > U'[Y(X)]$$

or, equivalently, for some number $u$,

$$U'[Y(X')] > u \quad \text{for} \quad X_2 \leqslant X' \leqslant X_2 + \delta,$$
$$U'[Y(X)] < u \quad \text{for} \quad X_1 \leqslant X \leqslant X_1 + \delta. \qquad \textbf{11}$$

Now substitute **10** into **9**,

$$E\{U[Y_2(X)] - U[Y_1(X)]\} = -\pi_2 \varepsilon \int_{X_1}^{X_1+\delta} U'[Y(X)]\varphi(X)dX$$
$$+ \pi_1 \varepsilon \int_{X_2}^{X_2+\delta} U'[Y(X)]\varphi(X)dX.$$

From (**11**), it follows that,

$$E\{U[Y_2(X)] - U[Y_1(X)]\} > -\pi_2 \varepsilon u \pi_1 + \pi_1 \varepsilon u \pi_2 = 0,$$

so that the second policy is preferred.

It has thus been shown that a policy cannot be optimal if, for some $X_1$ and $X_2$, $I(X_{1r}) > 0$, $Y(X_1) > Y(X_2)$. This may be put in a different form: Let $Y_{\min}$ be the minimum value taken on by $Y(X)$ under the optimal policy; then we must have $I(X) = 0$ if $Y(X) > Y_{\min}$. In other words, a minimum final wealth level is set; if the loss would not bring wealth below this level, no benefit is paid, but if it would, then the benefit is sufficient to bring up the final wealth position to the stipulated minimum. This is, of course, precisely a description of 100 per cent coverage for loss above a deductible.

We turn to the second proposition. It is now supposed that the insurance company, as well as the insured, is a risk-averter; however, there are no administrative or other costs to be covered beyond protection against loss.

*Proposition 2.* If the insured and the insurer are both risk-averters and there are no costs other than coverage of losses, then any non-trivial Pareto-optimal policy, $I(X)$, as a function of the loss, $X$, must have the property, $0 < dI/dX < 1$.

That is, any increment in loss will be partly but not wholly compensated by the insurance company; this type of provision is known as coinsurance. Proposition 2 is due to Borch (1960, sec. 2); we give here a somewhat simpler proof.

*Proof:* Let $U(y)$ be the utility function of the insured, $V(z)$ that of the insurer. Let $W_0$ and $W_1$ be the initial wealths of the two, respectively. In this case, we let $I(X)$ be the insurance benefits less the premium; for the present purpose, this is the only significant magnitude (since the premium is independent of $X$, this definition does not change the value of $dI/dX$). The final wealth positions of the insured and insurer are:

$$Y(X) = W_0 - X + I(X),$$
$$Z(X) = W_1 - I(X), \hspace{3cm} \textbf{12}$$

respectively. Any given insurance policy then defines expected utilities, $u = E\{U[Y(X)]\}$ and $v = E\{V[Z(X)]\}$, for the insured and insurer, respectively. If we plot all points $(u, v)$ obtained by considering all possible insurance policies, the resulting expected-utility-possibility set has a boundary that is convex to the northeast. To see this, let $I_1(X)$ and $I_2(X)$ be any two policies, and let $(u_1, v_1)$ and $(u_2, v_2)$ be the corresponding points in the two-dimensional expected-utility-possibility set. Let a third insurance policy, $I(X)$, be defined as the average of the two given ones,

$$I(X) = (\tfrac{1}{2})I_1(X) + (\tfrac{1}{2})I_2(X),$$

for each $X$. Then, if $Y(X)$, $Y_1(X)$, and $Y_2(X)$ are the final wealth positions of the insured, and $Z(X), Z_1(X)$, and $Z_2(X)$ those of the insurer for each of the three policies, $I(X)$, $I_1(X)$, $(I_2X)$, respectively,

$$Y(X) = (\tfrac{1}{2})Y_1(X) + (\tfrac{1}{2})Y_2(X),$$
$$Z(X) = (\tfrac{1}{2})Z_1(X) + (\tfrac{1}{2})Z_2(X),$$

and, because both parties have diminishing marginal utility,

$$U[Y(X)] \geq (\tfrac{1}{2})U[Y_1(X)] + (\tfrac{1}{2})U[Y_2(X)],$$
$$V[Z(X)] \geq (\tfrac{1}{2})V[Z_1(X)] + (\tfrac{1}{2})V[Z_2(X)].$$

Since these statements hold for all $X$, they also hold when expectations are taken. Hence, there is a point $(u, v)$ in the expected-utility-possibility set for which $u \geq (\tfrac{1}{2})u_1 + (\tfrac{1}{2})u_2$, $v \geq (\tfrac{1}{2})v_1 + (\tfrac{1}{2})v_2$. Since this statement holds for every pair of points $(u_1, y_1)$ and $(u_2, v_2)$ in the expected-utility-possibility set, and in particular for pairs of points on the northeast boundary, it follows that the boundary must be convex to the northeast.

From this, in turn, it follows that any given Pareto-optimal point (i.e., any point on the northeast boundary) can be obtained by maximizing a linear function, $au + \beta v$, with suitably chosen $a$ and $\beta$ non-negative and at least one positive, over the expected-utility-possibility set. In other words, a Pareto-optimal insurance policy, $I(X)$, is one which maximizes

$$aE\{U[Y(X)]\} + \beta E\{V[Z(X)]\} = E\{aU[Y(X)] + \beta V[Z(X)]\},$$

for some $a \geq 0$, $\beta \geq 0$, $a > 0$ or $\beta > 0$. To maximize this expectation, it is obviously sufficient to maximize

$$aU[Y(X)] + \beta V[Z(X)], \tag{13}$$

with respect to $I(X)$, for each $X$. Since, for given $X$, it follows from 12 that

$$dY(X)/dI(X) = 1, \qquad dZ(X)/dI(X) = -1,$$

it follows by differentiation of 13 that $I(X)$ is the solution to the equation,

$$aU'[Y(X)] - \beta V'[Z(X)] = 0. \tag{14}$$

The cases $a = 0$ or $\beta = 0$ lead to obvious trivialities (one party simply hands over all his wealth to the other), so we assume $a > 0$, $\beta > 0$. Now differentiate 14 with respect to $X$ and use the relations, derived from 12,

$$dY/dX = (dI/dX) - 1, \qquad dZ/dX = -(dI/dX).$$

$$aU''[Y(X)][(dI/dX) - 1] + \beta V''[Z(X)](dI/dX) = 0,$$

or

$$dI/dX = \frac{aU''[Y(X)]}{\{aU''[Y(X)] + \beta V''[Z(X)]\}}.$$

Since $U''[Y(X)] < 0$, $V''[Z(X)] < 0$ by the hypothesis that both parties are risk-averters, Proposition 2 follows.

## References

ALCHIAN, A. A., ARROW, K. J., and CAPRON, W. M. (1958), *An Economic Analysis of the Market for Scientists and Engineers*, RAND.

ALLAIS, M. (1953), 'Géneralisation des théories de l'équilibre économique général et du rendement social au cas du risque', in Centre National de la Recherche Scientifique, *Econometrie*, Paris.

ANDERSON, O. W., and STAFF OF THE NATIONAL OPINION RESEARCH CENTER, (1957), *Voluntary Health Insurance in Two Cities*, Harvard University Press.

ARROW, K. J. (1953), 'Les rôle des valeurs boursières pour la repartition la meilleure des risques', in Centre National de la Recherche Scientifique, *Econometrie*, Paris.

ARROW, K. J. (1962), 'Economic welfare and the allocation of resources for invention', in *The Role and Direction of Inventive Activity: Economic and Social Factors*, pp. 609-25, NBER.

BATOR, F. M. (1958), 'The anatomy of market failure', *Q. J. Econ.*, vol. 72, pp. 351-79.

BAUDIER, E. (1959), 'L'introduction du temps dans la théorie de l'équilibre general', *Les Cahiers Economiques*, December, pp. 9-16.

BAUMOL, W. J. (1952), *Welfare Economics and the Theory of the State*, Bell for the London School of Economics.

BORCH, K. (1960), 'The safety loading of reinsurance premiums', *Skandinovisk Aktuarichdskridt*, pp. 163-84.

BUCHANAN, J. M., and TULLOCK, G. (1962), *The Calculus of Consent*, University of Michigan Press.

DEBREU, G. (1959), *Theory of Values*, Wiley.

DEBREU, G. (1960), 'Une économique de l'incertain', *Economie Appliquée*, vol. 13, pp. 111-16.

DUBOS, R. (1959), 'Medical utopias', *Daedalus*, vol. 88, pp. 410-24.

FIELD, M. G. (1957), *Doctor and Patient in Soviet Russia*, Harvard University Press.

FRIEDMAN, M. (1953), 'The methodology of positive economics', in *Essays in Positive Economics*, pp. 3-43, University of Chicago Press.

FRIEDMAN, M., and KUZNETS, S. (1945), *Income from Independent Professional Practice*, NBER.

KESSEL, R. A. (1958), 'Price discrimination in medicine', *J. Law and Econ.*, vol. 1, pp. 20-53.

KOOPMANS, T. C. (1957), 'Allocation of resources and the price system', in *Three Essays on the State of Economic Science*, McGraw-Hill.

LITTLE, I. M. D. (1950), *A Critique of Welfare Economics*, Oxford University Press.

MUSHKIN, S. (1958), 'Towards a definition of health economics', *Public Health Reports*, vol. 73, pp. 785–93.

NELSON, R. R. (1959), 'The simple economics of basic scientific research', *J. Pol. Econ.*, vol. 67, pp. 297–306.

PARSONS, T. (1951), *The Social System*, Free Press of Glencoe.

PECK, M. J., and SCHERER, F. M. (1962), *The Weapons Acquisition Process: An Economic Analysis*, Harvard University Press.

SCHELLING, T. C. (1960), *The Strategy of Conflict*, Harvard University Press.

SHAPIRO, A. K. (1960), 'A contribution to a history of the placebo effect', *Behavioral Sci.*, vol. 5, pp. 109–35.

SOMERS, H. M., and SOMERS, A. R. (1961), *Doctors, Patients and Health Insurance*, The Brookings Institution.

STEVENSON, C. L. (1945), *Ethics and Language*, Yale University Press.

US DEPARTMENT OF HEALTH, EDUCATION and WELFARE, (1959), *Physicians for a Growing America*, Public Health Service Publication no. 709, Government Printing Office.

# 2 A. J. Culyer

## Is Medical Care Different? [1]

Extract from A. J. Culyer, 'The nature of the commodity "health care" and its efficient allocation', *Oxford Economics Papers*, vol. 23, 1971, pp. 189–211.

[...] Since economists began to turn their attention to matters concerning the efficient allocation of resources devoted to preventing, curing, and alleviating ill health round about the end of the 1950s, a whole new area posing intriguing new questions has been opened up. Many of the most fundamental of these problems have yet to be cleared up (for example, the definition of the 'product' of health care institutions and how it may be measured). The purpose of this article is to attempt to resolve just one of these difficulties, namely, whether the commodity 'health care', defined generically as the kinds of service provided by surgeons, physicians, nurses, hospitals, etc., is *different* from other commodities in particular and crucial ways such as to make some forms of organization of the health industry *intrinsically* inefficient and others intrinsically efficient. As is well known, this question has been the subject of frequent controversy over the last twenty years, a controversy that is today as lively as when it began, but a controversy, it is hoped to show here, that has been largely unproductive because it has been characterized on both sides by a surprising propensity to leap from certain interesting (and important) descriptive characteristics of health care to conflicting (and again important) policy prescriptions (see Arrow, Reading 1; Clark, 1957; Feldstein, 1963; Klarman, 1965, pp. 47–56; Mushkin, 1958; Titmuss, 1968; Weisbrod, 1961; Also see Lees, 1960, 1962, 1964; Jewkes, 1961, 1963; Lindsay, 1969; Lindsay and Buchanan, 1970). What is even more surprising, most of this discussion has been conducted at an entirely *a priori* level with the practical conclusions being inferred in an *ad hoc* fashion, without a proper

1. Acknowledgement is made to the Nuffield Provincial Hospitals Trust for a research grant to the Institute of Social and Economic Research, University of York, for research into the social and economic problems of health care provision. The Trust is not, of course, responsible for the analysis herein nor for the conclusions based upon it.

logical foundation. One reason for this may be that an explicit social welfare function has rarely been stated, though some contributions have been cast in a Paretian welfare economics mould[2] (see Arrow, Reading 1; Lindsay 1969b). There are, however, other more powerful reasons why different analysts' conclusions have not been the same, and it is upon these that we shall concentrate. A major purpose of this article is therefore to attempt to evaluate the policy implications that have been drawn for the appropriate organization of health care in terms of the Pareto criterion, i.e. changes which improve someone's welfare without placing a net harm on anyone else are deemed an improvement, while changes that yield net benefits to some and net harms to others cannot be evaluated in terms of whether society as a whole is better off.

Current orthodoxy is adequately summarized in an early article by Feldstein:

'the availability of private health insurance does not remedy the most basic defects of the market mechanism as a method of providing health care. Although it can permit some people with adequate foresight to escape from the precariousness of major medical espenses, . . . if medical care is allocated according to the patient's financial position rather than his medical condition, the nation's health-care resources will not be used as productively as possible' (1963, pp. 22–3).

The major reasons why this may not come about will be discussed later, but the diligent reader of the *a priori* health economics literature will search in vain for a clear alternative objective function. Feldstein, to be sure, in the article mentioned does ask '. . . should not health care be allocated to maximize the level of health of the nation instead of the satisfaction which consumers derive as they use health services?'[3] But even supposing that a satisfactory measure of the nation's level of health existed, the unconstrained maximization of such a level is an absurd objective

2. One conjectures that some at least of the differing views would explain the existence of the institution of which they disapproved as evidence of irrationality. But that is very unscientific and inconsistent with the corpus of economic analysis. For a recent attempt, and the only one to date to 'explain' the NHS, see Lindsay (1969b).

3. In theory, it is clear that neither the market nor the NHS-type institution is presumptively superior in achieving objectives, such as the satisfaction of some technically determined 'need', other than economic efficiency, see Cooper and Culyer (1970). In this paper, however, the maximization of social welfare according to indications given by the Pareto criterion is emphasized.

since it seems unlikely that the stage of negative (or zero) marginal returns would be reached short of incredibly large investments in health. Not that Feldstein suggests this objective, for he later prescribes that 'in making their decisions, doctors and health-care administrators should look for the *optimal* use of resources by weighing the benefits and costs of alternative programmes and methods of treatment' (1963, p. 25), and, indeed, much of his own subsequent work has been directed toward helping them to do just that. But a dilemma still exists, for if individual preferences are not to be counted, what are the benefits and costs to be weighed? If some benefit is foregone, no matter who loses it, is not a social cost incurred to the same value? It matters little whether the difference between benefits gained and necessary production costs is maximized, or whether production costs plus all *other* foregone benefits are minimized, optimal consumption remains the same since it is, quite rightly, independent of the accounting conventions used. By a roundabout route, therefore, it seems that the Pareto criterion may have been implicit in economists' analyses all the time. But if this was the case, the qualitative arguments for and against various market structures, as compared with the quantitative arguments for improving the workings of extant institutions, are without a logical foundation. This is partly because of a nirvana approach to the problem, i.e. comparing the actual operation of an existing system with the hypothetical operation of an ideal system (see Demsetz, 1969), but also partly because of a failure by some commentators to recognize that organizational reforms cannot abolish economic problems, though they may change their form.

### The characteristics of health care

There can be no doubt that health care is not the same thing as other economic goods. It has, moreover, some intriguing characteristics which appear to make for conceptual difficulties in defining the nature of an optimal allocation. Some are shared with education, another good frequently provided publicly, for example the direct involvement of the consumer in the production process and the difficulty of separating out consumption and investment elements and the very substantial cost that may fall on individuals giving rise to major distributional problems. Others, however, are probably unique in the extent to which they apply to health care compared with other goods or services. The purpose in this section is to examine these for the evidence they provide for public or private provision of health care (see Arrow, Reading 1; Klarman 1965; Mushkin, 1958; Boulding, 1966).

## Consumer rationality

Welfare economics makes two crucial assumptions regarding consumer rationality. The first is the normative judgement that the individual's own interpretation of his own welfare is the one that counts. The second is the non-normative (but also untestable) assumption that choices reveal preferences. Our purpose is neither to defend nor criticize these assumptions but to discover whether health care characteristics conflict with them.

Three arguments concerning rationality have been put forward which are alleged impediments to the optimization of welfare in open markets for health care. These are: (a) Many consumers, though sick, do not desire treatment and may even be ignorant of their sickness; (b) the mentally sick fit oddly into a 'consumers' sovereignty' model; (c) patients requiring emergency treatment are frequently not in a position to reveal their preferences.

1. The first of the alleged impediments has been well documented. Spectacular evidence for the truth of this proposition was discovered in the famous 'Peckham experiment' of 1935–9, where 64 per cent of the persons examined had identifiable disorders but were unaware of them. In 1964, for example, it has been estimated that there were 150,000 unknown diabetics in Britain (Israel and Teeling-Smith, 1967 , pp. 43–56). It also appears that the problem has similar dimensions in other countries. Such evidence appears to violate a fundamental and necessary condition for the attainment of an optimum through open markets. Such an inference, however, neglects two important problems. First, the problem of ignorance is not a problem characterizing markets only. Knowledge must be economized in all social systems, and by using patient ignorance as a stick with which to belabour private medicine, attention is diverted from the more important problem of assessing the *optimal* amount of ignorance. There is little evidence that post-war British patients are any less ignorant of their state of health than their pre-war patients were or that a nationalized health care system devotes more resources to preventing sickness than other systems (Office of Health Economics, 1970). This, of course, is not evidence for or against the efficiency of any particular system of provision, but it is evidence for the view that the description of a theoretical optimum does not tell

one how it may be achieved. Secondly, the inference ignores the possibility that the degree of ignorance measured in experiments such as that at Peckham may, in fact, be optimal. If information about one's health is costly to collect, it may be irrational to dispel all ignorance. I.e. it is perfect information, rather than ignorance, that is *a priori* more likely to be inconsistent with the postulates of welfare economics. The fact that one set of individuals sees a social benefit in reducing the ignorance of others is a problem of externalities, to which we shall return later, but it does no damage to the conclusions here that the observation of ignorance is not sufficient to infer inefficiency in resource allocation and that the specification of an optimal distribution does not indicate the most appropriate form of social organization for attaining or approaching that optimum.[4] What is required if a specific institutional arrangement is to be changed is a behavioural theory of how individuals operating within the framework of constraints implied by that form of organization can be expected to act compared with their behaviour under an alternative form. This, however, is a problem of positive economics, to which attention has only relatively recently been turned, and to which a satisfactory answer has yet to be reached (see Newhouse, Reading 9; Weisbrod, 1965; Culyer, 1970).

2. A similar conclusion must hold with regard to patients who, though knowing that they are sick, fail to demand treatment. Given their preferences, information, fears, etc., there is no *a priori* reason for supposing that they are behaving irrationally, nor that they would behave differently under an alternative system. On the other hand, if there exists another set of individuals who would prefer them to receive more care than they choose, then there may again be marginally relevant externalities which should be taken into account in describing the nature of the optimum. The point here, however, is not that the individuals in question are behaving irrationally, violating any of the postulates of utility theory by, for example, acting inconsistently with their own preferences, but that they are behaving inconsistently with

4. This is viewed as a problem in externality theory since it seems clear that for any behavioural result to appear, those who are 'too' ignorant or myopic must in some way affect the behaviour generating function (i.e. the utility) of another set of individuals. The latter usually describe their resulting behaviour as being in the interests of the former, which it may indeed be (Culyer, 1972), though there are some difficult conceptualizations required in order to show this and it may be almost impossible in practice to distinguish such cases from others involving outright coercion.

the preferences of an entirely different set of individuals (see footnote 4).

3. Similar conclusions hold with respect to the emotionally disturbed, children, and emergency cases. If there is evidence that these individuals are actually behaving irrationally or are not in a position to choose, then it must follow that welfare economics, based as it is on an assumption of rationality, has nothing at all to say about their subjective utility maximization. It cannot therefore be used to assess alternative forms of provision. On the other hand, welfare economics can be used to describe the characteristics of an optimum if there exists an *external* demand for the care of such people. Since the problem of external demands emerges as a general problem in health economics its discussion is, however, postponed until a later point in this paper. It is, however, dangerous to overstate the degree of irrationality in the behaviour of patients, and the discussion here is not intended to lend support to any presumption that individuals, even those who are emotionally disturbed, are in general irrational in matters of personal health care.[5]

*Uncertainty*[6]

Four points in particular have been raised, which may affect the ability of an open market to satisfy the necessary optimal conditions, all arising from various aspects of patient uncertainty about various dimensions of health care services: (*d*) Patients frequently will not be able to calculate the cost they will incur in receiving medical treatment; (*e*) they are frequently ignorant about the quality of the care they receive; (*f*) fair insurance may not be obtainable; and (*g*) moral hazard prevents an optimal insurance pricing structure.

4. Consumers who seek medical care usually do so before they know how much cost they will be incurring. In the face of this uncertainty it is clearly possible that they may take decisions which

5. In some cases, especially in emergency care, where the demand curve is quite inelastic and the costs of the appropriate treatment not 'too' high, it seems quite reasonable to assume that others may make proxy decisions, where the individual in question cannot do so himself, without fear of severe welfare losses anywhere. Such is implicit in the Hippocratic oath and is common to *all* medical care systems. It is a matter (almost) entirely apart from the externality question.

6. The major items in health economics literature on uncertainty and insurance, chronologically, are Arrow (Reading 1), Lees and Rice (1965), Arrow (1965), Pauly (1968), and Crew (1969).

subsequently they may come to regret. They may, for example, take too much care and discover they have run up a bill higher than they would have been prepared to pay before consultation; or they may take too little if they overestimated the probable cost and the appropriate treatments are highly indivisible (e.g. having embarked upon a cheap course, an expensive and more effective course would add too much to the cost given the wealth effects that have already happened as a result of treatment already received; or that alternative courses are mutually incompatible, e.g. having embarked upon a cheap course the expensive course would not be medically feasible). Partly, the problem here is one that has already been met, namely how one can tell whether the optimal amount of information about the relevant choice parameters has been obtained. Under a zero pricing system, such as one may imagine the 'ideal'[7] National Health Service to be, the optimal amount of information about direct costs for any patient to collect will normally be zero, since the costs of his choices are spread over the whole of society and the burden upon him is effectively zero, though the collective burden of the decisions of the rest of society clearly is not zero. In this system, the cost of care falls on an individual not as a result of his own individual choices but as a result of the choices of others through the payment of a (hidden) tax-price. The result of society-wide risk pooling is thus to reduce to negligible proportions the incidence upon him of the costs implied by his own choices while reducing to quite a low level the uncertainty about the costs that will be thrust upon him by the rest of society. The 'ideal' NHS system may therefore appear to have two major built-in allocative inefficiencies. The first of these derives from the pooling element. As Arrow has shown, insurance requires a maximum degree of risk discrimination for its full social benefit to be realized, while pooling implies no discrimination. Thus, under conditions of uncertainty, options on future consumption would be purchased some of whose expected benefit exceeded expected cost at the margin (where the premium exceeded actuarially predicted cost) and some of whose expected benefit fell short of expected cost at the margin (where the premium was less than the actuarially predicted cost) (Arrow, Reading 1). The second derives from a zero price implying excess demand and a failure to satisfy the

7. The 'ideal' NHS is characterized by zero pricing for all health care services, public ownership of all non-human inputs, and general fund tax-financing.

necessary condition that expected marginal valuation should equal marginal cost. Neither of these two objections, however, can be regarded as sufficient to show the *relative* inefficiency of the NHS. First, the maximum discrimination requirement is a condition relating to a hypothetical world of zero transaction, contract and information costs. All real world institutions have degrees of pooling built into them as a means of economizing on the costs of collecting enough information for the 'correct' premiums to be found. The comparison is properly one between different conceivable real world institutions, where second-best solutions must be discovered. At least, such solutions may be second-best by comparison with a hypothetical ideal, but they may be first-best in terms of what can actually be done. This is clearly not a matter to be settled by *a priori* reasoning since the correct degree of pooling depends upon the costs of administering various pooling/discrimination mixes – an empirical matter. There is also an alternative argument which asserts that pooling as under the NHS is actually more efficient than risk discrimination. Risk discrimination requires that individuals in groups having a higher incidence of sickness should pay higher premiums since they impose higher social costs. With pooled risks in the NHS, however, the premium takes the form of a tax-price which, to the extent that the NHS is financed out of general funds and the tax-system is progressive, divorces the premium from the individual's risk and relates it instead to income. Since the poor would tend to be less discriminated against under this system than one in which risk discrimination was the rule, there may be some social benefit from such a form of organization relative to one in which pooling was less prominent. This argument is an important one to which we return later. At this point, however, it is observed that whatever merit the argument may have, it is not related to the matter of optimizing cost uncertainty. Instead it concerns the incidence of absolute costs. It is therefore not relevant to the discussion of this section.

The second objection to the NHS system is also derived from comparing the real world with a hypothetical ideal instead of a realistic, or conceivable, alternative. In any known health care system, however, there is some response to the problem of the uncertainty of costs which incorporates insurance or pooling elements by which all fail the test of comparison with a hypothetical ideal. The reason for this is that so long as the tax-price (or premium) does not exceed the expected value of consumer's surplus, the operation of a zero price for *use* of the service (as under the NHS or even a full insurance system with risk discrimination) will ensure that individuals will, under either type of institution, try to adjust so that their marginal valuations become zero. Any differences between alternative institutions may arise because of differences in behaviour that are implied about how individuals can adjust by, for example, coinsurance in the market, or by political voting processes in the NHS case, which reduce total supply below the rate of consumption implied by zero marginal valuations. These are, however, more or less empirical questions about the *processes* by which preferred positions are attained and have very little to do with the specification of an optimal solution. Before a judgement about the relative merits of the market or the NHS can be reached one therefore requires far more information about these processes and about how the excess demands under either institutional framework are *actually* removed. Currently, we lack even a satisfactory positive theory of managerial behaviour as a framework in which such an empirical investigation could be conducted. (see Newhouse, Reading 9; Weisbrod, 1965; Culyer, 1970). Thus, at the microeconomic level, one's preference for one system or another will depend upon how resources in excess demand are actually rationed out. Since a prime health service supplying agency, the hospital, is characteristically non-profit in either system, there must be substantial initial uncertainty about any behavioural differences between them, which further whittles away any *a priori* case favouring either one over the other. This problem is additional to another concerning the determination of the *size* of the excess demand, which in the case of the NHS requires some theory of public expenditure (since marginal valuations are not, in practice, equated with zero) and in the market case requires analysis of the means used to reduce the effects of moral hazard.

5. Uncertainty about the quality of care received by consumers is more important in the health services than in many other areas of economic life, since the patient is frequently prevented, in the nature of his case, from shopping around and learning about the quality of the service of rival suppliers by trial and error. Even if second opinions are feasibly obtainable, as they frequently are, the patient may not be able to weigh one against the other. The typical case, however, is probably that second opinions are obtainable but that they are not sought because of the mystique associated with the medical profession and the assumption that 'the

doctor knows best'. The difference in the amount of information available to doctors on the one hand and to patients on the other is not of the same type as occurs with most other goods and services. Typically the producer knows more about the technical methods by which a product (in this case, say, a course of treatment) is supplied. In the case of medical care, however, an additional differential exists in that the doctor will usually also have a substantially greater idea of the usefulness to the patient of alternative 'products', whereas with other commodities the consumer is presumed to know this better. As the purveyor of a service, this puts the doctor in a special position since he presumes to tell the patient what he needs as well as supplying those needs. In an ideal world, as Arrow has pointed out (Reading 1), one can conceive of devices which would enable such risks to be insured optimally. One possible scheme (Arrow, Reading 1, p. 39) would be to pay doctors by results so that they had an appropriate incentive for using their superior information as efficiently as possible, with the doctor transferring the risk of failure to insurance agencies. The reasons why such mechanisms do not operate are, however, easy to identify. The major one must certainly be the enormous costs of discovering whether treatment had been 'successful'. How successful is a treatment that saves a person's life but renders him permanently disabled? How does one measure a treatment that relieves, but does not eliminate, a particular set of symptoms? How successful is a treatment that prolongs a life for two months, or three, or four? Instead of this kind of mechanism for reducing the costs of uncertainty for the patient, most societies have evolved what is usually called 'the doctor–patient relationship', the special trust relation between doctors and patients which gives the medical profession a high social status in the community as trustworthy and impartial. It is the same ethic, one may argue, that calls for an absence of any obvious commercialism in the physician's dealings with his patients. It is an ethic which is as old as Hippocrates, and one which appears to be commonly shared across different societies and across different institutional frameworks, in both the market-type health systems and the NHS. Whether a periodic bill from one's family physician or the periodic spectacle of an entire profession threatening disruptive action in support of a pay claim is more conducive to this special relationship is difficult to say, and there seems to be no obvious grounds for *a priori* choice between alternative institutions here.

6. A common complaint against health care that is organized in a market is that actuarially fair insurance is not available, apart from the problems due to pooling elements, because charges are loaded by administrative costs. Clearly, if marginal social costs are incurred in administering insurance, a price for insurance which ignored them would imply a state in which social welfare could be increased: assuming a negative sloped demand curve for risk avoidance, too many people would be insured. The absence of an actuarially 'fair' price cannot therefore be held to be an inefficiency of the market save in comparison with the hypothetical ideal world where administrative costs are absent. The existence of self-insurance is not a sufficient condition for sub-optimality. The relevant comparison is, as has been emphasized above, between conceivable real world institutions. In practice, one suspects that a pooling system with compulsory membership will provide lower unit administrative costs than a voluntary risk-discriminatory insurance system, though the matter is an empirical one and one's suspicions are not always well founded. The problem is more complicated than this, however, since both compulsion and pooling imply social losses to be offset against any cost reductions, so the conceptual argument is less unambiguous than might appear and the empirical exercise would involve some quite heroic cost-benefit efforts.

7. The problem of moral hazard, which has previously been alluded to, arises with some forms of insurance because the consumer of medical care is confronted with a marginal cost at the point of receiving care that is less than the true marginal social cost of provision, hence leading to some loss of welfare. If an individual would consume $X$ 'units' of medical care if he contracted a particular sickness (and had to pay the full cost) his behaviour changes when he insures against the costs, whatever they may amount to, of that contingency. Ignoring transaction costs etc., with unit costs of providing care at $c$, he might expect to pay an actuarially fair premium of $p(cX)$, where $p$ is the probability of falling sick. Being insured, however, the marginal cost of further treatment (e.g. more days convalescing in hospital, more physician visits, hiring a more eminent physician) is zero to him, leading him to consume $X'$ 'units' of care where $X' > X$, at a cost to the insurance company of $p(cX')$, assuming constant costs per unit of care. The actuarially fair price therefore rises, leading to a reduction in the number of insured persons, i.e. an increase in the number of uninsured risk-averse persons. In

addition, each insured person incurs a dead-weight loss on all extra-marginal units of care consumed beyond the point at which marginal valuation equals marginal social cost. The problem is similar to that faced by the NHS-type organization, which has zero user prices and which satisfies demands in excess of the optimal amount. There are, however, differences in the way the two types of system distribute their excess burdens. In the market, the excess burden can be avoided by self-insurance, but the self-insured also lose, of course, by virtue of being confronted with a range of premiums which, although they may reflect the full social costs incurred by the insurance company, do not reflect the lower premia that would exist if moral hazard were absent. In the NHS the excess burden is incurred by all, and some individuals' dead weight utility loss may exceed, with compulsory 'insurance', the utility gain from risks avoided. It does *not* follow that because the market permits individuals to escape the excess burden (though at a cost the NHS is inherently relatively inefficient compared with a market system, since both types of system have developed mechanisms by which moral hazard can, so to speak, be economized. In the market, for example, a fixed indemnity scheme places a limit on the extent of any deadweight loss from moral hazard; a policy containing deductibles, in which the insured person agrees to pay for the first $X$ units of care, will affect the moral hazard in consumption beyond this level only to the extent that the payment of the deductible has an income effect on his demand, so long as net consumer's surplus remains positive (assuming health care to be a superior good), but it will reduce insurance prices; coinsurance, under which the insured person contracts to pay some proportion of the costs of care, will reduce, though not normally eliminate, moral hazard through substitution and income effects; prepayment removes the moral hazard altogether. In the NHS, the mechanism is effectively almost equivalent to the fixed indemnity type of insurance policy with, however, the amounts to be supplied in any contingency being taken altogether out of the hands of the individual patient and decided by the medical profession working within the resource constraints determined by public policy. While there is far less freedom for an individual to adjust in the way he most prefers under the NHS type system,[8] it does not necessarily follow that his net position is inferior since the total social deadweight

8. Third-party control of the rate of consumption when an insured individual falls sick is not, of course, restricted only to the NHS. Market

loss incurred depends on how effective these various methods, and combinations of methods, are at minimizing it. As before, the *a priori* argument could go either way.

One thing, however, does seem clear: it is most unlikely that full insurance of all uncertain medical expenses can be optimal. The market economizes on moral hazard by offering a variety of different contracts at different prices; the NHS economizes with a variety of non-price rationing devices. In both systems moral ✓ hazard is present in unknown degrees.

## Externalities

The final set of characteristics of health care that may have implications for the form of organization suitable for producing and distributing the services are all conveniently grouped together as problems of external relationships. These are: (*h*) cases of communicable diseases where the benefit from an individual's immunization accrues to others in society beside himself (or alternatively, the external costs of not being immunized); (*i*) the problem of ensuring that sufficient capacity is available for those who do not currently require, say, hospital beds but who value the existence of capacity sufficient to ensure them a place should they require it at some later date; (*j*) finally, and possibly most important in health care, is the problem alluded to previously concerning individuals who, though possibly behaving perfectly rationally, may not consume sufficient health care in the opinion of other individuals in society. This may arise either because of a low income level or because of uninsurability due to chronic and costly illness, or for other reasons such as myopia, social milieu, or any of the many factors that shape a person's preferences and circumstances.

8. The problems involved in the case of communicable disease and other environmentally harmful effects fall into the well-understood category of events known as physical externality. They are twofold. First is the question of how to internalize a marginal external diseconomy such as may be imposed by an individual's failure to be immunized, upon the rest of society in the form of a higher probability that they will contract the disease. Second, there is the problem of who should pay for the marginal (public) benefit produced when a suboptimal situation is rectified. There

___
forces in the USA are also supplemented by institutional controls by insurance agencies.

appears to be general agreement among economists that this activity is most appropriately subsidized under government auspices and financed out of general taxation (see Lees, 1967; Weisbrod 1961). This solves the free-rider problem[9] while at the same time reducing, usually to zero, the user cost of the service and hence encourages its use. When coupled with various non-price rationing devices, such as restricting the subsidized service to particular classes of the population, especially those that are particularly at risk, there seems to be a consensus that a practical approximation to the optimum is attained. It is noteworthy, however, that this is a shared judgement about the facts of the situation, and there are cases of public health policy, especially where the externality relation is confined quite closely in a geographical location, where it may plausibly be argued that private initiatives in the market eliminate relevant marginal externalities. Again, therefore, the *a priori* case is inconclusive and the fact that this area of health economics has been relatively free from *a priori* controversy may fairly be attributed to the contexts in which most of the discussions have taken place, that is within wealthy developed countries of fairly dense population and efficient communications networks. When dissident voices have been raised the context has been within less developed countries where a realistic bound can be set on the geographical extent of the externality, for example a malarial swamp containing or adjoining a rubber plantation but surrounded by an unpopulated region. In such cases it is clearly possible (though it is not certain) that the costs and benefits of an eradication programme may be sufficiently internal to one commercial organization that a financial appraisal yields a solution that is as satisfactory at the margin as a more comprehensive analysis of all the side-effects (Perlman, 1964).

9. The problem of ensuring optimal option capacity has been identified only relatively recently in the literature (Weisbrod, 1964). Individuals cannot be sure when they will require medical treatment and new capacity can be created only in finite time. If, therefore, hospital bed capacity were fully utilized all the time

9. The 'free rider problem', called on p. 68 'prisoners' dilemma', refers to a situation in which each individual would reach a privately optimal situation if others provide the public good or service while he enjoys a free ride: i.e. fails to contribute to the cost while still enjoying the benefit. Even if he recognizes that the same situation faced by each individual will imply zero production of the public good and he joins in some cost-sharing voluntary contract with other potential beneficiaries, he faces an incentive to break the contract.

there would be no means of taking additional cases whose demand arises unexpectedly and urgently short of discharging patients early who are already occupying space. Clearly, removing existing occupants to make room for new ones is a method of ensuring the efficient use of existing capacity, and it is one practised in all countries. Equally, however, this procedure has social costs, the avoidance of which constitute a benefit to be set against the costs of providing spare capacity. The criticism of a market mechanism is that one does not pay directly for one's 'share' or 'option' in this capacity and hence the market is likely to provide a suboptimal, though usually a positive, amount. The market, however, is not restricted to trading in the form of fees for specific items of service, which would certainly be an inadequate method (compared with the hypothetical ideal) for producing capacity that was essentially a public good in its technical characteristics, for where potential gains from trade exist between resource owners and potential demanders, there is clearly a motive for either side to invent a mechanism by which such gains may be mutually exploited and shared. Two such mechanisms exist in the market, one being the prepayment method of insurance discussed above, whereby subscribers purchase an option on the capacity of hospitals or groups of hospitals (Lindsay, 1969a), the other takes the form of voluntary charitable activity to assist hospitals in providing more capacity. It does not follow, therefore, that state provision or subsidy is a necessary condition for optimality. The correct policy must be inferred from the actual performance of the current system (whichever it is) in relation to an objectively specified capacity. Qualitative *a priori* arguments give no guide to policy since all the known alternatives appear to supplement immediate demands for use with indirect demands which move capacity in the correct direction, but one does not know whether they move it far enough, or too far, nor whether one method is less costly to operate than another.[10]

10. According to Weisbrod's original argument, one would expect occupancy rates in American hospitals to be too high for optimality. Oddly enough, Titmuss, a stern critic of the North American system of medical care, points to higher occupancy rates in *British* hospitals as compared with American ones as evidence of large-scale waste in the USA (1968, p. 254). In a reply, Lees, a stern critic of the NHS, demonstrated that American hospitals have, in fact, the higher occupancy rate and thereby lent support to the inference to be drawn from Weisbrod's (chronologically later) paper! (Lees, 1964). The rates in both countries have been around 80 per cent during the last decade. For some intensive econometric study of the British

10. At several previous points of the discussion in this paper there was a postponement of the analysis concerning what many, including the present author, will regard as key problems in health economics. The first of these concerned policy toward those who are not 'sufficiently' concerned with their health and those who are too poor to be able to implement any concern they may have by actual consumption. The most common approach to these problems has hitherto been to regard health care as a 'merit' good on the one hand, with 'imposed' choice being implemented in some way (Musgrave 1959, pp. 6–16; Head, 1966, 1–29) and, on the other, to stipulate certain criteria for evaluating the properness of any given income distribution. Both ideas have had troubled histories. In the second case economists have, when discussing allocative efficiency, been careful only to evaluate compensated changes as either social gains or losses because of a general methodological reluctance to introduce interpersonal utility comparisons. When the question of income distribution arises a separate criterion is used clearly involving such comparisons and conceptually quite inconsistent with the previous approach. For some years welfare economics thus limped along in this uneasy harness. In the first case, that of merit goods, it has now been demonstrated that replacement of voluntary with imposed choice must, in general, cause an uncompensated welfare loss which also cannot be evaluated using the Pareto criterion (McClure, 1968). More recently, however, it has been realized that all cases of apparent merit wants need not involve uncompensated changes in individuals' positions, for to enable consumption by one set of individuals to take place may, under certain circumstances, constitute a social good for which other individuals may be prepared to pay. In other words, it becomes possible to view some forms of consumption subsidy as a part of a general Lindahl–Bowen voluntary exchange theory of public finance. Similarly, the state of distribution of income may be considered as a social good (or bad), and for the same reason: individuals' utility functions are not independent of other individuals' consumption patterns, nor of the overall level of others' consumption. The development of the formal theory of voluntary distribution, while having some aspects that are dissimilar from the usual externality analysis, is in principle not different. It is even possible to merge the theory of merit wants and of voluntary

data on occupancy, length of stay, case-mix, and utilization of capacity, consult Feldstein (1967).

redistribution by viewing the taxing (or prohibition) of some demerit goods as a *quid pro quo* offered the relatively rich in exchange for whatever redistribution is agreed at the political level.[11] In these ways, the range of problems that can be analysed with the Pareto criterion is widened as well as a whole new range of possible applications of positive economics being opened up. One is no longer required necessarily to work with mutually inconsistent normative assumptions in order to discuss important issues such as the welfare of the poor, and the range of problems in which personal preferences of the economist are more prominent than the relatively neutral Paretian prescriptions is narrowed.

This approach requires the dropping of the assumption of selfishness in human behaviour, with alternative institutions analysed in terms of an assumption of altruism, or interdependent utility functions.[12] In particular, assume that of two classes of individual, rich and poor, the relatively low consumption of health services by the poor in the open market imposes external disutilities on the rich.[13] A two-person Marshallian model can assist in setting out the essence of the problem.[14]

11. The theory of Pareto-optimal income distribution is developed in Hochman and Rogers (1969) and Musgrave (1970). The same conceptual approach is applied to merit wants in Culyer (1972) and to health care by Cooper and Culyer in a forthcoming textbook of health economics (Penguin, 1973).

12. Selfishness in this context is defined to mean utility functions of the form $U^A = U^A(a^A, b^A, ..., z^A)$; $U^B = U^B(a^B, b^B, ..., z^B)$. Altruism implies utility functions of the general form $U^A = U^A (a^A, b^A ...., z^A; a, a^B, b^B, ..., z^B; a^C, ...)$; $U^B = U^B(a^B, b^B, ..., z^B; a^A, ..., z^A; a^C, ...)$; ... .

13. The textual discussion of interdependent utility functions is couched expositionally in terms of the 'rich' and the 'poor', terms which are intended, however, as *portmanteaux*, representing also relationships between the 'sensible' and 'foolhardy', rational and irrational) etc.

14. Three observations are in order to avoid confusion and to spotlight one limitation of this approach. The first is that a two-person model is as satisfactory a method of handling the problem as any partial equilibrium framework of analysis. The model enables distribution, in money or in kind, to be analysed between the two as a familiar 'gains from trade' problem. In generalizing from two to $n$ persons, however, the model does not permit normative analysis of the preferences of any third party regarding distribution between any two. If $A$ and $B$ voluntarily redistribute between themselves, $C$ may receive an external benefit, but cases where $C$ prefers more redistribution than $A$ and $B$ are mutually prepared to effect cannot be evaluated unless $C$ compensates $A$ and/or $B$ for any welfare loss they may suffer in satisfying $C$'s preferences. Secondly, redistribution between $A$ and $B$ will occur only if the one (usually, presumably, the wealthier) receives an external disutility from the other's condition. If the poorer

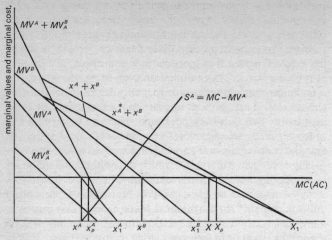

Figure 1

In Figure 1, $MV^A$ and $MV^B$ are the Marshallian demand curves of $A$ (poor) and $B$ (rich) for units of medical care. If both individuals are selfish, the open market result produces a result where $A$ consumes $Ox^A$ and $B$ consumes $Ox^B$, with a total demand (= supply) of $X$. This paradigm of the market must clearly be suboptimal if $B$ thinks that it is unjust that $A$ receives so little care (Strictly, if $A$ imposes a Pareto-relevant marginal externality on $B$. See Buchanan and Stubblebine, 1962). Denote $B$'s demand for more care for $A$ by $MV^B_A$. $X$ (medical care) now takes on public good characteristics in that a unit of $X$ consumed by $A$ is also 'consumed' (indirectly) by $B$, and society's marginal valuation curve for $A$'s care is now given by the vertical summation of $MV^A$

individual receives an external disutility due to the wealth of the relatively rich person, but the rich individual experiences no corresponding disutility from the relative poverty of the poor man, there is no scope for *mutually* beneficial exchange, nor could any transfers between them be evaluated without invoking interpersonal utility comparisons. Finally, as Lindsay (1969b) has shown, the social good could be analysed in terms of a demand for equality *per se*, rather than, as here, a demand for the raising of someone else's consumption. The major disadvantage of the Lindsay approach is that while it 'explains' the NHS, it appears not to have other implications to provide corroborative evidence of its validity. For some empirical work on equality in the NHS see Cooper and Culyer (1970), Gough (1970), and Rein (1969).

and $MV_A^B$. The Pareto optimal amount of $A$'s care is now $x_p^{A}$,[15] and the total optimal amount for society is $X_p$, for the optimum allocation to $B$ remains (in the Marshallian case) $x^B$. Now it is clear that even in the market place there are various means by which $A$ can induce $B$ to increase his consumption. If $B$'s utility gain from a rise in $A$'s consumption from $x^A$ to $x^A_p$ exceeds the cost of subsidizing the price necessary to induce $A$ to consume $x^A$, an across-the-board subsidy is one way. Alternatively, $B$ could compensate $A$ for his marginal losses beyond $x^A$ by offering him bribes to move up the curve $S^A = MC - MV^A$, which is $A$'s 'supply' curve of his own consumption to $B$, until $B$ is in equilibrium at $MV_A^B = MC - MV^A$, which is an alternative statement of the necessary condition for optimality.[16]

The distribution problem can thus be seen as a problem of internalizing externalities, and the market clearly has means by which charitably inclined persons can assist those less well off than themselves. The relevant policy question is, of course, whether the market devotes sufficient resources to this end; that is, whether there exists at the current rate of consumption by $A$ any divergence between marginal social value and marginal social cost. Note that at $x_p^A$, the fact that both $A$ and $B$ value increments in $A$'s consumption positively does *not* imply that he should have more, since no one is prepared to pay for additional consumption —beyond this point marginal opportunity cost exceeds the summed marginal values in use—and the continuing existence of a marginal externality is not therefore a sufficient warrant for further subsidy. Does the market fail? The answer at the *a priori* level is clearly ambiguous. The perfect market clearly will not. By contrast, the 'ideal' NHS, producing a solution where $A$ consumes $x^A_1$ and $B$ consumes $x^B_1$ is definitely non-optimal. In practice the market is not perfect and neither is the NHS ideal,

15. Pareto-optimal $x^A$ consumption is thus where $MV^A + MV_A^B = MC$. The form of utility function assumed is $U^A = U^A(a^A, b^A, ..., x^A, ..., z^A)$ and $U^B = U^B(a^B, b^B, ..., x^B, ..., z^B; x^A)$, where $x$ is medical care. The general Samuelsonian condition for optimal allocation of a public good is

$$\frac{\delta U^A}{\delta x^A} \Big/ \frac{\delta U^A}{\delta a^A} + \frac{\delta U^B}{\delta x^A} \Big/ \frac{\delta U^B}{\delta a^B} = fx/fa,$$

where $a$ is the numéraire good and $fx/fa$ is the marginal rate of transformation. $MV^A + MV_A^B = MC$ is the Marshallian equivalent of this necessary condition.

16. For further discussion of the welfare economics of consumption subsidies see Pauly (1970). Buchanan (1968) makes extensive use of Marshallian geometry in his discussion of the supply and demand of public goods.

so if the question about the alternative merits of the two is to be resolved, it can be done only by empirical studies, which would involve in many cases impossible cost-benefit efforts, though where substantial divergences between marginal social benefits and costs are suspected general indications of the directions for change may be obtainable.

Perhaps the major difficulty inhibiting the market from satisfactorily internalizing externalities in health care consumption is the prisoners' dilemma that individuals typically find themselves in where the externality is felt by many people. Suppose that a hundred members of the community believe that public harm is inflicted by other people's behaviour which they regard as myopic; and that they each consider the merits of forming a private charity to subsidize some aspect of health care which will be sold at less than cost thereby increasing the consumption of 'myopic' citizens. Each one of the 100 stands to gain £20 worth of utility from the activities of the group, but membership requires each member to contribute £5 if the costs of the programme are to be covered. Each charitably inclined person clearly may either join or not join the group. Each individual's problem may be set out in the following pay-off matrix, assuming there is a 50 per cent chance in his view that others will join.

|  | Other individuals | | Individual's expected gain |
|  | Join | Not join | |
| Join | $(\frac{1}{2}) 20 - 5 = 5$ | $(\frac{1}{2}) 0 - 5 = -5$ | 0 |
| Individual | | | |
| Not join | $(\frac{1}{2}) 20 - 0 = 10$ | $(\frac{1}{2}) 0 - 0 = 0$ | 10 |

With each individual seeking to maximize his expected gain the net result will obviously land the community in the south-east cell of the matrix with the result that the externality remains uninternalized. This in an extreme example, highlights the inadequacy of private charity. Changing the expected reaction of others will not affect the result, though if each individual believes that his own decision may affect the decisions of others, different results may be obtained (Buchanan 1968, ch. 5). Such, however, might be the situation supposed to exist by supporters of the view that open markets are a less satisfactory way of allocating resources than the government.

The outcome of the private charity case was unsatisfactory since everyone stood to gain from a situation in which everyone else joined the club. Now suppose that the political mechanism is to be used instead of voluntary charity. This introduces two new elements: (1) A group of people who feel no externality and who are opposed to the relief programme, (2) a rule saying that if the majority party favours the programme *everyone* must pay tax to help finance it, so that (assuming an electorate of 500 people) a uniform tax-price of one pound will be imposed. Now consider the problem of the pro-programme individual. With his vote the chances of the pro-programme party winning are, let us assume, 60 per cent in his estimation.

| | *Pro-programme party* | | |
|---|---|---|---|
| | *Wins* | *Loses* | *Individual's expected gain* |
| Individual votes for or against pro-programme party | | | |
| For | $(20-1)0.6 = 11.4$ | $(0-0)0.4 = 0$ | $11.4$ |
| Against | $(20-1)0.598 = 11.362$ | $(0-0)0.402 = 0$ | $11.362$ |

Rational choice for each pro-programme individual is now to vote for the pro-programme party since this strategy maximizes his expected gain (ignoring the complications arising from his need to trade-off several policies offered in a package-deal by each party). The outcome, however, depends on who gets a majority. If the pro-programme party wins the externality is internalized, but the existence of the minority having also to pay the tax-price imposes external harm on them. Without careful assessment of the facts in actual cases, which will frequently, one may hazard, not be possible, it is not clear whether the gainers could compensate the losers and still be better off. The problem here is that the only valid voting test for Pareto optimality is one based on consensus, yet no rational society will normally choose this voting rule, so *a priori* conclusions again cannot be reached about the desirability of the two methods of organization. The problem has been identified clearly in the literature of 'political economy', where it is well understood that the only valid political rule for testing welfare propositions requires a full consensus of all affected individuals before any change is made (Buchanan, 1959), yet the theory of constitutions predicts (in its positive form) that the rules adopted for making collective decisions will be various kinds of majority rule, and (in its normative form) recommends such rules to maximize social welfare (Buchanan and Tullock, 1965). It is possible that a majority decision is not in conflict with one reached by consensus, especially if vote-trading of various forms takes place, but it is not, unfortunately, the case that such decisions must necessarily correspond with the consensus view; hence the agnosticism of *a priori* reasoning.

## Conclusions

The major omission of this paper has been a discussion of monopoly in the production of health services. The omission is deliberate since it is difficult to see how any useful comparative theoretical discussion can as yet proceed on the workings of monopoly in health services. The reason for this is simple—the typical monopoly in the health field, whether it be a local GP, a hospital, a health insurance agancy, or the NHS itself, is characteristically a non-profit organization, and the analysis of such institutions is still unfortunately only embryonic.[17] A policy relevant debate can therefore only begin when a set of theoretical propositions for non-profit institutions comparable with those of the received theory of the firm can be derived. Such a complement to standard theory is clearly necessary if systematic comparisons are to be made of the relative desirability of alternative institutions.

Health care has several characteristics which in their degree and combination make it 'different' from other goods. The conclusion of this article is that an itemization of its characteristics tells us nothing about the most efficient method of producing or allocating it. There are two fundamental reasons for this. First, observation of market 'imperfection' is not sufficient to infer inefficiency even by comparison with the hypothetical ideal. It has to be established whether the imperfection is Pareto-relevant.

17. The suggestion by Kessel (1958) that the medical profession behaves as if it were a price-discriminating, wealth-maximizing cartel is illuminating for some purposes but misleading for others. For example, it does not follow necessarily that the AMA trust should be broken, for reasons suggested by Arrow (Reading 1) and mentioned above (p. 58). In any case it seems odd, *a priori*, that the presumptively utility maximizing individuals who are private doctors, or who run non-profit hospitals, should seek to maximize only *one* argument (i.e. wealth) in their utility functions.

Second, choice of institutions is never a choice between an imperfect one and a perfect one. Instead, one lives in a world of second best where each case has to be assessed on its own merits. The major reason for this is that the institutions through which resource allocation and distribution are accommodated to individuals' preferences are all costly to operate. On the usual assumption of wealth and utility maximizing behaviour, the explanation of why an open market may have spillover effects, i.e. unexploited gains from trade, must be that the institutions (to define rights, organize contracts, identify persons affected, etc.) required to internalize such effects must be too costly in total terms relative to the value expected to be gained from them. In the real world, therefore, even 'Pareto-relevant' externalities may be inefficient to remove. An open market with externalities is not therefore necessarily 'really' inefficient. But what of publicly owned enterprises? Unless it can be shown that the costs of internalization are lower with this form of organization and, moreover, that they are not accompanied by other inefficiencies, it does not follow that this alternative is superior in welfare terms. But, as we have shown, the public enterprise solution *does* have its own inefficiencies. Furthermore, we do not know what the relative transactions costs are under either institution. Choice between them must therefore be based on quantitative study of these decisive factors. Thus, even if the NHS *is* inefficient, it is not obvious from *a priori* considerations that an institutional change could be made which would increase efficiency. Neither is it obvious, *a priori*, that the market can be improved on by the government taking over production and distribution. Many health economists have overstated their case. The general conclusion, that these matters are fundamentally empirical and, moreover, in many cases quantifiable only in principle, seems to have two major implications. The first is that a far more extensive use of cost-effectiveness and cost-benefit analyses to improve *extant* institutions and to improve understanding of their general efficiency is required. The second is that we need a well-developed positive theory of non-profit institutions from which implications comparable to those of the received theory of the firm can be derived. An increase in the use of positive economics in this field would be an important step in the right direction if those socially undesirable effects that can be identified are to be removed.

Economic theory enables one to predict with more or less accuracy the consequences of various market institutions for the allocation of resources. By contrast, analysis of allocation under political mechanisms is still in its infancy. One might conjecture that this accounts for two characteristic reactions of economists to the problems raised by suspected non-optimal allocations. On the one hand, knowing much about the ways markets can be expected to operate, the tendency is to seek reform by returning enterprise to the market itself. On the other hand, knowing how imperfectly markets operate, compared with a hypothetical ideal, there is a tendency to suppose that the government could not do it *less* well. If the argument of this paper is correct, neither of these views is tenable. The heady atmosphere of grand designs has to be replaced by the mundane, but ultimately more fruitful, ground of systematically applied economics—cost-benefit, cost-effectiveness and output budgeting to improve the efficiency of allocation within extant institutions; statistical and econometric estimation of production and demand functions to improve long-run planning and forecasting; and systems analysis and positive economics to assess the consequences of different institutional frameworks of health care. In this scheme of things the role of welfare economics is to provide an appropriate theoretical base on which to build empirical studies and not to prejudge the facts.

## References

ARROW, K. J. (1965), 'Uncertainty and the welfare economics of medical care: reply (the implications of transactions costs and adjustment lags)' *Amer. Econ. Rev.*, vol. 55, pp. 154–8.

ARROW, K. J. (1968), 'The economics of moral hazard: further comment', *Amer Econ. Rev.*, vol. 58, pp. 537–9.

BOULDING, K. E. (1966), 'The concept of need for health services', *Milbank Memorial Fund Q.*, vol. 44, pp. 202–21.

BUCHANAN, J. M. (1959), 'Positive economics, welfare economics, and political economy', *J. of Law and Econ.*, vol. 2, pp. 124–38.

BUCHANAN, J. M. (1968), *The Demand and Supply of Public Goods*, Rand McNally.

BUCHANAN, J. M., and STUBBLEBINE, W. C. (1962), 'Externality', *Economica*, no. 29, pp. 371–81.

BUCHANAN, J. M., and TULLOCK, G. (1965), *The Calculus of Consent*, University of Michigan Press.

CLARK, J. M. (1957), *Economic Institutions and Human Welfare*, Knopf.

COOPER, M. H., and CULYER, A. J. (1970), 'Some economic aspects of the performance of the NHS', in *Health Services Financing*, BMA.

CREW, M. (1969), 'Coinsurance and the welfare economics of medical care', *Amer. Econ. Rev.*, vol. 59. pp. 906–8.

CULYER, A. J. (1970), 'A utility-maximizing view of universities', *Scottish J. of Pol. Econ.*, vol. 47, pp. 349–68.

CULYER, A. J. (1972), 'Merit goods and the welfare economics of coercion', *Public Finance*, vol. 25, pp. 546–72.

DEMSETZ, H. (1969), 'Information and efficiency: another viewpoint', *J. of Law and Econ.*, vol. 12, pp. 1–22.

FELDSTEIN, M. S. (1963), 'Economic analysis, operational research and the National Health Service', *Oxford Econ. Papers.*, vol. 15, pp. 19–31.

FELDSTEIN, M. S. (1967) *Economic Analysis for Health Service Efficiency*, Amsterdam.

GOUGH, I. R. (1970), 'Poverty and health – a review article', *Soc. and Econ. Admin.*, vol. 4, pp. 211–23.

HEAD, J. G. (1966) 'On merit goods', *Finanzarchiv*, NF Band 25, pp. 1–29.

HOCHMAN, H. M., and ROGERS, J. D. (1969), 'Pareto optimal distribution', *Amer., Econ. Rev.*, vol. 59, pp. 542–55.

ISRAEL, S., and TEELING-SMITH, G. (1967), 'The submerged iceberg of sickness in society', *Soc. and Econ. Admin.*, vol. 1, pp. 43–56.

JEWKES, J., and S. (1961), The *Genesis of the British National Health Service*, Oxford University Press.

JEWKES, J., and S. (1963), *Value for Money in Medicine*, Oxford University Press.

KESSEL, R. A. (1958), 'Price discrimination in medicine', *J. of Law and Econ.*, vol. 1, pp. 20–53.

KLARMAN, H. E. (1965), *The Economics of Health*, Columbia University Press.

LEES, D. S. (1960), The economics of health services', *Lloyds Bank Rev.*, vol. 56, pp. 26–40.

LEES, D. S. (1962), 'The logic of the British National Health Service', *J. of Law and Econ.*, vol. 5, pp. 111–18.

LEES, D. S., *et al.* (1964), *Monopoly or Choice in Health Services?*, Institute of Economic Affairs.

LEES, D. S. (1967), 'Efficiency in government spending social services: health', *Pub. Fin.*, vol. 22, pp. 176–89.

LEES, D. S., and RICE, R. G. (1965), 'Uncertainty and the welfare economics of medical care', *Amer. Econ. Rev.*, vol. 60. pp. 140–54.

LINDSAY, C. M. (1969a), 'Option demand and consumer's surplus' *Q. J. of Econ.*, vol. 83. pp. 344–6.

LINDSAY, C. M. (1969b), 'Medical care and the economics of sharing', *Economica*, no. 144, pp. 351–62.

LINDSAY, C. M., and BUCHANAN, J. M. (1970), 'The organization and financing of medical care in the United States', in *Health Service Financing*, MMA, pp. 535–85.

MCCLURE, C. E. (1968), 'Merit wants: a normatively empty box', *Finanzarchiv*, NF Band 27, pp. 474–83.

MUSGRAVE, R. A. (1959), *The Theory of Public Finance*, McGraw-Hill.

MUSGRAVE, R. A. (1970), 'Provision for social goods in the market system', paper presented at the 1970 Conference of the International Public Finance Association in Leningrad.

MUSHKIN, S. J. (1958), 'Toward a definition of health economics', *Pub. Health Reports*, vol. 73, pp. 785–93.

NEWHOUSE, J. P. (1970), 'Towards a theory of non-profit institutions: an economic model of a hospital', *Amer. Econ. Rev.*, vol. 60, pp. 64–74.

Office of Health Economics (1970), 'International health expenditure', *OHE Information Sheet*, no. 9.

PAULY, V. (1968), 'The economics of moral hazard: comment', *Amer. Econ. Rev.*, vol. 57, pp. 531–7.

PAULY, V. (1970), 'Efficiency in the provision of consumption subsidies', *Kyklos*, vol. 23, pp. 33–55.

PERLMAN, M. (1964), 'Some economic aspects of public health programs in under-developed areas', in S. J. Axelrod (ed.), *The Economics of Health and Medical Care*, University of Michigan Press.

REIN, M. (1969), 'Social class and the utilization of medical care services', *Hospitals*, vol. 43, pp. 43–54.

TITMUSS, R. M. (1968), 'Ethics and economics of medical care', in *Commitment to Welfare*, Allen & Unwin.

WILLIAMSON, E. (1964), *The Economics of Discretionary Behaviour*, Prentice-Hall

WEISBROD, B. (1961), *The Economics of Public Health*, University of Pennsylvania Press.

WEISBROD, B. (1964), 'Collective-consumption services of individual-consumption goods', *J. of Econ.*, vol. 78, pp. 471–7.

WEISBROD, B. (1965), 'Some problems of pricing and resource allocation in a non-profit industry – the hospitals', *J. of Business*, vol. 38, pp. 18–28.

# 3  Cotton M. Lindsay

## Medical Care and Equality

Cotton M. Lindsay, 'Medical care and the economics of sharing',
*Economica*, N.S., no. 144, 1969, pp. 531–7.

This paper provides an economic explanation of the observed
widespread support of direct public provision of medical care. It
is based on a characteristic of the relevant market different from
characteristics which underlie various arguments in support of
public provision. Thus Arrow (Reading 1) has resorted to particular uncertainty elements in the demand and supply of medical
services to justify government intervention. Weisbrod has developed the implications of an option demand characteristic which
indicates that purely private provision of health facilities may be
'sub-optimal' (1964, pp. 471–7). Pauly (1967) has explored the
role of externalities of consumption in the demand for medical
care.

Each of the characteristics noted has its own implications for
the required adjustment in the structure of the medical market.
There remains, however, an aspect of demand bearing similar
implications for the medical market which has received scant
attention from economists. That aspect is the apparently universal
desire and willingness to share. It is the attitude often expressed
that everyone should have 'equal access' to the medical resources
available, that medical need and not economic status should
determine eligibility for medical care; that high income or wealth
should not entitle one to better or more care. This argument
runs throughout the literature of medical economics, but it has
never to my knowledge been examined formally for its economic
as opposed to its normative content. This paper attempts to fill
this void.

### A theory of sharing

For simplicity in introducing the model it will be assumed initially
that everyone has the same 'medical needs' (whatever that may
mean). The egalitarian attitude under discussion holds that the
amount of care made available to anyone should be based strictly

on 'medical need' and not on 'economic status'. We may therefore infer from this that what is desired among individuals demonstrating the same 'medical need' is *more equal* treatment. Such a desire might be formalized into a utility function with the following characteristics:

$$U^j = U^j(x^j{}_1, x^j{}_2, ..., x^j{}_n, e_1) , \qquad\qquad 1$$

where[1] $\quad e_1 = -\sum_{i=1}^{s} \left| \bar{x}_1 - x^i{}_1 \right| .$

In other words, the individual would value, in addition to quanties of the $n$ private goods available, the degree of equality with which one of these goods (i.e. medical care) is distributed. He would obtain positive satisfaction from a redistribution in shares which reduced the dispersion in individual holdings.[2] This may be seen more clearly with the aid of Figure 1 which assumes (a) a community of two persons of differing incomes, (b) where demand for the good in question is normal, and (c) where the supply is perfectly elastic. Schedules $D_1$ and $D_2$ are individual demand schedules of the poorer and the richer man, respectively, yielding consumption quantities $OA$ and $OB$. The value of the $e_1$ term in this case is clearly $AB$ by our definition. If the wealthy individual has a utility function as described in expression **1**, he will positively value a reduction of $AB$ (an increase in $e_1$). Similarly, in the large number case the individual would value a reduction in the total variation in consumption shares.[3]

It might be argued that separate treatment of this aspect of

1. The expression defining $e_1$ is given a negative sign simply to facilitate discussion. It is convenient to use $e_1$ to describe the degree of equality of given shares. Thus as the absolute value of $e_1$ falls, and the dispersion in shares lessens, we may describe the process interchangeably as an 'increase in equality' or a 'rise in $e_1$'.

2. The degree of equality in shares (the $e_1$ term) may, of course, be measured in a number of ways. A good intuitive case might be made for choosing the standard deviation which weights extreme values more heavily. The method chosen was selected arbitrarily for expositional convenience in the analysis which follows.

3. This approach is similar to that developed in Buchanan (1965, pp. 1–14), where separate utility function arguments were employed representing the size of the group consuming each item. This approach also bears a similarity to, though it remains fundamentally different from, that found in the studies of Leibenstein (1950, pp. 183–207); Duesenberry (1949, ch. 4); and Baumol (1952, pp. 83–94). These treat the case in which the quantity demanded of a particular good is affected by the quantities consumed by others. As will become clear, this approach is unnecessarily restrictive.

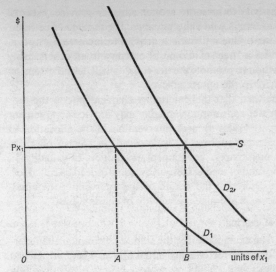

Figure 1

demand is unnecessary since it seems to concern only the parameters governing the wealthy individual's valuation of the good itself. To include these considerations as a separate argument in the utility function may seem redundant. For example, consumers prefer apples with flavour. Yet it is not necessary to include flavour as a separate argument in the utility function. It is a characteristic governing the value placed on apples themselves. This argument does not apply to the current example for two reasons: (a) the provision of greater equality itself yields external economies; and (b) there are means of obtaining a rise in the value of the $e_1$ term (i.e. a subsidy) which are completely independent of the quantity of the good desired or purchased privately.

The nature of the external economies which arise in the provision of greater equality may be noted by referring again to the simplified model used above. As long as only one individual in the community has the altruistic attitude described in expression (1), no problem is created. The individual may proceed to adjust to his own valuation of greater equality by producing the private equilibrium amount (see below). The amount thus produced will satisfy Paretian optimality conditions. If, however, more than one such individual exhibits these egalitarian preferences, private adjustment will not lead to the welfare frontier. Individual unilateral activity to promote greater equality provides external economies to others who value equality. The familiar 'free-rider' effect is present. One individual's activity to increase his own $e_1$ value provides a 'free' extension of equality to all others. Only collective action to promote greater equality will permit extension of this activity to the optimum level.

It appears then that this externality characteristic in the provision of greater consumption equality may provide an argument for some possible government intervention in the allocation of medical resources. Given a widespread incidence of these egalitarian preferences, government promotion of equality in shares of the fund of medical resources would indeed be called for. In order to determine the nature of the intervention required, however, we must examine the activity of sharing itself.

### The means of sharing

This leads to an examination of the second exceptional characteristic of the demand for equality noted above. There are indeed several methods which might be employed alternatively or jointly to produce the desired extension of equality in consumption of the good in question. These may be illustrated with reference to Figure 1. The inequality in shares consumed may clearly be reduced by either inducing the poor individual to consume more than $OA$ or by inducing the wealthy individual to consume less than $OB$. So far as the $e_1$ term in the utility function alone is considered, the means chosen is a matter of indifference. It is simply equality as such that is desired. Further examination reveals, however, that the options available for inducing either are broader still. There are four alternatives which a wealthy individual might employ to promote the desired extension of equality.

*1. The burnt-offering method.* The wealthy individual might purchase the full amount $OB$ which his private demand dictates and simply destroy (or at least not use) a portion of this amount. In so far as the amount he actually consumed was nearer $OA$, greater equality in consumption would have been served.[4,5]

4. Though this method may seem trivial, it is certainly not without historical (even biblical) precedent.

5. It may be objected here that the wealthy individual would re-enter the market to purchase more of the good bringing his holding back up toward his original private consumption level. The final reduction in his holding would then result only from the income effect of the initial loss. This objection is invalid. It ignores the fact that this reduction results from his demand for equality and would leave him at private adjustment equilibrium.

*2. The gift method.* Greater consumption equality could be achieved if the wealthier individual purchased the full amount $OB$ and transferred a portion directly to the poorer.[6] Clearly this method would attack the existing inequalities from both ends.

*3. The abstention method.* The wealthy individual might achieve greater equality in distribution of the good by simply refraining from purchasing the full amount $OB$ in the market.

*4. The subsidy method.* Finally, the wealthier individual might promote greater equality in consumption of the good by continuing to consume at his private level $OB$ while offering a subsidy to promote extended consumption by the poorer.

As noted above, an individual responding to the preferences described would be indifferent among units of equality produced via any of the four methods listed. This does not imply, however, that he would employ the methods indifferently. On the contrary, acting rationally, he would seek to promote equality to the point where his marginal evaluation of a unit of equality was equal to the marginal subjective cost of that unit. In so doing he would strive to employ the least-cost methods of producing that quantity. In examining the individual decision-calculus regarding how much equality he would produce as well as which methods he would elect to employ, it is therefore necessary to specify clearly the cost implicit in each method.

### The costs of sharing

The subjective cost of promoting equality in consumption is simply the value to the individual (doing the promoting) of the item or activity surrendered in the process.[7] The difficulty of identifying this cost lies in defining a unit of equality. As noted above, the selection of the definition adopted here is arbitrary. The complete analysis to follow may be rejected on the grounds that this definition is not acceptable. In that case, however, at least the guidelines for the applicable analysis are established in the following. One need only fit in the preferred definition.

6. It is assumed here that some means is found to prevent the poor from readjusting their holdings in response to this transfer. Such a readjustment would reduce the second half of the result of the transfer to its income-effect proportions.

7. It will facilitate discussion to focus attention at first on the *primary* effect of this activity. As noted above, individual unilateral promotion of consumption equality results in external economies to others who value it. These secondary effects will be brought into the discussion at a later point.

The definition chosen does have certain convenient properties which recommend it. For example, it is clear that in a group of any size, the sacrifice of one unit of the good in question via the burnt-offering method will produce a single corresponding unit of equality for the individual concerned.[8] All subsequent sacrifices, as well, produce equality on a similar one-for-one basis. It is therefore quite simple to construct a marginal cost schedule for producing equality via this method utilizing Figures 1 and 2. The cost to the individual concerned of the first and subsequent units of equality produced is the value of the corresponding unit of the good in question which is sacrificed. Assuming he has originally purchased his full private demand quota $OB$, the cost of the first unit will be $P_{x_1}$, the market price of the commodity. Furthermore, the marginal cost schedule will simply be a reflection of the leftward portion of the demand curve. This is shown in Figure 2 as schedule $S_1$.

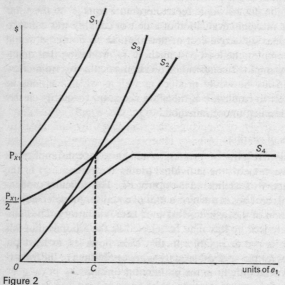

Figure 2

The cost functions of the remaining three methods may be derived in a similar fashion. The marginal cost function of method 2, the gift method, differs from that of method 1 in only one respect. In giving the good to a poor man rather than destroying it,

8. The external effect of his activity on others is ignored for the moment as noted.

the individual makes a double incursion in inequality. He increases the size of the poor man's holding while at the same time reducing the size of his own. The transfer of one unit of the good in this fashion produces twice as much equality (increasing the value of $e_1$ by two). The cost of producing equality via this method is therefore exactly half the cost of the burnt-offering method. The marginal cost schedule for the gift method is thus shown in Figure 2 as $S_2$, having exactly half the slope of $S_1$ and a $y$-intercept of $P_{x_1}/2$.

The derivation of the cost of the abstention method must be approached somewhat differently. Although it produces equality in the same one-for-one proportions as method 1, the cost of this method clearly is less. The individual who restrains his consumption in this manner has not actually devoted resources to goods he cannot use. He has free income which he may devote to other uses. The cost of producing a unit of equality in this manner is therefore only the consumer surplus sacrificed in the failure to consume the item. This is represented in Figure 1 by the area under the demand curve $D_2$ above the market price $P_{x_1}$. Clearly the individual's marginal cost schedule for producing equality via the abstention method is identical to $S_1$ but shifted downward by the value of the constant $P_{x_1}$. This is shown in Figure 2 as schedule $S_3$.

The cost of producing equality via the subsidy method is the cost of inducing a poor individual to purchase more of the good (or, alternatively, of inducing some other wealthy individual to purchase less. This possibility is arbitrarily ignored). Each unit of the good he is thus influenced to add to his normal consumption increases $e_1$ by one unit. Since we have assumed a perfectly elastic supply of medical care at price $P_{x_1}$, the marginal cost of producing equality can never rise above this amount.[9] There is reason to believe, however, that over some range of output the cost may indeed be less. This may be illustrated once again with reference to Figure 1. Conceptually, at least, in the two-person case the wealthier individual might induce the poorer individual to consume additional units by offering to bear the portion of the price of the marginal units which exceeded the latter's valuation of them. In other words, given the poorer individual's demand schedule $D_1$, the subsidy required would be the amount represented by the area between supply schedule $S$ and $D_1$.[10]

9. It is further assumed that the good in question is never supplied in such quantity to the poor that it takes on a nuisance value.

10. The actual administration of such a subsidy scheme might prove

The analysis becomes much more complicated as the number of individuals involved is increased above two. The slope of the marginal cost curve may be steeper or flatter depending on the relative proportions of those subsidizing and being subsidized. It is unnecessary to deal with these complications, however, as the essential characteristics for our purpose still appear manifest. Whatever the number, in so far as one additional unit of consumption produces one unit of equality, the maximum marginal cost of producing equality via the subsidy method will remain $P_{x_1}$, the price of a unit of the good itself. Furthermore, even in a large-number setting, the marginal cost of inducing the first units of increased consumption is likely to be quite small. The marginal cost schedule for the subsidy method of achieving consumption equality would therefore resemble $S_4$ in Figure 2. It rises from a point near the origin to a plateau at the rightward extremity.

We now have cost schedules for each method of individual unilateral promotion of equality of consumption. However, before we may proceed to a discussion of the decision calculus used in selecting among these methods, two additional factors must be considered. We must examine the implications of a non-separability characteristic in some of the methods of producing equality, and we have yet to consider the external effects generated by this activity.

It will be recalled from the earlier discussion that inequality may be attacked from two sides. The large holdings may be reduced, or the small holdings extended. However, we have considered three methods, methods 1, 2 and 3, which all involve a reduction of the large holding. It is clear that one may not give up the same unit to be simultaneously destroyed, given to the poor, and not purchased at all. One may not therefore operate simultaneously on the lowest portions of two of the three cost curves. Efforts to combine the various methods in least-cost proportions must be wary of this. If, for example, a significant quantity of the good has been sacrificed via the burnt-offering method, the cost of producing one unit of equality via the gift method is no longer only $P_{x_1}/2$, but something more. The individual concerned must therefore choose among these three discrete methods rather than attempt to combine them.

The second factor remaining to be examined is the effect of the

more costly than a flat-rate subsidy over the full range of consumption of the good. For this reason costs may be significantly higher than depicted. For a thorough analysis of these problems see Pauly (1970).

external economies generated in the process. This interaction of private and collective adjustments where such effects are present has been examined exhaustively by Buchanan (1968). He shows that by moving an activity which produces external effects from the private sector to the collective sector, individual production frontiers are shifted. This can be shown as follows. Any individual acting alone who produces one unit of the good provides a windfall gain to all others who value it. These others will then adjust their own production downwards in response to this windfall, yielding a net output to the original individual of less than one. On the other hand, if these production decisions are made collectively, the result is reversed. One individual agrees to produce one unit only if all others produce some amount as well. By incurring the same cost as in the individual-production case above, the individual in effect produces a net output of many times more than one unit via the collective process.[11] He will clearly be led to extend his activity when it is 'collectivized'.

The essential characteristic of this process for the selection of least-cost methods of producing equality is that this increase in productivity will apply equally to all methods. Given our assumption of community indifference among methods, the manner in which the individual agrees to produce equality in the collective process will be irrelevant to the decisions of others regarding the quantity they agree to produce. The effect of the external economies produced is therefore that of a scalar applied to the production functions (or cost functions) of the various methods available. In Figure 2 this will have the effect of reducing the slopes of the marginal cost functions by a uniform factor. The overall effect therefore will be identical to a change in the scale of the horizontal axis. In so far as the *relative* positions of the marginal cost schedules are unaffected by the externality aspect, the analysis may proceed. We need only assume that the required adjustment in the scale of the horizontal axis has been made.

### The selection process

Having established the effects of the external economies generated in the production of equality, we may now observe the process of selecting the least-cost techniques for producing the desired level. Since the introduction of externalities has altered nothing essential

11. This discussion ignores the possibility of strategic behaviour in the collective decision process. Such behaviour is deemed to be unlikely in a large-number political setting.

here, Figure 2 may still be used for this exposition. The most obvious step in this selection is the elimination of the burnt-offering method as an economical method for producing equality. Clearly it would be less costly to extend production via the subsidy method $S_4$ to *any level* than to produce even one unit via the former. It is also obvious that the subsidy method will be employed to some extent. Since the marginal cost schedule for this method extends from near the origin, it follows that at least some portion of the total is likely to be produced via this approach.

Whether method 2 or 3 is combined with method 4 to produce the desired level requires closer scrutiny. The decision between the two appears ambiguous. We recall that the non-separable property of these two methods dictates that only one be employed. Yet the two schedules intersect, seemingly indicating that the method selected may depend on the quantity desired. Small quantities appear less costly via the abstention method while production of large quantities appears more economical via the gift method.

This ambiguity is removed by noting the location of the intersection itself. It is easily shown that it lies at precisely the point where both schedules reach the market price of the good in question.[12] It will never pay to produce a quantity of equality greater than $OC$ via either of these methods, since marginal additional units are always available at cost $P_{x_1}$ via the subsidy method. The chooser will therefore select the method which produces quantities less than $OC$ with the lower average cost.[13] Since $S_3$ intersects

12. This is shown by recalling the relationships between the marginal cost functions. From our definitions we note the following:

$$S_1(e_1) = 2S_1(e_1) ,$$ 
2

and

$$S_1(e_1) = S_3(e_1) + P_{x_1}.$$
3

Substituting 3 in 2 and re-arranging terms, we get

$$S_3(e_1) = 2S_2(e_1) - P_{x_1}.$$
4

At the point of intersection $S_2(e_1)$ will equal $S_3(e_1)$. Thus subtracting $S_2(e_1)$ from both sides and setting the results equal to zero, we get

$$S_3(e_1) - S_2(e_1) = S_2(e_1) - P_{x_1} = 0 ,$$
5

which simplifies to

$$S_3(e_1) = S_2(e_1) = P_{x_1}.$$
6

13. The actual decision processes are complicated by the necessity to choose a discrete system to be combined and adjusted marginally with a third. This requires that the chooser be governed by both marginal and

$S_2$ from below at $OC$, it is clear that $S_3$ will be chosen. The least-cost 'package' of methods will therefore be a combination of subsidy with restraint on the size of individual shares (i.e. rationing).[14] The proportions in which the two methods would be combined are illustrated in Figure 3.

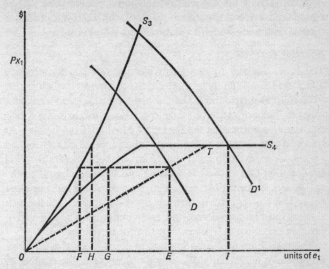

Figure 3

In Figure 3 the diagram contains the marginal cost schedules for the two selected methods facing a 'typical voter' in the political process. It is assumed that the scalars resulting from external effects have been applied to these marginal cost curves. This means that the quantities reflected as produced at the various marginal cost levels are the total quantities which the collectivity would produce subject to general agreement. The dotted schedule $OT$, the horizontal sum of the two marginal cost curves, represents

average cost values in this decision. The ultimate quantity produced via the method selected is determined by marginal considerations while the choice between the two methods themselves must be decided on average cost grounds.

14. It is interesting to note that this analysis confirms speculations of James Tobin made well over a decade ago in which he suggested that rationing might be justified by 'egalitarian' preferences where 'the arguments in the consumers' utility functions were not absolute physical quantities but . . . were amounts relative to the consumption of others'. See Tobin (1952, p. 549).

the locus of least cost combinations. Assuming that the voter's marginal evaluation curve for consumption equality is $D$, he would favour a programme producing $OE$ equality. Such a programme would entail a subsidy measure which produced amount $OG$ and a rationing measure which produced $OF$.[15] Alternatively, if his marginal evaluation schedule were $D'$, he would favour a total programme of $OI$ of which $OH$ was produced through rationing and $HI$ was produced via a subsidy.

### Selecting the system

The basic analysis to this point has suggested a two-pronged attack on the inequality of shares of the commodity which results from market distribution. On the one hand, tax-supported subsidies to the poor are to be made to promote an extension of their consumption increasing the degree of equality 'from below'. At the same time restraint on the level of consumption is to be applied via rationing, extending equality 'from the top'. Before the final step may be taken towards drawing conclusions relevant to the real world, however, two remaining considerations must be dealt with. The costs of administrative overhead implicit in the two systems must be considered, and, more important, the convenient assumption of equal 'medical need' must be relaxed.

The relaxation of the assumption of equal medical need poses no problems analytically. We may simply increase the number of $e_1$ terms in expression **1** to include all the relevant states of health. The individual as a member of the collectivity is then assumed to face a trade-off situation with regard to the degree of equality he wishes to produce among the various states. The actual choice calculus involved in this process seems completely straightforward. The difficulty arises in conjunction with the second consideration raised above. The costs of administering either a subsidy or a rationing system along the lines suggested may severely constrain the actual options open in this regard. The mere tasks of defining clinically-identical states or of identifying individuals in such states appear a practical impossibility. Coupled with the fact that individuals would almost daily be shifting from one state to another, this would seem to rule out either the standard ration-

15. It is quite essential to note that while he would favour this level in the context of the political decision-process, he is motivated privately by 'free rider' incentives to reduce his own activity below the level shown. The necessity to employ the coercive powers of the state for enforcing restraint on consumption (rationing) and levying taxes to support the subsidy programme is evident.

ing or subsidy approach keyed to this characteristic. Resort to some second-best alternative programme clearly is suggested.

Among the alternatives which might be considered is a single-source programme on the order of Britain's National Health Service. It is surprising how well this system seems tailored to the essential requirements derived from the analysis above. Clearly it attacks the problem of unequal consumption from both ends. On the one hand, since it is financed almost totally from general revenues which in turn are obtained through progressive taxation, the element of subsidy to the poor is retained. Second, since virtually all citizens are participants in the National Health Service programme which is required to administer 'equally' to all, the ability of the wealthy to purchase extraordinary amounts of care is clearly circumscribed. The physicians themselves are charged with the responsibility of dispensing care in accordance with their own appraisals of 'medical need'.

It might be argued that individuals are free to purchase any quantity of private medicine in Great Britain, and hence that there is no real restraint on consumption. But closer examination will prove the contrary. Private medicine, though it was not forbidden by the National Health Service Act, was isolated by insuring that its use was a substitute for rather than a complement of state medicine.[16] The individual desiring care is therefore effectively forced to choose either public or private medicine. By offering Health Service medicine at virtually no cost, the *relative price* of private medicine is made much more costly. This increase in relative price clearly acts as a restraining factor on the private purchase of medicine.

It is difficult in fact to conceive of another practical means of introducing the required restraint into the distribution of medical care. As noted above, a rationing scheme is not practical here. There is no restraint characteristic in the subsidized national health-insurance schemes found in America and other countries, and it is difficult to conceive of one being introduced. Therefore, in communities and countries where egalitarian feeling is strong and a spirit of national sharing is general, a national health service may indeed be the most efficient means of satisfying these wants. Aneurin Bevan, the principal architect of, and the first Minister of Health under, the National Health Service may indeed have

16. For example, private patients of general practitioners are not entitled to prescription drugs at nominal cost as are Health Service patients. Private patients of consultants must pay the full cost of their hospitalization.

had keen vision in 1948 at the advent of the new experiment when he remarked,

The picture I have always visualized is one, not of 'panel doctoring' for the less well off, nor of anything charitable or demeaning, but rather of a nation deciding to make health-care easier and more effective by pooling its resources – each sharing the cost as he can through regular taxation and otherwise while he is well, and each able to use the resulting resources if and when he is ill (1948, p. 24).

## Conclusion

The foregoing has provided a possible theoretical foundation upon which the institutional characteristics and structure of the British National Health Service *may* be justified. No attempt has been made to analyse the structure itself to determine whether the desired results predicted of the programme are in fact achieved. Such an examination might reveal factors not considered here which act to thwart the egalitarian aims of the Health Service. For example, to a certain extent medical care is clearly rationed among individuals on the basis of the opportunity cost of the time spent 'waiting' for service rather than on the basis of the doctor's evaluations of the relative 'medical needs' of competing patients. Furthermore, the ability of doctors to make consistent evaluations of 'medical need' – indeed, the ability of the profession to establish abstract guidelines for the use of individual physicians in rendering the decisions – seems questionable. These are operational issues, however, which may only be resolved satisfactorily by examining the performance of the system in being.

A more fundamental question regarding the appropriateness of the structure of the National Health Service is whether the British people do in fact have preferences similar to those described above which are sufficiently intense to justify the approach suggested. Only if a large segment of society believes that medical care should be distributed equally among men of all stations, and is willing to bear the costs of implementing these beliefs, is such a programme justified. No attempt has been made in this study to quantify or test for the existence of such preferences. Indeed, the results of any such attempt are likely to be of limited value. All the problems associated with the measurement of demand functions for public goods are present here.[17] This may well be one of

17. For a systematic review of these and related problems see Buchanan, (1967, part 1). Information obtained through opinion surveys in 1963 and 1965 sponsored by the Institute of Economic Affairs casts some

those situations in which the politician's sensitive ear may read the preferences of his constituents better than the econometrician with his computer. In any case, the politician has made his reading and acted accordingly. He apparently feels that the provision of medical care is indeed a special case calling for unique treatment by governments. In view of the foregoing, it would appear that the *onus probandi* has fallen to the economist to prove him wrong.

doubt on the dominance of the egalitarian attitude among the population at large. Well over half of those participating in the survey felt that universal state provision of medical care should be discontinued. On the other hand, more than two thirds of those questioned stated that they would prefer the current National Health Service regime to state distribution of vouchers worth 70 per cent. of the cost of comprehensive private insurance coverage. See Seldon (1958, pp. 13–19).

## References

BAUMOL, W. J. (1952), *Welfare Economics and the Theory of the State*, Bell for the London School of Economics.

BEVAN, A. (1948), Letter in *Lancet*, July 3rd, p. 24.

BUCHANAN, J. M. (1965), 'An economic theory of clubs', *Economica*, vol. 32, pp. 1–14.

BUCHANAN, J. M. (1967), *Public Finance in Democratic Process*, University of North Carolina Press.

BUCHANAN, J. M. (1968), *The Demand and Supply of Public Goods*, Rand McNally.

DUESENBERRY, J. (1949), *Income Saving and the Theory of Consumer Behavior*, Harvard University Press.

LEIBENSTEIN , H. (1950), 'Bandwagon, snob and Veblen effects in the theory of consumer demand', *Q. J. of Econ.*, vol. 44, pp. 183–207.

PAULY, M. V. (1967), 'Efficiency in public provision of medical care', Ph.D., Department of Economics, University of Virginia.

PAULY, M. V. (1970), 'Efficiency in the provision of consumption subsidies', *Kyklos*, vol. 23, pp. 33–5.

SELDON, A. (1958), *After the NHS*, occasional paper 21, IEA.

TOBIN, J. (1952), 'A survey of the theory o frationing', *Econometrica*, vol. 20, p. 549.

WEISBROD, B. A. (1964), 'Collective-consumption services of individual-consumption goods', *Q. J. of Econs.*, vol. 78, pp. 471–7.

# Part Two
# Improving Decisions

Part Two considers the empirical side of health economics.
The Readings that have been chosen are directed at specific
problems, or types of problem. They illustrate the variety of
problem in which economic analysis has a part to play and also
illustrate which problems appear to be *primarily* economic in
nature and which require substantial non-economic research
inputs and interdisciplinary co-operation.

Mushkin (Reading 4) provides a survey of the methodology
of the theory of investment in human capital as it has been
applied in health economics, discussing the differences between
education and health investments, some of the techniques which
can be used and some of the results that can be obtained.
Fuchs (Reading 5) examines the vexed problem of the output
of health services which are so frequently, in common with
other public activities, confused with their *inputs*.[1] In particular,
Fuchs relates his discussion to the feasibility of measuring the
contribution of health services to national output, i.e. their
productivity. Fuchs is unable to press as far in this direction as
economists of education have, but in the course of his
discussion he raises many of the problems that are likely to
arise and identifies precise areas for future research. Yett
(Reading 6) applies economic theory to the problem of the
American nursing shortage where traditionally the rather rigid
'ratios approach' of manpower forecasting has applied. His
paper is a clear example of how theory and the facts can be
explicitly stated and combined to produce useful conclusions
for public policy. Feldstein (Reading 7) tackles the task of
developing a model of the health care sector to show how
hospitals, doctors etc., local and central governments, insurance
agencies and patients interact to determine the pattern of
services produced, the resources used up, the patients who

receive care, the prices paid, and so on. The successful outcome of aggregate models of this kind would enable policy makers to predict the consequences throughout the system of any change made within it which, given the great interdependence of health services of all kinds, is clearly an important if ambitious, matter. Reading 8 is a study by Herbert Klarman *et al.*, of a specific disease showing how cost-effectiveness (a variety of cost-benefit analysis) can help to decide which form of treatment is best adopted. It is especially at this level, where the problem is primarily a medical one, that the economist's contribution has to be regarded as one contribution among many. For example, any calculations the economist may propose to do will depend upon medical knowledge of treat-ments, the natural history of the disease, and so on.

All the papers in this section show (a) the method and (b) its application, in attempts to improve the efficiency of resource allocation. For many, efficiency in the allocation of health resources is of little interest, but, in fact, it is of paramount importance. Greater efficiency implies better health, more health services *and* more of other things (such as education).

1. A different approach to this problem is explored in the articles by Culyer, Lavers and Williams (1971) cited in the Further Reading.

# 4 Selma J. Mushkin

## Health as Investment

Selma J. Mushkin, 'Health as an investment', *Journal of Political Economy*, vol. 70, 1962, pp. 129–57.

A theory of human capital is in the process of formulation. The primary question is 'What is the contribution of changes in the quality of people to economic growth?' The academic economists first raised the question after their research showed that production in developed economies had been increasing much faster than could be explained by inputs of physical capital and additions to the labor force (Fabricant, 1959; Solow, 1957). But the wide interest which the question has aroused indicates much more than academic curiosity. It reflects the desires and aspirations of people throughout the world – people anxious to add weight to their demands for action against disease and illiteracy by showing that such action is not only humanitarian, but will make a major contribution to economic growth as well. Though research on the return to investment in people is barely getting started, even the most tentative conclusions have been widely quoted. Preliminary indications that the rate of return on investment in people is high have been seized upon in a growing number of countries as justification for including investment in people in economic development programs.

In 1961 two important international conferences were held on investment in people as a facet of economic development (World Health Organization and Pan American Sanitary Bureau, October; OEEC Policy Conference, October). One of these discussed health programs, the other education. Given the climate of thought today it seems difficult to imagine that only four years ago authorities writing on economic development, with few exceptions, omitted consideration of investments in people. A footnote in one such volume may be cited as illustrative. In explaining the omission, the authors write, 'once one leaves the *terra firma* of material capital and branches out into the upper ether of human capital there is endless difficulty in finding a resting place (Bauer and Yamey, 1957, p. 27).

Research leading toward a theory of human capital formation has been largely pioneered by Professor Theodore W. Schultz and supported by the Ford Foundation's Fund for the Advancement of Education. This work centers on investment through education. Basic economic research on investment through health programs is receiving far less attention, and sustained financial support for such research is even at this time uncertain. But out of the work that Schultz has done and the work of others whom he has encouraged has come a better understanding of the economic processes that apply to health programs as well as to education. The far more intensive work on education as an investment suggests that it may be useful to start this paper with a comparison of health and education as types of investment. The first part of this paper, therefore, states briefly some of the similarities between the two programs, as well as characteristic differences between them.

The second part deals with capital formation through health care and returns to investment in health. Some empirical work on specific diseases has been done; work has also been done on the overall problems of disease. Although I do not review these specific empirical studies, I attempt to summarize the basic assumptions underlying their estimates and to point to examples of the 'payoff' on investment in eradication of disease.

Throughout I address myself to the economic effects of health programs – public and private, curative and preventive. Promotion of health patently involves more than health services and the related commodities used in the provision of these services. It includes food, housing, recreation and clothing. Although they contribute importantly to health, the present inquiry is limited to investment in health services and their component commodities. It appears necessary, however, in the present context to include water supplies among the investments in health. Environmental health programs, including safe water supplies, are largely responsible for the rate of decline in death rates in the United States between 1900 and 1917. In this period the overall age-adjusted death rates decreased at 1·074 per year, a higher rate of decrease than took place in the subsequent period 1921–37. Diseases that can be controlled through sanitation and safe water supplies – typhoid, diarrhea, and dysentery – are among the major diseases today in the underdeveloped countries which give a high priority to investment in water supplies and sanitation.

# I  Education and health: similarities and differences

The concept of human capital formation through both education and health services rests on the twin notions that people as productive agents are improved by investment in these services and that the outlays made yield a continuing return in the future. Health services, like education, become a part of the individual, a part of his effectiveness in field and factory. The future increase in labor product resulting from education or from health programs can be quantified to an extent useful for programming purposes. While there are apparent limitations to such measures, these limitations can be identified.

## Complementary content of investment

Health and education are joint investments made in the same individual. The individual is more effective in society as a producer and as a consumer because of these investments. And often the return on investment in health is attributed to education.

The interrelations between health and education are many, as suggested by the illustrations which follow. Some types of health programs essentially depend upon education in personal hygiene and sanitation. On education falls responsibility for training of health personnel (both professional and ancillary) to provide the health services. A child's formal schooling is impossible unless he is well enough to attend school and to learn. Loss in days of schooling due to ill health, which in the United States in 1958 averaged 8·4 days per school year, reduces the effectiveness of investment in education. And death of children of school age adds to the cost of education per effective labor-force member. A lengthening of life expectancy through improved health reduces the rate of depreciation of investment in education and increases the return to it. An increase in productive efficiency through improved education, on the other hand, increases the return on a lifesaving investment in health.

It is a fairly simple bit of arithmetic to determine the differences in human capital formation through education, given the mortality experience of the early 1900s and today. Differences in years of work expectancy on the average between two periods will change the value of lifetime income differentials between the high-school and the college graduate, for example. It is also simple arithmetic to compute the value of future earnings, on the average, of a death postponed to old age when the number of years of schooling approximates the norm of the early 1900s and the norm of today. But far more difficult is the problem of assessing the loss to the country from the early death or incapacity of a would-be inventor, scientist, or political leader. What would have been the loss if Einstein had died during the flu epidemic following the First World War, or had Keynes' last work been his *Treatise on Money*?

Educational levels determine to a large extent the seeking out of health services and the selection of appropriate kinds of services. A large body of information exists pointing to a high correlation between use of health services and educational status (Koos, 1954). And one of the major health problems that confronts public health officers is education of groups in the community to use available public services, for example, Salk vaccine. Delays in seeking care, due to ignorance, intensify disease problems and convert cases that could be prevented or controlled into serious disabilities or premature deaths (Bergsten, 1960)

Health services are similar to education, too, in that they are partly investment and partly consumption, and the separation of the two elements is difficult. An individual wants to get well so that life for him may be more satisfying. But also when he is well he can perform more effectively as a producer. What part of the expenditure made to cure his illness is a consumption expenditure, and what part is an investment in a producer? The type of issue involved is familiar to those who have been working on investment in education.

As consumer goods, both education and health are extra-ordinary. They are not sought simply to satisfy human wants but are essential ingredients of human welfare. The distinction I have in mind was made several years ago by Munoz-Marin, the governor of Puerto Rico, when he proposed an 'Operation Serenity' through which society 'would use its economic power increasingly for the extension of freedom, of knowledge, and of understanding imagination rather than a rapid multiplication of wants'. Levels of education and health are implicit components of a standard of living (WHO, 1957; UN-ILO and UNESCO, 1954). When man does not have sufficient vitality to function normally, other consumption loses its significance, and without education the distinctive qualities of the human being are lost.

Returns to investment in both health and education accrue in part to the individual who makes the investment and in part to other individuals. Purchase of health services for the prevention of contagious and infectious diseases, such as smallpox, poliomyelitis, and whooping cough, benefits the community as a whole. Curative health services, such as those for the treatment of tuberculosis or syphilis, help prevent the spread of the disease; thus an individual's purchase of services for his own care benefits his neighbors. By his improved health status and by that of his neighbors the productivity of the economy is increased.

Health, like education, is being financed largely out of current consumption funds. Denison (1962) has pointed out that whether the individual spending for education thinks of himself as consuming or investing is not so important as whether the resources used for financing the services have come from consumption funds or investment funds. He emphasizes that funds used for education – both public and private – largely reduce consumption and thus make a positive net contribution to economic growth. Educational outlays, assuming this diversion of funds from consumption to investment, increase the total volume of investment even if the rate of return on educational investment is considerably lower than that on investment in physical capital. Denison's observations on the sources of educational funds apply by and large to sources of health funds as well. But here we have the perhaps curious juxtaposition of circumstances that funds, at least in the United States, are withdrawn from alternative investments primarily to finance those health-service costs that most clearly could be classified as consumption – costs of major medical incidents that lead to disabling chronic illness and to death.

It must be remembered that health and education services in most countries are financed in part through the public sector of the economy and in part through the private sector. The mixture of public and private varies widely, however, from nation to nation, and the mix may not be the same for health as it is for education within a nation. Expenditures for health in the United States amount to more than $25 billion; expenditures for education also are about $25 billion. But public outlays for health account for less than 25 cents of each $1 spent; and private outlays for the remaining more than 75 cents. In the case of education the proportions are reversed; about 80 cents of each $1 of educational costs is publicly financed and about 20 cents privately financed.

## Differences between health and education

There are these important similarities between health and education as investments. But the differences between them necessitate different approaches to the problem of measurement of human capital. As I see the differences, they are:

1. Health programs increase the numbers in the working force as well as the quality of labor's product. Education chiefly affects quality of the producers. The people added to the work force through a reduction in number of deaths and in disability provide a direct measure of the units of labor resulting from improvement in health status. By valuing these added workers at the present value of their future earnings, the capital stock in health status can be determined. This is analogous to valuing physical capital, such as real property, on the basis of its rental income. But as indicated below, the health-program content of this health status is difficult to disentangle from other factors affecting health of a population. And valuation of changes in quality of the work force attributable to health programs presents an additional problem.

The number of potential workers that may be added through health programs is especially large in the non-industrial nations. Average life expectancy at birth in many nations of Asia and Africa – nations that include almost two thirds of the world population – was until recently about thirty years. This may be contrasted with almost seventy years of life expectancy achieved in the United States. Large increases in life expectancy for these non-industrial nations can be brought about quickly and with fairly small direct outlays. Spraying with DDT, immunization with BCG, and treatment with penicillin have yielded dramatic results in reduced mortality from malaria, tuberculosis, syphilis, and yaws. An intensification of programs to control these diseases could reduce death rates rapidly.

2. Units of quality change through human capital formation by health programs cannot be defined as tidily as units of education embodied in the labor force. There is no quality unit comparable to that of the number of years of schooling, devised by Schultz (1961) as a measure of educational stock in the labor force. To assess the quality changes resulting from the health-program content embodied in the labor force, a positive measure of health status would be required. The most frequently used indexes of health status, however, are negative – death rates and morbidity rates that reflect changes in numbers rather than quality. There are two other types of indexes in use: first, measures of the relative availability of health facilities, for example, the number of physicians or the number of hospital beds per 1000 population.

Second, the number of services rendered is used, for example, the number of children vaccinated or the number of births in hospitals.

Some indicators of change in health status exist, but they have a limited use; for example, in the United States and Great Britain children in each age group are taller today than their fathers and grandfathers were at the same age. Puberty comes at an earlier age. More recently work has been done on physical fitness, which may have some application in the future to the measurement of work capacity of a population. Physiological tests have been developed of the individual's total ability to perform prolonged physical work. 'For all practical purposes, this means the ability of the cardiopulmonary system to take up, transport, and give off oxygen to the muscle tissue for the performance of physical work' (Hettinger, *et al.*, 1961; Rodahl, *et al.*, 1961). Muscle strength, oxygen uptake, and pulse responses have been combined in a series of tests.

At present, it is difficult to disentangle the effects on the health status of the population that are attributable to health programs from those attributable to better nutrition, better housing, better working conditions, and higher incomes. Sickness is a cause as well as a consequence of poverty. Tuberculosis, for example, is closely related to housing conditions. 'Lung block' in New York City conveyed the image of this association. Indeed, Lowell after a detailed study of the tuberculosis problem in New York City, wrote: 'if optimum benefits are to be realized in mastering tuberculosis progress in medicine and public health, they must be accompanied by comparable and parallel socioeconomic improvements in living conditions' (Lowell, 1956). Communicable diseases generally have a higher rate of incidence among the poor than among the rich. Conditions of poverty give rise to the easy transmission of infectious diseases; thus improved living standards contribute importantly to reduction in prevalence and incidence rates. The improvement in health status in the past six decades in the United States is in part the result of health services that brought the infectious and contagious diseases under control. (In part, too, it is the result of the growth in the economy.) For example, of 100 white males born in 1900–1902, seventy-nine reached age fifteen and thirty-nine will reach sixty-five years of age. In 1958, out of 100 white males born, ninety-six will reach age fifteen and sixty-six will reach age sixty-five. Isolation of some of the major factors responsible for prolonging life would help to identify the contribution of health programs as well as the contribution of specific aspects of health programs such as sanitary control of the environment, widespread immunization, better medical care and community health services. But we are a long way from identifying the contribution of health programs.

3. Closely related to the problem of measuring quality changes attributable to health programs is the question of assessing earning differences. In assessing the private return to investment in education, one begins with data on differentials in earnings according to years of schooling. Average differences in lifetime incomes of high-school and college graduates, for example, corrected for differences in ability and other factors, serve as an index of return to higher education. We now have no similar indexes of differences in income associated with gradations in health. More particularly, we have no indexes of differences in earnings reflecting such gradations.

The National Health Survey provides information on the time lost from work because of temporary sickness. Bergsten (1960), analysing the results of this survey, shows an inverse relation between family income and time lost from work. While persons (usually working) in families with income under $2000 lose an average of 10·8 days a year from work due to illness and injury, those with income of $7000 or more lose only 5·9 days. Data on differences in sickness rates by income class, however, reflect the interaction of illness and income.

We have some negative measures that indicate the market's evaluation of risk of sickness and death and potential loss in earning due to permanent impairment. Rates under workmen's compensation laws reflect differences in the risk of death and injury in different occupations. If a correction is made for the effects of statutory limits on benefit payments, workmen's compensation rates should reflect the 'charge' for the risks of death and disability. Rates levied in the states vary widely for different employers depending upon their industrial accident experience. For certain types of iron and steel erection in the construction industry, for example, rates are in the neighborhood of 20 per cent of wages, while in the same state, large retail trade outlets pay premium rates in the neighborhood of only 0·5 per cent. If workmen's compensation charges, as adjusted, can be used to measure the risk of death and disability, it may be possible to use premiums paid for extra occupational risks – or 'hazard pay' – as an index of the market evaluation of the risk of continuing debility. Hazard pay is paid to persons in occupations such as airplane pilots, undersea divers, and longshoremen handling dangerous cargoes. And injury rates become one of the many factors considered in wage negotiations even when separate hazard premiums are not paid.

4. Educational investment is a developmental process, which ferrets out and encourages native talent. It proceeds step by step from one level to another, transmitting a cultural environment by building on the existing store of knowledge. Health programs seek basically to prevent a hostile environment from killing and crippling. They seek to stay the natural forces of biological selection.

Peoples throughout history have invested in health; even the most primitive of peoples have invested in a selectivity process whereby those most fit for their environment survived. The survivors developed immunities to the diseases of their environment, but the price of these immunities (the investment in health) was the early deaths of the less fit with the consequent loss of their net productive contribution. In some early cultures an even larger investment was made in the selectivity producing a health status through the killing of the disabled and the weak.

Many underdeveloped countries or regions within these countries have progressed in health programs little beyond sustaining a natural death rate – a rate reflecting the early deaths of those unable to withstand the dangers of a hostile environment. And while modern medicine has been brought into such regions and has lowered death rates, modern civilization in some remote places has destroyed the earlier investment of the people in these places in building immunity to disease. New diseases have been brought in.

In a modern economy biological selection is no longer an acceptable method of investing in health, not only because our humanitarian instincts rebel against it, but because it costs too much. The cost of foregoing the productive contribution of those who would die early is now too great. In our present economy, in the United States and other industrially developed nations, physical strength of the human hand is not often used in the production processes. People with so-called impaired lives can and do make great contributions to our national output. Brain power and other human capabilities and talents are far more important than physical stamina. In replacing the physical energy of people by inanimate power, and crude natural products by synthetic substitutes, mankind has altered the nature of its investment requirements, both human and physical.

The significance of the difference between education and health as an investment lies in the range of choices to be considered in the regions of the world that are in the twilight of a cultural transition from the ancient to the modern. The choice in the case of health is not between some investment and no investment; it is between investment in biological selection and investment in modern public health measures or in other measures that indirectly promote health.

One word of further qualification is needed so that I will not be misunderstood. Biological selection does not necessarily result in a strong and virile and creative people; it results only in the survival of those best able to withstand the rigors of their physical and biological environment.

These then are some important differences between health and education investments. Some of the differences are pertinent only to consideration of health programs in the underdeveloped nations; others to industrialized countries.

## II Measuring capital formation through health care

In its simplest form the economic resources (labor and commodities) devoted to health care represent in some part an investment in health. In some part, that is, the health outlays improve the labor product and continue to yield a return over a period of years. The labor product created by this care and savings in health expenditures in the future, if any, as a consequence of reduction in disease is the yield.

Just as the stock of physical capital may be measured in a number of different ways, so the stock of health capital in people may be variously measured. This human capital formation by health care for a population may be counted, for example, at cost – the cost of environmental and curative health services embodied over their life spans in each of the age cohorts in the present labor force. Cost for this purpose may be set at the cost of acquisition of the health services in the years they were acquired; they may be determined on a replacement cost basis, or at constant prices prevailing in a base year.

At today's prices if we valued the health care received by persons currently in the labor force, for example, we might arrive at a figure of, let us assume, about $250 billion. Is the yield on this $250 billion stock $12 billion, $25 billion, or of what order of magnitude? What, in other words, has been the money value of the annual labor product added as a consequence of the health investments made?

A study of the stock of health-program capital on a cost basis stimulated by the Exploratory Conference on Investment in Human Beings is in progress. This study has not progressed sufficiently to describe fully its scope nor patently to yield findings. Some preliminary and very partial figures may illustrate the possible quantities, however. Medical care costs of child-bearing in 1957–8 averaged $272 (Health Information Foundation, 1961); the health costs for an infant and child (at 1957–8 prices) come to about $45 a year. If we include all medical care expenditures for a child up to age eighteen, the average child uses more than $1000 in health and medical services.[1] To produce a labor force member aged eighteen at today's quantities and quality of health care and at today's prices, accordingly, upward of $1000 is spent in health resources alone. For the seventy-three million persons in the labor force of 1960 this would mean a $73 billion stock of health care up to age eighteen when valued on replacement costs basis, without adjustment for losses due to early death. At pre-First World War quantities and quality of health care and medical prices prevailing then, the health stock in a labor force of 1960 size (counting costs only up to age eighteen) would have been about $5·5 billion before addition of costs lost through these earlier deaths prior to age eighteen. Data on *per capita* expenditures for health care are shown in Table 1.

The capital stock of health services may also be measured as the present value of the added labor product acquired through health programs, that is, the stock may be valued at the present value of the future earnings generated through the health programs. In some health programs, the labor product added is contingent on the services received by a specific individual, and on his death or retirement the capital value of health services is lost. Accordingly, the future earnings to be valued for the present period are limited by survival and retirement rates.

The present value of future labor product created by health care becomes a second measure of capital value. The question that is being asked in this measurement of investment is: 'What is the expected return from the health care which in turn determines its value?'

1. These figures are approximate and may be revised substantially when additional research is done.

## Table 1 Health-care expenditures, selected years, 1914 to 1958–9

| Year | Amount (in millions) | Per capita | As percentage of gross national product |
|------|------|------|------|
| 1914* | $1091 | $11 | 2·7 |
| 1921* | 2024 | 19 | 2·7 |
| 1927* | 3030 | 25 | 3·1 |
| 1956* | 18,358 | 109 | 4·4 |
| 1928–29† | 3650 | 30 | 3·6 |
| 1939–40† | 3915 | 30 | 4·1 |
| 1949–50† | 12,365 | 83 | 4·7 |
| 1956–57† | 21,027 | 125 | 4·9 |
| 1958–59† | 25,196 | 145 | 5·4 |

* Compiled from United States Bureau of Census (1960). Includes personal consumption expenditures and also public outlays for health programs, federal, state, and local.

† From Merriam (1960, p. 43). Includes industrial-in-plant services and philanthropy as well as personal health expenditures and public outlays for health programs.

The cost in terms of health-program expenditures and, in turn, in terms of resources devoted to health care may be greater or less than the capitalized value of the added labor product created through improved health status.

This measure of the capitalized expected income over the productive life span of the new labor product added through a health program takes account of the depreciation on the investment by the loss of labor product through retirement and death. There are types of health programs, however, which yield returns into perpetuity. The asset created in the main does not depreciate. The value of the health services continues beyond the life span of the individuals for whom the services initially are provided. For example, complete eradication of malaria or of typhoid from an area means that individuals of succeeding generations are not subject to these diseases. In instances where there is a return into perpetuity, in effect the labor product added through a health program may be capitalized without allowance for depreciation, that is, for retirements from the labor force and deaths.

As this brief summary of measures of capital formation through health programs suggests, a central problem in assessing yields and investment in health is the measurement of labor product added through health care.

## Labor product measurement [2]

The resource gained as a result of prevention or cure of sickness is human labor. In order to value the gain in dollars it is necessary to estimate the output added. There are two types of questions – one in the future; the other in the past. If there were no sickness how much would those persons who are now sick have produced? How much has been added to national income by health care – by the prevention and therapy measures now in use for specific diseases?

The effect of sickness upon the amount of human labor available for productive purposes can be summarized under three headings: (1) deaths (loss of workers); (2) disability (loss of working time); and (3) debility (loss of productive capacity while at work).

Essentially there are two stages in calculating the output added: (a) estimating the gain in productive work time and (b) assigning a money value to the output that this added work time represents. The result is then a dollar figure which represents the value of the gain in output attributable to reduction in deaths, disability and debility. In other words, it would be a rough estimate of the increase in output attributable to eradication of a specific disease or improvement in health status.

*Conceptual problems.* An estimate of gain in work time due to elimination or cure of a specific disease involves the assumption that if it were not for the disease those persons in the productive age groups stricken by the disease would have been working. In fact, where there is unemployment or substantial underemployment, improved health may result in more unemployment rather than more output. One obvious reason for using the simplifying assumption of full employment is that, unless we do, we cannot arrive at any definite concept of what the resource gain is. Apart from this, however, the fact that production losses resulting from poor health cannot be realized in an unemployment situation should be attributed to unemployment, not to ill health. Unemployment has its own cost, which in effect may cancel out reductions in the cost of sickness, but for analytical purposes it is necessary to distinguish between the two. We therefore measure the gains of disease eradication or cure in the assumed absence of

2. The discussion of labor product measurement which follows is, with minor exceptions, from Mushkin and Collings (1959, pp. 795–809).

costs of unemployment, recognizing, however, that unemployment itself may have an effect on the incidence of illness.[3]

There is another assumption implicit in the view that gains in production due to reduction in death, disability, and debility of workers can be attributed to a particular disease, namely, that persons who die from, or are disabled by, the disease would otherwise be in good health. Here again, it is possible that persons saved from one disease may promptly die of another, and their production thus be lost in any case. It seems reasonable enough to disregard this possibility for clearly defined diseases that strike primarily at persons of working age; but it is less reasonable if the disease, or treatment required to overcome it, weakens the patient by making him more prone to other ailments, and if the disease strikes mainly at persons who are constitutionally weak in any case, as with the diseases of old age. In these cases, the gains in production from prevention or cure can less clearly be identified as an effect of a single disease. The result of disregarding the presence of multiple diseases is an overestimate of the gains from eradication or control of any single disease. At some later stage in refinement of the concepts, a methodology must be developed to deal with this multiple-disease problem.

Moreover, the assumption that side effects of other diseases may be disregarded in order to measure the direct effects of the disease in question means that the gains from prevention or cure of each disease, taken individually, cannot be added together to make a meaningful total of gains from prevention or cure of all diseases.

In practice, the three categories of gains due to reductions in death, disability and debility need closer definition; and it may be necessary to subdivide them further to make them correspond to available data.

Death is unambiguous in meaning, but cause of death is sometimes not. In estimates of gains from prevention or cure caused by a particular disease, deaths from multiple causes may need to be treated differently from those caused by the disease in question

3. However, it is desirable to make an allowance for frictional unemployment, that is, the essential unemployment that exists even at full employment levels as when persons change jobs or are temporarily laid off. It is also desirable to allow for absenteeism over-employment, which is normal absence of workers from jobs because of vacations, bad weather, and temporary sickness. These adjustments may be applied to the final estimate of productive work time added due to prevention or cure of a disease in terms of a full-time equivalent number of man-years.

alone. Disability caused by sickness may be partial or total, and it may be short-term or long-term. Cases of long-term disability, especially when total, may be found primarily in institutions, and thus it may be convenient to subclassify again into institutional and non-institutional populations and use data available on institutional cases to measure a part of the disability caseload.

The division between disability and debility, furthermore, will not be clear-cut in many cases. For example, a blind person may be excluded altogether from the work force (total disability) or he may find some sheltered employment where his contribution to production is small (debility). He may also become a scientist, a writer, or a musician, where his contribution is average or above average, reflecting effects of neither disability nor debility.

The impact of diseases which cause debility, or loss of working efficiency, is no simple matter to define or to measure. In its broadest dimension, a measure of gain in output due to reduction in debility by prevention or cure of a disease requires formulation of a standard of output in the absence of the disease, from which shortcomings may be measured. While work on this concept is going forward, there still remain difficulties in applying the notion in terms of added product per unit of work time.

*Working time added.* The gain in resources through prevention or cure of disease and reduction in death, disability, and debility must, for the first stage of the estimate, be stated in terms of units of productive work time added. The second stage, to be dealt with later, is to assign a value to these units. In the case of reductions in death and long-term disability, the gains will take the form of periods of added time on the job, and these may be converted into equivalent units of full-time work added. Debility, defined as reduced productive efficiency per man, too may be converted into full-time equivalents. For convenience, the following discussion will refer to man-years as the units of productive work time.

How the equivalent of the full-time work force is defined operatively is of central importance to the estimate. A decision must be made on the age limits within which persons who contract disease will be considered as productive workers. In the United States, the age of entry into the work force is usually considered as fourteen years. This starting age is largely an historical carry-over in definition which has been perpetrated for comparative purposes in spite of the trend toward later entry into the work force. The retirement age varies widely among different groups and in different areas; the average age of retirement for the United States is estimated at present at sixty-eight years of age for men (Myers, 1957–8, pp. 337–50)

The consequence of this limitation of work-force participation is to count the resource gain from reduction in death, disability, and debility of children and the retired aged as zero when measuring annual output gains. This is consistent with the definition, since persons outside the work force are not considered to contribute anything to production in the year in question. For a capital formation analysis, however, infant and childhood deaths represent a future loss to society and must be allowed for, although the time interval between death and anticipated entry into the work force may be such that the present value of the future loss of working time is small.

The importance of the retirement-age assumption will vary with different social and economic settings. In some economies, the urgency of production for survival leaves little room for retirement prior to death or total disability; with higher productivity and industrial advances, cessation of work activity becomes feasible before extreme old age is reached. In an industrial community, therefore, it seems reasonable to exclude retired persons who cease to contribute to production, but in others retirement may be disregarded.

Whatever age limitations are set upon the productive work force, further qualification is necessary because not all persons of productive age are actually engaged in production. At full employment, only a certain proportion of the members of each age group will be productively employed, and the gain in man-years of work attributable to reduced deaths and disabilities among these persons alone should be counted in the estimate of work time added. Here again, this implies that death or disability of a person not in the active work force occasions no loss of productive resources.

Special problems arise in the case of women working in the home. Such women are not normally included in standard definitions of the work force, and their product, unlike that of paid domestic workers, is not included in the national economic accounts. Thus defined, their death or disability is not an economic cost – reductions in the number of such deaths in a year not an economic gain. However, this is highly anomalous; it implies that the national product is increased if every wife does housework for pay for the family next door and lowered if every man marries his cook. The only alternative is to impute some value to the services of housewives in the home, thus imputing an economic gain to reduction in their deaths or disabilities. Although proposals have been advanced for broadening the concept of production used for national product purposes to include such non-market services, no generally agreed way to do so at present exists (Copeland, 1957, pp. 19–95). To simplify the estimate and to follow an approach consistent with national product accounting it seems desirable to omit the valuation of housewife services.

A related problem concerns the method of counting deaths and disabilities among unpaid family workers. In the United States and several other countries, unpaid family work is included in the national product accounts, in effect requiring a prorating of income among the working members of the family. In this case, there is a basis for allocating a value to the services of such a worker. The importance of this problem obviously varies in different social settings, but in countries where a large proportion of production is carried on on farms and in other family enterprises it would be clearly advisable to count the gains from reduction in deaths and disabilities among those who work within the family unit without money wages.[4]

In estimates over a life span, work-life tables developed by the Bureau of Labor Statistics may be applied which identify the remaining years of work life at each age group. Estimates of work-life years have been developed for 1940 and 1950 for both men and women; and historical changes in the pattern of work-life expectancies have been estimated for 1900 and projected to the year 2000 (US Department of Labor, 1950, 1956; Garfinkle, 1955, pp. 297–301).

Data on deaths are collected by the National Vital Statistics Division of the United States Public Health Service. Data on absences from work due to sickness are collected as part of the National Health Survey and published as *Health Statistics* (Series B). A total of 371 million days of work loss by persons 17 years and over were reported for 1960 by those working or who had a business during the two previous weeks. The comparable figure

4. Further problems arise in connection with part-time workers. The gain in productive work time from reduction in a given impact of disease among these persons will be less than that among full-time workers, and this gain will have to be converted to a full-time equivalent for purposes of the estimate. The most practical solution to these definitional problems may be to use existing concepts of 'work force' and 'labor force' (converted to full-time equivalents) to estimate the gain in working time from prevention or cure of disease.

for 1961 was 365 million days. Assuming an average of 250 working days a year for each full-time worker (5 days a week for an average of 50 weeks), the 5·6 average work days lost per person in 1960 is equivalent to a 2·24 per cent loss of working time on the average due to sickness and injury. These figures exclude persons who withdraw from the labor force due to illness; some of these former workers are in institutions, others at home. When adjusted for withdrawals from the labor force, the 2·24 per cent work-time loss may be doubled to about 4·5 per cent. This 4·5 per cent figure sets the upper limit of the potential gain in work time from eradication of the disabling effects of disease and injury.

Absence from work due to disability is in part a result of the physical or mental condition of the individual but it reflects other factors affecting decisions to be absent from work. These decisions change with an individual's knowledge about health care, the institutional arrangements for social protection against wage loss, the net income consequences of the decision, and the nature of an individual's job and his employment relationships. A total of $0·7 billion was excluded from income taxable under the federal income tax as sick leave and insurance compensation for wages lost due to sickness in 1959.

Estimates on numbers of workers at work on a day but suffering some restriction in their usual activity may be derived from information collected by the National Health Survey.[5] The conversion of such information to full-time equivalent workers, however, poses additional difficulties.

Several different yardsticks of the effect of debility on worker efficiency have been used. Several others have been discussed. These include:

1. Output in a plant with recorded information on number of machines in operation, before and after disease control work is instituted (Ezdorf, 1916, pp. 614–29).

2. Wages earned on a piece-rate basis by those with a disease and those free of the disease (Fisher, 1909).

3. Wages of workers in an area with a high disease prevalence compared to wages of similar workers in areas free of the disease.

4. Output on a farm in which a disease problem is controlled, measured against output of a control group of workers.

5. Laboratory tests of work energy of groups of workers afflicted

5. We are a long way, however, from having data on work time lost through debility comparable to that on disability.

with a disease, measured against work capacity of a normal control group.

There are records of studies of increased worker output after disease control is instituted. The control-group type of experiment has been discussed and a beginning toward such experimentation has been made. Demands from the control groups for treatment in an area with a high rate of endemic disease have been met, and I am told that no experiment has been carried through to definitive findings. The laboratory approach to the problem of work energy grew out of a meeting with the productivity analysis staff of the Department of Labor and – though implementation has been considered – no steps toward it have been taken.

The alternative to these case studies is to compile mass data on output and on disease prevalence among workers and to analyse the data to find the effects of pertinent variables, including the extent of the disease.[6]

*Gain in output.* The previous stage in the computation has resulted in an estimate of the productive man-years added by reduction in deaths, disability and debility from sickness. This in itself may prove a useful piece of political arithmetic, but in most cases it will be desirable to translate this into dollar cost by assigning a value to the man-years added to production.

In the available studies on losses from illness, two essentially divergent approaches have been used in assigning a value to each unit of labor work time. The first is to value each unit by an amount equivalent to total product per worker; the other is to use earnings as a measure of labor product per worker.

6. Gains in working time due to reduction in debility from diseases now virtually eradicated have played a role in the economic growth of the United States. An analysis of the effect of reduced debility due to control of malaria and hookworm in the South would, I think, yield added perspective on the relative economic growth rates of the South and other sections of the country. Irving Fisher, writing in 1908 on the prevalence of hookworm disease in the South stated: 'The disease is remarkable not so much for its fatality . . . as for the chronic incapacity for work which it produces. For this reason, the hookworm has been nicknamed the "germ of laziness".' In the same report Fisher noted that there were probably three million cases of malaria – another debilitating disease – in the United States, mostly in the South. In the early 1930s it was estimated that at the height of the malaria season there were 6·8 million cases of malaria in the South – a figure well over one hundred times the number of annual deaths from malaria reported then.

The first of these assumes, as Fein has indicated, 'that all of the national product (income), and therefore any gains in national product, are attributable to labor rather than to some combination of joint factors of production, land, labor, capital, etc. Although it may indeed be true that if there were no labor there would be no product, it is equally true that if there were no capital there would be very little product' (Fein, 1958). The total-product-per-worker approach was used by Reynolds in his study of the cost of road accidents in Great Britain and also in the National Planning Association study on the costs of tuberculosis in the United States (Reynolds, 1956; National Planning Association, 1948).

The second alternative – to use earnings as a measure of the output attributable to labor – is more appropriate for purposes of estimating labor product added. Earnings, in this case, must be distinguished from income, which includes returns on property or capital; earnings consist only of wages and salaries (or equivalents for the self-employed). These wages and salaries are paid in direct return for productive services and correspond to the individual's contribution to production. The estimate of labor product added put in these terms thus measures the gain in production attributable to labor.

Average earnings multiplied by the number of man-years added as a result of the prevention or cure of disease yields the dollar estimate of resource gain. We are now in a position to define the result more closely. It is, essentially, an estimate of the money value of the labor product lost as a result of death, disability and debility. The prevention or cure of these provides a labor product that is added and gives an estimate of added income flow, or it can be converted into an estimate of capital formation through health programs by capitalizing this annual added labor product attributable to health care.

### Reduction of deaths and economic growth

Health programs use economic resources – men and materials; they also create economic resources. Viewing expenditures for health programs as an investment helps to underscore the contribution of health programs to expansion of income and economic growth. As the earlier discussion on the measurement of added labor product indicates, reductions in deaths are easier to quantify than reduction in disability or debility.

I attempt here to estimate the contribution to economic growth resulting from the enlargement of the work force through reductions in death rates over the past decades. The first question for which an estimate is sought may be put this way: how large would the 1960 work force be if death rates of earlier decades had prevailed and other factors remained unchanged? The second question: what is the value of the work force added by reduction in deaths, in terms of both the annual added product and the capital value of the future stream of earnings of the additional workers?

Denison (1962) analyses the potential contribution to economic growth rates of a series of labor-market and other measures, including improved health status of the population. He assumes, as a first approximation, that a given percentage change in the size of the labor force produces a constant percentage change in output. This constant return to scale assumption is modified so that over the twenty-year period ahead (1960–80) a 1 per cent rise in inputs of each of the factors of production – labor, land and capital – is assumed to yield a 1·09 per cent rise in output. A 1 per cent rise in number of workers, other factors held constant, is assumed to yield an 0·843 per cent rise in national output.

Within this framework, Denison assesses the effects of a reduction in the death rate on the rate of economic growth. He shows the maximum change in rate of growth that is attributable to the change in the number of workers, assuming no one died in the two decades of the 1960s and 1970s before reaching age sixty-five. Under this extreme assumption the labor force in 1980 would be 4·8 per cent larger than is now projected, and the national income would be 4 per cent higher; averaged over the twenty-year period this would mean an 0·20 percentage point rise per annum in the growth rate. If death rates were reduced 10 per cent, which would be 'an extraordinary achievement', the growth rate would be increased by 0·02 per cent.

He applies a similar analysis to the loss of work days through illness and injury, as reported in the National Health Survey, and adds the loss attributable to the population in mental and tuberculosis institutions. Together the work loss of the institutional and non-institutional population for 1958 amounted to 4·4 per cent of work time. A reduction of one-fourth in this lost time, Denison estimates, would increase labor output by 1·1 per cent by 1980 and total national income by 0·9 per cent; the 1960–80 growth rate would be raised by 0·05 per cent.

While the contribution to economic growth of the sizable changes in mortality and morbidity assumed by Denison is not large percentagewise, a 1·5 per cent rise in the labor force by 1980 (1·1 per cent disability and 0·4 per cent deaths) converted to absolute amounts would be the equivalent of well over $5 billion.

*Addition to employment and national income.* Denison estimates the effect of improvement in education of the labor force on the national income over an historical period, but he does not apply his analysis to historical trends in health status. It is possible, however, to estimate employment increases attributable to the improvement in life expectancy over the past decades and to estimate the growth in employment and national income resulting from this improvement. One method is to estimate the size of the work force in 1960 under the hypothetical condition of death rates of early decades and to compare the actual work force in 1960 with these hypothetical estimates.

Table 2 **Additional persons in work force in 1960 attributable to improved life expectancy, by age and sex** (in thousands)

| Sex and age group | Average number employed 1960 | Persons employed in 1960 who would not have survived to 1960 if mortality experience were that of year designated | | | | | |
|---|---|---|---|---|---|---|---|
| | | 1950 | 1940 | 1930 | 1920 | 1910 | 1900 |
| Male | 44,484 | 235 | 864 | 2245 | 3647 | 7081 | 8743 |
| 14–24 years | 6695 | 3 | 47 | 292 | 576 | 998 | 1192 |
| 25–34 years | 9759 | 10 | 98 | 332 | 859 | 1532 | 1923 |
| 35–44 years | 10551 | 24 | 179 | 496 | 876 | 1783 | 2279 |
| 45–54 years | 9182 | 55 | 220 | 542 | 808 | 1322 | 1772 |
| 55–64 years | 6106 | 79 | 208 | 397 | 427 | 995 | 1130 |
| 65 years and over | 2191 | 64 | 112 | 186 | 101 | 451 | 447 |
| Female | 22,195 | 75 | 474 | 1285 | 2362 | 3464 | 4467 |
| 14–24 years | 4457 | 4 | 32 | 178 | 348 | 611 | 740 |
| 25–34 years | 3871 | 4 | 46 | 147 | 368 | 585 | 743 |
| 35–44 years | 5046 | 10 | 91 | 257 | 515 | 817 | 1080 |
| 45–54 years | 5055 | 19 | 116 | 313 | 581 | 698 | 1006 |
| 55–64 years | 2884 | 26 | 124 | 260 | 392 | 519 | 643 |
| 65 years and over | 882 | 12 | 65 | 130 | 158 | 234 | 255 |

Sources: Based on estimates by Dr Monroe Sirken, of the National Vital Statistics Division, United States Public Health Service, of 1960 white labor force by age, assuming specified changes in mortality experience. Estimates presented above apply mortality experience of white males and females to total employed persons and make no allowance for added births due to increased numbers in child-bearing ages.

Estimates of the number of persons in civilian employment in 1960 who survived to that year because of improved life expectancy are shown in Table 2. These estimates are computed by applying to the 1960 employed population, by age and sex, the ratio of the number of survivors in earlier decades (per 100,000 born) to the actual number surviving to these ages in each generation (per 100,000). In developing these estimates, the mortality experience of white males and females is applied to all employed persons and no allowance is made for the added births due to the increased number in the child-bearing ages; nor is a correction made for immigration. Educational levels and employment patterns are assumed to be the same for the additional survivors as for others.

The employed population in 1960 would have been over thirteen million less than it was if death rates had not declined since 1900; it would have been six million less if death rates had declined from 1900 to 1920, but had remained at the 1920 rates thereafter. Reductions in mortality rates made possible these additions to the work force and also added their labor product. The labor product added by the additional thirteen million survivors, when valued at average earnings of 1960, amounts to a more than $60 billion addition to national income. The six million additional survivors, attributable to the decline in mortality since 1920, added almost $28 billion to the nation's output of goods and services (Table 3).

Stated differently, the labor force in 1960 was about 25 per cent higher than it would have been if 1900 mortality rates continued unchanged throughout the sixty-year period 1900–1960, and about 10 per cent higher than it would have been if 1920 mortality rates had continued from 1920 to 1960. The decline in mortality rates in the 1950s increased the 1960 labor force by an amount equivalent to a ·05 per cent rise per annum in employment, but not all of the gain for the first years of life is reflected as yet in the labor force and will not be until about 1970.

National income was increased by an amount equivalent to a 0·3 per cent rise per annum due to the decline in mortality rates from the 1900 level (assuming, as does Denison, that a 1 per cent rise in number of workers, other factors held constant, yields a 0·73 per cent rise in national income for this period). The decline in death rates in the past sixty years thus accounts for over 10 per cent of the overall 3 per cent growth rate in the economy.

An alternative analysis of the effect of declining death rates on

**Table 3 Estimated effect on growth of work force and national income of improved life expectancy from 1900 and other years as designated to 1960**

A. Additional civilian work force and labor product (in millions)

| | Work force in 1960 if mortality rates had continued unchanged since | Additional work force in 1960 attributable to reduced mortality rates | Value of added labor product in 1960 |
|---|---|---|---|
| 1960 | 66·7 | | |
| 1950 | 66·4 | 0·3 | $1390 |
| 1940 | 65·3 | 1·4 | 6489 |
| 1930 | 63·2 | 3·5 | 16,222 |
| 1920 | 60·7 | 6·0 | 27,810 |
| 1910 | 56·2 | 10·5 | 48,668 |
| 1900 | 53·5 | 13·2 | 61,182 |

B. Percentage increase in civilian work force and labor product

| Increase in 1960 attributable to reduction in mortality since | Percentage by which 1960 work force raised | Percentage by which 1960 national income raised | |
|---|---|---|---|
| | | Total | Per annum equivalent |
| 1950 | 0·5 | 0·4 | 0·04 |
| 1940 | 2·0 | 1·5 | 0·07 |
| 1930 | 5·6 | 4·0 | 0·13 |
| 1920 | 9·9 | 7·2 | 0·18 |
| 1910 | 18·8 | 13·7 | 0·26 |
| 1900 | 24·7 | 18·0 | 0·27 |

economic growth may be made. In the figures presented above, the base in each case is the actual civilian work force in 1960 compared to the hypothetical 1960 civilian work force. A set of estimates similar to those presented here for 1960 may be developed for each of the earlier decades. These additional estimates would permit comparison of the growth of employment under conditions of varying mortality.

For example, Denison estimates employment in 1957 at an index of 144·1 with 1929 as 100. If 1930 death rates had continued unchanged throughout the twenty-eight years between 1929 and

1957, the index of employment in 1957 would have been 136·7 and not 144·1. The difference, 7·4 percentage points, is attributable to the decline in death rates. Accordingly, 20 per cent of the *rise* in employment in the twenty-eight year period (1929–57) is due to lower death rates. A 20 per cent employment increase, assuming labor inputs account for 73 per cent of the total factor income, again results in about a 15 per cent rise in national income.

These figures assume, as I have indicated, that other things remained unchanged. Hours of work, educational investments, labor productivity, immigration policies, and labor-force participation rates, among other factors, undoubtedly were influenced by the decline in mortality but the purpose here is to consider the effect of the single factor – the decline in deaths – on employment and national income. Not all of the decline in deaths is, of course, a consequence of medical advances and improved health care. Productivity increases, which have enlarged earnings, reflect technological progress and improved education of the labor force, both formal education and on-the-job training. While it is difficult to assess the role of health programs in the over-all lengthening of life expectancy, such an assessment can be made for specific diseases over a relatively brief span of years, and when new therapies can be identified as the cause of a decline. Dauer estimates that 1·1 million lives were saved in the period 1938–52 as a result of the use of antibiotics and chemotherapy in pneumonia and influenza cases (Dauer, 1955). Given the age distribution of the saved lives and also labor-force participation rates, I calculate that the labor force in 1952 was almost 0·5 per cent higher than it would have been had the new therapies not been used. The national income in 1952 was as a consequence enlarged by well over $1 billion.

*Capital formation.* The future earnings stream created by the additional workers and their labor product may be capitalized and converted to a capital stock figure. Persons at work in 1960 who would not have survived to that year if mortality experience of earlier decades had prevailed contributed to national output in 1960, but they also continue to work during their remaining lifetimes. The present value of the future earnings of these additional workers at different ages is shown in Table 4. The estimates of the assets created by improved life expectancy are presented in Table 5, based on the estimated additions to the civilian work force

Table 4 **1960 discounted value of future earnings at selected ages, males and females***

| Age | Males | Females |
|---|---|---|
| 20 | $89,270 | $49,460 |
| 30 | 101,394 | 50,931 |
| 40 | 88,170 | 44,982 |
| 50 | 62,179 | 33,380 |
| 60 | 30,200 | 16,131 |
| 65 and older | 12,003† | 6141† |

* Computed by Mr Robert J. Myers, chief actuary of the Social Security Administration, on the basis of United States Life Tables for 1959, using average earnings by age in 1960 estimated from 1960 average income data (Census Bureau) as indicated in text; and applying a net discount rate of 5 per cent per annum. (See text for discussion of the net discount rate.)

† Based on three years' earnings at age sixty-six average earnings rate.

(Table 2). While the additional survivors reflect the improved health status of the work force, the added earnings reflect the composite effects of many factors contributing to the trends in earnings. Among these factors are increased educational levels of the work force and improved industrial organization and techniques.

The question answered by the figures presented is: what is the

Table 5* **Capital value in 1960 of labor product added by improved life expectancy, 1900–1960** (in billions)

| Change in mortality experience since | Capital value in 1960 added by | | |
| | All additions to employment† | Added male workers | Added female workers |
|---|---|---|---|
| 1950 | $12·0 | $10·0 | $2·0 |
| 1940 | 65·3 | 51·0 | 14·3 |
| 1930 | 194·7 | 151·4 | 43·3 |
| 1920 | 365·9 | 280·1 | 85·8 |
| 1910 | 649·2 | 519·3 | 129·9 |
| 1900 | 820·5 | 652·0 | 168·5 |

* Based on Tables 2 and 4. Represents the 1960 value of the future lifetime earnings of persons added to the 1960 work force by changes in mortality experience, discounted by 5 per cent. (See text for underlying assumption on trend in average earnings and interest rate.)

† Totals may not add due to rounding.

value of product that will be contributed after 1960 by the additional workers when we view this product as a capital asset? Or stated somewhat differently: how large a holding would be required to yield a sum equivalent to that of the added labor product over a period of years comparable to that of the work life expectancy of the additional workers?

The asset value in 1960 of the added labor product attributable to the workers added to the work force by the reduction in mortality rates since 1900 is $820 billion. Or it would require a capital stock of $820 billion to replace the product equivalent of the additional workers. The reduction in death rates since 1930 contributed to the creation of a capital asset of over $190 billion.

In developing these estimates the years of work-force participation beyond 1960 for the additional workers in each age-sex group is computed based on 1959 United States Life Tables for men and for women, without an allowance for any further gain in life expectancy. Retirement at age sixty-eight is uniformly assumed for both men and women. Average future earnings by age and sex are estimated from 1960 Census data.[7] These average earnings by age and sex are adjusted upward to a full-time earning base, an adjustment made so that the average of earnings is conceptually the same as the additional employment figures.

It is also assumed that average earnings continue to rise in the future as they have in the past decades. (A composite rise in earnings of 3 per cent per annum is assumed.) Uniform gains in average earnings each year are assumed for all age groups, although a more precise formulation may suggest relatively higher gains in productivity at the younger ages because of their longer period of education. Earnings from 1960 to the end of their working life of those persons added to the 1960 civilian work force through improvement in life expectancy over the past decades are discounted at an arbitrary interest rate of 8 per cent, a rate used in recent studies of returns on educational capital.

The growth in earnings and the discount rates are essentially combined in the mechanics of the estimating procedure. A 5 per

7. The 1960 earnings by age are derived from a free-hand plotting of cross-sectional curves of 1960 average earnings by age groups. The average earnings figures, in turn, were derived from average income figures by age and sex for 1960 as estimated by the Census Bureau. The conversion of average income to average earnings by sex and age is made on the basis of the ratio of median earnings by age to median income by age in 1951, the latest date for which these data appear to be available.

cent *net* discount figure is used (that is, an 8 per cent discount rate, less a 3 per cent increase in average earnings per annum). Different sets of assumptions could be substituted without altering the estimates shown in Tables 4 and 5. For example, a 7 per cent discount rate and a 2 per cent rise in earnings per annum would also indicate a net figure of 5 per cent, as would a 5 per cent interest rate without allowance for future increases in earnings.

Net discount rates other than 5 per cent, however, will affect the rapidity of the decline involved in placing a present value on earnings far in the future. The influence of different interest rates on valuing future earnings is illustrated in Weisbrod's study in which he uses alternatively interest rates of 4 and 10 per cent – these being based, respectively, on the cost of long-term government borrowing and the rate of return on corporate investment (Weisbrod, 1958).

The estimates considerably overstate the magnitude of capital formation through improved health care. Not all the gains in life expectancy originate in medical advances and health programs. And gains in productivity are mainly attributable to non-health factors such as improved education and technology. However, the estimates make no allowance for any reductions in disability or debility. The overstatement of the effect of health programs on improved life expectancy is not necessarily balanced by the omission of any gains from reduced disability and debility. Data are not readily available by which to assess this problem. Far more research is needed before we can measure the shares of added capital values attributable to health care, research that would yield data on the capital formation due to reduced disability and debility.

### Earlier studies

Two concepts of a system of measurement of human assets created through health programs may be identified in the work that has been done. The first is the measurement of the costs of rearing a child, or of developing a productive labor force, an investment that is lost if premature death occurs. The second is a capital stock measure of the present value of future work that may be gained through eradication or control of disease. A third line of inquiry has been followed in the measurement of the contribution of health programs to annual output and to economic growth.

*Developmental-cost concept.* The developmental-cost approach compares the lost investment in the rearing of a child who dies before making his full contribution to production with the investment required to enable him to make that contribution.

The developmental-cost approach was used by Richard Contillion in his essay on *The Nature of Commerce in General* published in 1755, and by Quetelet, a social statistician who wrote in 1835:

In his early years, man lives at the expense of society; he contracts a debt which he must one day discharge; and if he dies before he has succeeded in doing so, his life will have been a burden rather than a benefit to his fellow citizens (Sand, 1952, p. 584).

Edwin Chadwick, while serving as secretary to the Poor Law Commission, was struck with the extent to which sickness produced poverty. For the first time a group of physicians systematically studied environmental conditions resulting in preventable illness. Chadwick's report in 1842 on the *Sanitary Conditions of the Laboring Population of Great Britain* created an urgent demand for environmental sanitation measures; it also established the idea of health programs as an integral part of economic policy. Fein quotes Chadwick as writing: 'The economist for the advancement of his science may well treat the human being simply as an investment of capital . . .' and cites Chadwick's detailed money estimates of the value of individuals based on the costs of rearing a child, taking account of the factor of death before he became productive and the number of his productive years (Fein, 1961).

The investment in bringing up a child has been measured for a number of purposes, including (a) farm family budgetary needs, (Tarver, 1956) (b) indemnity insurance (Dublin and Lotka, 1946), (c) the setting of amounts of family allowances (Henderson, 1959), and (d) assessing child welfare levels (Ogburn, 1919). This concept recurs in analyses of economic development. For example, Singer writes:

Thus it may be said, perhaps somewhat paradoxically, that one of the troubles of underdeveloped countries is not so much that there is not enough investment but rather that *there is too much unproductive investment*. Practically all investment . . . is investment in the feeding and bringing up of a new generation for productive work. . . . If that is included as investment – as it should – it may well be found that investment in underdeveloped countries is much higher in relation to national income than in the more developed countries, with their low birth rates and low death rates, perhaps even higher on a per capita basis. The trouble is that so much of this investment is unproductive because high death rates prevent the repayment, with interest, of the capital sunk in the younger generations[8] (Singer, no date).

In this development-cost concept, health programs are not the sole measure of investment; the yardstick used is the total cost of rearing a child. Essentially, it is the child that is viewed as an asset to yield a future return, and all the cost of upbringing, including food and clothing, are included in the investment outlays. The child's production after it is grown to adulthood is counted as the yield on the investment.

*Capitalized earnings.* The second system of measurement had its origins primarily in insurance and actuarial theory. In one study it was used to compare the value of life insurance in force with the total value of insurable individuals (Woods and Metzger, 1927). Dublin and Lotka, demographers and actuaries rather than economists, contributed the major work on the methods of evaluating the capital represented by man. For their purposes of insurance claims and indemnity of families they define capital value of man as the present and discounted value of future earning power of the wage earner, reduced by the costs of birth, upbringing and maintenance during a working life and retirement (Dublin and Lotka, 1946).

8. H. W. Singer. However, Coale and Hoover (1958), state that the thesis developed by Singer and others on developmental investment is fallacious. If more children are enabled to survive to their adult years, they say, there will not only be more workers but also more parents and the increased numbers of parents will produce more children, if birth rates remain unchanged. In fact, Coale in other research studies has shown that the rise in the number of children is somewhat greater than the rise in the number of workers. The argument is advanced to the point of concluding that, since the proportion of children rises slightly with typical mortality improvements, the economy 'wastes' *more* (not less) of its substance on non-productive resources as a consequence of improved mortality.

Health care which reduces mortality, however, also raises the output of workers in a nation by increasing the vitality of these workers; many diseases with high prevalence rates in underdeveloped nations – diseases such as malaria, yaws, trachoma, schistosomiasis, and bilharziasis – moreover, are chiefly cripplers of mankind rather than killers. Enterline and Stewart, applying an age cohort analysis similar to that used by Coale and Hoover, estimate that less than a 20 per cent rise in productivity per worker over a seventy-five-year period (a percentage equivalent to less than a quarter of 1 per cent rise in productivity per annum) would be needed to achieve an advancing level of real income *per capita* at the same time as life

In their study Dublin and Lotka trace the thinking on man's capital value through the works of Sir William Petty, Adam Smith, William Farr, E. Engel, Irving Fisher, J. M. Clark, and others. Petty, in his *Political Arithmetic* measured the value of the whole population by determining their total earnings and capitalizing these earnings so as to derive the equivalent capital sum, which would yield such earnings, if invested at a given rate of interest. He wrote of the *per capita* values he set forth, 'from whence we may learn to compute the loss we have sustained by the plague, by the slaughter of men in war, and by sending them abroad' (Dublin and Lotka, 1946, p. 9).

William Farr in his 1853 article in the *Journal of the Statistical Society* and in his later volume on *Vital Statistics* (1885) computed the economic value of a human life by discounting the value of future earnings taking account of average life duration at different ages. Farr deducted from these earnings the discounted value of maintenance costs, including the cost during the period of childhood dependence and 'helpless old age'. Farr applied his estimates of human values to problems of public policy, including tax policies, as well as health programs, as did Petty before him.

Beginning with Chadwick's studies, health workers have repeatedly applied the concepts of the value of a human life to problems of health program expenditures. Hermann M. Biggs expressed the health administrator's concern in his slogan coined almost four decades ago for New York City's health department: 'Public health is purchasable; within natural limitations a community can determine its own death rate.' Valuation of human life and the economic effects of health programs through reduction in deaths and disability have been measured for a series of disease problems over many decades.

---

expectancy is increased from thirty years at birth to sixty-eight years at birth – the level in the highly industrialized nations of the world. A less than 20 per cent rise in productivity over a seventy-five-year period would compensate for the combined effects of (a) the larger number of births due to increased numbers in the child-bearing ages, (b) the increased proportion of dependents in the population, and (c) the increased investment in physical capital goods required to maintain a consistent ratio of marginal capital to workers. I conclude on the basis of information about the debilitating effects of disease on worker productivity that the wastes in the investment in children resulting from high mortality rates can be prevented and economic growth advanced rather than delayed by improving health conditions. (A more detailed, although preliminary, analysis of this problem was included in an earlier draft of this paper.)

At the beginning of this century, President Theodore Roosevelt by executive order called for the co-operation of executive agencies in the work of the National Conservation Commission chaired by Pinchot. 'The problem of conserving natural resources is only one part of the larger problem of conserving national efficiency. The other part relates to the vitality of our population.' In carrying out the work of the National Conservation Commission, Irving Fisher wrote his *Report on National Vitality: Its Wastes and Conservation*. Fisher points up the relation between health and conservation of physical assets indicating that in its broadest view health is the primary form of wealth. 'Without enlarging or insisting upon this concept, it is obvious that by the conservation of health we may ultimately save billions of dollars of wasted values' (Fisher, 1909, p. 125).

Fisher's estimates of disease-cost include (a) a cost of premature death measured according to Farr's method of determining the present value of net future earnings, (b) the loss of working time of those in the working ages who are sick, and (c) the cost of medical attendance, medicine and nursing. The cost of illness, including loss of wages and cost of care is set at $1 billion. Fisher also estimates the human assets of the United States' population of over 85·5 million people (1907) at $250 billion, 'which, though a minimum estimate, greatly exceeds value of all other wealth'. The current value of net future earnings which could be gained by eliminating preventable deaths, Fisher estimates, would add another $1 billion.

Fisher draws on studies made during the early 1900s on the economic cost of tuberculosis, hookworm, typhoid, malaria and smallpox. And during the next decades, additional studies were made on special disease problems and on the costs of preventable deaths (Dublin and Whitney, 1920; Williams, 1938, pp. 148–51; Lees, 1918; Cummings and White, 1923; Ashford and Igdravidez, 1911). These studies fell into disrepute in the health field and interest lagged. The reasons for this can be found in part in the use of aggregate estimates of costs of preventable deaths and disabilities in the arguments in favor of a national health insurance program (Ewing, 1948), a program about which even now there continues to be much political controversy. Some of the objections to these studies are familiar to those doing research in investments in education – one is the 'crass' valuation of human life.

Nevertheless, in three health-program areas cost-benefit estimates have been applied effectively. Occupational health programs have been urged in terms of the 'payoff' in reduced absences and workmen's compensation premiums (Klem and McKiever, 1950; Klem, *et al.*, 1950; Bachman, *et al.*, 1952; University of Michigan Survey Research Center, 1957). Extension of vocational rehabilitation services has been advocated in terms of tax payments by those rehabilitated, amounting to many times the cost of rehabilitation. And health-research agencies have pointed to economic gains through improved health far in excess of the medical research outlays (National Health Education Committee, 1959). 'When the capital value of human beings is once recognized, the tremendous importance of movements for conserving and lengthening life is better appreciated' (Woods and Metzger, 1927).

The origin of recent economic research on the value of human capital created by health care lies in the development of public expenditure theory and the emphasis given to cost-benefit analysis. The economist, in attempting to identify an objective function for decisions on expenditures, has evaluated benefits from programs in the social welfare field.

The allocation of economic resources is generally determined in the market by the preferences of consumers for work, leisure, and income. These preferences, as expressed in the market, are a guide to optimum use of resources. But there are a number of reasons why consumer preferences are not a wholly reliable guide to optimum use of health resources, even when the word 'optimum' is used in this special sense.

First, the consumer would prefer to avoid both illness and the purchase of health services. An individual's purchase of some medical services is of benefit to others. Purchases by some consumers, for example, of influenza vaccination during an epidemic prevent further spread of the disease. The value of the medical services to each consumer does not depend upon his consumption of medical services alone but upon decisions of his neighbors as well. Those who make no purchases of influenza vaccine also benefit. Thus, the social value of medical services is far larger than the private marginal value to those making the investment in themselves. Individual decisions of a consumer are therefore inadequate as an efficient guide to the optimum allocation of resources for health purposes. For these individual decisions tend to undervalue health services and result in an underproduction of these services.

Second, some health services entail processes which have in them 'indivisibilities' which do not lend themselves to pricing on the market so that society's preference for them cannot be adequately valued on the markets (Clark, 1926). Air and water pollution control, fluoridation of water supplies, and mosquito control are examples of these services. Furthermore, the price system for individual services is not applied to all cases: (a) the medically indigent are not excluded from care when they are sick, and (b) public safety and health sometimes require direct provision of health services and the removal of the individual from the community. Public hospital services for the mentally ill and for persons with tuberculosis are examples of services that are outside the price–market system.

Third, the allocation of health resources is determined by a mixture of private market decisions and administrative decisions. 'Administrative decisions' include those decisions made by the government, by private non-profit agencies, and by professional organizations. Decisions concerning some health facilities (the size of a general hospital, for example) are made by voluntary agencies. In many communities, the Visiting Nurses Association determines the availability of part-time nursing care. In some places the content and quality of rural health services are determined by a regional organization associated with a medical school. The principles underlying these administrative decisions and the way in which they influence the allocation of health resources need to be explored.

Emphasizing that much health care is provided outside of the market mechanism and that the market test of efficiency is not applied, Weisbrod states the economic problem as follows:

With all of the many health-promoting activities that could be carried on, with all of the many demands upon limited public health funds, administrators of public health action programs . . . are sorely in need of some meaningful, scientifically defensible standards against which to appraise contending expenditure proposals. The economist should be able to contribute to the establishment of such standards by specifying, within limits, the social benefits from alternative health programs (Weisbrod, 1958).

Weisbrod outlines a procedure to aid in the making of rational choices among alternative public health projects and to establish a framework for estimating the social benefits of improved health. He applies this method to selected disease problems in the hope that the procedures will assist in establishing priorities among public health projects.

Drawing heavily on the work of Dublin and Lotka, Weisbrod assesses the comparative costs of three diseases – cancer, tuberculosis and poliomyelitis. He includes in each case, in addition to the direct cost of medical resources devoted to the care and treatment of the diseases, the loss of manpower through death and disability. He measures the economic value of a life saved by the present value of future average gross earnings, less consumption of a person at age $n$, taking account of the remaining years of work-force participation of males and of females at each age and making allowance for frictional unemployment. He defines earnings and consumption more precisely than Dublin and Lotka do, and he neatly formulates and measures 'earnings of a housewife' and 'consumption by an added member of a family'. The costs of disability are measured as the product of the number of new cases of disability at each age group, the average time lost from production and the average annual earnings. As Weisbrod suggests, the resultant ranking of diseases according to monetary losses leaves out non-monetary losses such as the psychological burden carried by the victim's family. A study by Laitin, limited to the costs of cancer, applies a similar method (Laitin, 1956).

Fein, in the only recent study by an economist that was published under the auspices of a health agency, makes explicit some of the underlying assumptions (Fein, 1958). In addition to estimating the cost of mental illness in the United States as it affects each year's output, he calculates the present value of the loss in future earnings of persons hospitalized for mental illness in a year, basing this calculation on the number of their remaining years of work expectation and their average earnings. But he refrains from comparing his estimates with others on different diseases. Suggesting that it would be both interesting and useful to make such comparisons, he emphasizes the lack of comparability of the existing estimates as to concept and statistical adequacy so that they in fact measure different things (see Table 6 for illustrations of the different methods currently in use). Fein emphasizes instead the interrelation of direct outlays for mental illness, defining such outlays to include medical care costs and transfer payments and the indirect costs due to losses in economic production.

A series of studies on highway accidents include the cost of impairment and loss of human life. The Eleventh International

Table 6 **Illustrative estimates of earnings loss due to deaths and disabilities from specific diseases used by private research organizations**

| Disease | Earnings loss (in billions) |
| --- | --- |
| Arteriosclerosis and hypertension: | |
| One year's added work for persons 25–64 years times median family income, 1957 | $1·1 |
| Heart disease: | |
| Man-years lost in a year times median family income, 1957 | 3·2 |
| Cancer: | |
| Man-years lost in a year times median family income, 1957 | 0·6 |
| Mental illness: | |
| Work lost by resident patients in mental hospitals and through absence of non-hospitalized patients (1952 and 1954) valued at average earnings | 0·7 |
| Arthritis and rheumatism: | |
| Basis of computation not fully stated | 1·2 |
| Blindness: | |
| Cash transfer payments | 0·09 |
| Cerebral palsy: | |
| Estimated on basis of cash assistance required to maintain those not self-supporting | 0·2 |

Source: Compiled from National Health Education Committee (1959).

Road Congress, after review of the problem of human costs of highway accidents as part of cost-benefit analysis of highway construction, concludes:

However repellent it may be to assess human life, it does not seem that such a valuation can be dispensed with.... Decisions attribute unconsciously in each case a value to human life and suffering. It seems preferable to make this more conscious and systematic (see Thedie and Abraham, 1961, pp. 589–95).

Thedie and Abraham, French engineers, in an interesting analysis of the capital value of man point out, 'every day decisions are taken. A crossroad is laid out, but a sharp turn remains. Some hospitals are built. Why not more? Certain sums are spent on medical research. Why not larger or smaller amounts?' Thedie and Abraham, while refining the methods of measurements used in an earlier study by Reynolds (1956) on human costs of highway accidents, draw on his classification of costs and add to them. Their objective is to find a rule making it possible to decide on a certain investment or to refuse it.

In Reynolds' estimates of economic cost he attempts to assess the net loss in output of goods and services due to death or injury and the expenditures necessitated by the accident, including medical-care expenditures. Thedie and Abraham question the omission of evaluation of a human life that makes no contribution to production. They argue that it does not follow that because the death of an individual costs the community nothing (in terms of production), no attempt should be made to avoid the death. The value of a human life without regard to whether the person is a producer or not, they suggest, should in fact be the outcome of a collective decision concerning the expense that the nation is willing – as a moral judgment – to undertake, to save one of its members. In addition, they reject Reynolds' view that pain and suffering cannot be evaluated. They classify moral (non-economic) losses due to accidents as follows: (a) affective injury to the family from the loss of one of its members, (b) affective injury to the nation from loss of one of its citizens, (c) loss of capacity to enjoy life caused by an accident, (d) pain and suffering of the accident victim. Last, they include a value for 'the desire to live' on the part of a person whose life is threatened and they suggest a term for this injury, 'the price of living'. They include these 'non-economic' losses and 'value' them by using the amounts determined by the courts as compensation in accident cases.

Cost-benefit analysis more recently has been extended to water-supply systems with a measurement of benefits from reduction in disease as part of the analysis (Pyatt and Rogers, 1961). Pyatt and Rogers include the costs of waterborne diseases with a view to developing a method that would be applicable to decision-making in the construction of municipal water systems. They define the money value of a man at a particular age as the stream of his future earning discounted to the year of evaluation, less future consumption also discounted to the year of evaluation. While the general outlines of the Weisbrod method are followed, the formulae for computation are revised to fit the types of data available.

These authors set forth the benefit-cost ratio, taking account of reduced mortality and morbidity for a period of fifty years – the estimated life of a water-supply system. Taking account of the minimum exposure to the water-supply system of children born in the year 2010 they lengthen the study period to 2010, plus seventy-five years, the length of life expectancy of those born in the last year of useful life of the water-supply system.

*Contribution to national income.* A still different approach is followed in several studies of the problem of the economic contribution of disease eradication and control – an approach designed to illustrate the yield from health expenditures in terms of annual labor product added, rather than the human assets or human capital added. These studies are concerned with the change in size of an annual income flow and with economic growth rates.

In an earlier article Frank Collings and I emphasized the usefulness of estimates of annual labor product gains through disease control as a basis for health program planning (Mushkin and Collings, 1959). The labor-product change attributable to eradication of mental illness is the subject of the Fein inquiry (1958). A similar method is used in a study of the costs of peptic ulcers and ulcerative colitis. The total economic cost of these two ulcerative disorders in the nation is measured by Blumenthal in terms of annual loss of earnings due to disability and death. The costs of medical care for those disabled by ulcerative disorders are added. Blumenthal places the costs of $0·5 billion and contrasts this with the $5 million being spent for research on these diseases (Blumenthal, 1959).

A Public Health Service study of the economic benefits of murine typhus control also uses an income flow analysis to tell a success story of a public health program (Hill and Saunders, 1960). Estimates are made of the average losses that would have been incurred by (a) the economy at large, (b) the individual's own family, and (c) the tax assessor, if 1944 incidence rates of murine typhus had continued into 1958. Estimates are made showing the loss from non-fatal and also from fatal cases, assuming alternatively that losses may be valued in terms of gross product per worker and of average earnings (with self-employed persons assumed to have the same average earnings as wage and salary workers). The figures are developed on a one-year basis over a thirteen-year period. The authors conclude that the earnings gained through the working time 'saved' far exceed the cost of the disease eradication. The additional taxes paid on the added annual earnings were about five times as large as expenditures for typhus control in the years for which expenditure data were available.

The murine typhus study is especially noteworthy. It illustrates the types of adjustments that are necessary in morbidity and mortality statistics before these statistics can be used for economic analysis. The work done strongly suggests the need for a team approach to the study of the costs of individual diseases. A team consisting of a biostatistician and a physician, as well as an economist, would help to improve the quality of the studies.

The staff of a subcommittee of the Senate Committee on Government Operations, in a 1961 report of its findings and recommendations on the budgeting and accounting of health expenditures, emphasizes the need for measurement of the economic costs of disease. While the task is not easy

it is both possible and desirable if the nation is in the future to allocate its health resources – men, money and material – on as objective a basis as possible. . . . It is the staff's judgment that it would be in the interest of the US Government to develop in cooperation with private authorities, a sound economic-statistical framework for estimating the toll of disease and disability (US Congress, 1961).[9]

9. United States Congress, Report of the Senate Committee on Government Operations Made by Its Subcommittee on Reorganization and International Organization, *Coordination of Federal Agencies' Programs in Biomedical Research and in Other Scientific Areas* (87th Cong., 1st sess., Senate Report 142 (Washington, 1961)).

### References

ASHFORD, B. E., and IGDRAVIDEZ, P. G. (1911), *Ucinariasis in Puerto Rico: A Medical and Economic Problem*, 61st Congress, 3rd Session, Washington.

BACHMAN, G. W., *et al.* (1952), *Health Resources in the United States: Personnel, Facilities and Services*, Brooking's Institution.

BAUER, P. T., and YAMEY, B. S. (1957), *The Economics of Underdeveloped Countries*, Cambridge University Press.

BERGSTEN, J. W. (1960), 'Volume of physician visits, US, July 1957 – June 1959', *Statistics from the US National Health Survey*, Series B–19, also Series B–10, July 1957–June 1958, Washington.

BLUMENTHAL, I. S. (1959), *Research and the Ulcer Problem*, Rand Corporation.

CLARK, J. M. (1926), *Social Control of Business*, University of Chicago Press.

COALE, A. J., and HOOVER, E. M. (1958), *Population Growth and Economic Development in Low Income Countries*, Princeton University Press.

COPELAND, M. A. (1957), 'The feasibility of a standard comprehensive system of social accounts', in *Problems in the International Comparison of Economic Account*, NBER.

CUMMINGS, J. C., and WHITE, J. H. (1923), *Control of Hookworm Infection at the Deep Gold Mines of Mother Lode, California*, Department of the Interior, Bureau of Mines Bulletin, no. 139.

DAUER, C. C. (1955), 'A demographic analysis of recent changes in mortality, morbidity and age group distribution in our population', Paper given at the Institute of Medical History, June 2nd, New York Academy of Medicine.

DENISON, E. F. (1962), *The Sources of Economic Growth in the United States and the Alternative before us*, Committee for Economic Development.

DUBLIN, L. I., and LOTKA, A. J. (1946), *The Money Value of a Man*, Ronald Press.

DUBLIN, L. I., and WHITNEY, J. (1920), 'On the cost of tuberculosis', *J. of the Amer. Stat. Assoc.*, vol. 17, December.

EWING, O. R. (1948), *The Nation's Health: A Report to the President*, Federal Security Agency.

EZDORF, R. H. von (1916), 'Demonstrations of malaria control', *Pub. Health Reports*, vol. 31, pp. 614–29.

FABRICANT, S. (1959), *Basic Facts on Productivity Change*, occasional papers, no. 63, NBER.

FEIN, R. (1958), *Economics of Mental Illness: A Report to the Staff Director, Jack R. Ewalt*, Basic Books.

FEIN, R. (1961), 'The interaction of health and economic development', paper delivered at the Third Annual Conference of the Society for International Development, April, 28–29th.

FISHER, I. (1909), 'Report on national vitality: its wastes and conservation', *Bull. of One Hundred on National Health*, no. 30.

GARFINKLE, S. (1955), 'Changes in the working life of men, 1900–2000', *Monthly Labor Rev.* vol. 78, pp. 297–301.

Health Information Foundation (1961), *Progress in Health Services*, vol. 10, news letter, New York.

HENDERSON, A. (1959), 'The cost of children', *United Nations Department of Economics and Social Affairs Population Studies*, vol. 3, pp. 130–50.

HETTINGER, J., *et al.* (1961), 'Assessment of physical work capacity: a comparison between different tests and maximal oxygen intake', *J. of Appl. Physiol.*, vol. 16, p. 1.

HILL, E. L., and SAUNDERS, B. S. (1960), 'Murine typhus control in the United States: a success story of the public health practice', United States Public Health Service, Draft.

KLEM, M. C., and McKIEVER, M. F. (1950), *Small Plant Health and Medical Programs*, Public Health Service Publication, no. 15, Washington.

KLEM, M. G., McKIEVER, M. F., and LEAR, W. J. (1950), *Industrial Health and Medical Programs*, Public Health Service Publication, no. 15, Washington.

KOOS, E. L. (1954), *The Health of Regionville: What the People Thought and Did about It*, Columbia University Press.

LAITIN, H. (1956), 'The economics of cancer', unpublished doctoral dissertation, Harvard University.

LEES, F. S. (1918), *The Human Machine and Industrial Efficiency*, Longman.

LOWELL, A. M. (1956), *Socioeconomic Conditions and Tuberculosis Prevalence in New York, City, 1949–51*, New York Tuberculosis and Health Association.

MERRIAM, I. (1960), 'Social welfare expenditure, 1958–9', *Soc. Security Bulletin*, November, p. 43.

MUSHKIN, S. J., and COLLINGS, F. d'A. (1959), Economic costs of disease and injury', *Pub. Health Reports*, vol. 74, pp. 795–809.

MYERS, R. J. (1957–8), 'Some implications of a retirement test in social security systems', Proceedings of the Conference of Actuaries in Public Practice, vol. 7, pp. 337–50.

NATIONAL HEALTH EDUCATION COMMITTEE (1959), *Facts on the Major Killing and Crippling Diseases in the United States Today*, NHEC.

NATIONAL PLANNING ASSOCIATION (1948), *Good Health is Good Business: A Summary of a Technical Study*, planning pamphlet no. 62, NPA.

REYNOLDS, D. J. (1956), 'The cost of road accidents', *J. of the Royal Stat. Soc.*, vol. 119, pp. 393–408.

RODAHL, K., *et al.* (1961), 'Physical work capacity', *Archives of Environ. Health*, vol. 2, pp. 23–24.

SAND, R. (1952), *The Advance to Social Medicine*, Staples.

SCHULTZ, T. W. (1961), 'Education and economic growth', in N. B. Henry (ed.), *Social Forces Influencing American Education*, University of Chicago Press.

SINGER, H. W. (n.d.), 'Population and economic development', and 'Some demographic factors in economic development', meeting no. 24, United Nations.

SOLOW, R. W. (1957), 'Technical change and the aggregate production function', *Rev. of Econ. and Stats.*, vol. 39, pp. 312–20.

TARVER, J. D. (1956), 'Costs of rearing and educating farm children', *J. of Farm Econ.*, vol. 38, pp. 144–53.

THEDIE, J., and ABRAHAM, C. (1961), 'Economic aspects of road accidents', *Traffic Engineering and Control*, vol. 2, pp. 589–95.

UN-ILO and UNESCO (1954), 'Report on international definition and measurements of standards and levels of living', Committee of Experts (E/CN/179), UN.

UNIVERSITY OF MICHIGAN SURVEY RESEARCH CENTRE (1957), *Employee Health Services*, University of Michigan.

US CONGRESS (1961), Co-ordination of Federal Agencies', Programs in Biomedical Research and in other scientific areas, 37th Congress Report, p. 142, Washington.

US DEPARTMENT of LABOR (1950), *Tables of Working Life: Length of Working Life for Men*, Bulletin No. 1001, Washington.

US DEPARTMENT of LABOR (1956), *Tables of Working Life: Length of Working Life for Women*, Bulletin no. 1204, Washington.

WEISBROD, B. A. (1958), *The Nature and Measurement of the Economic Benefits of Improvement in Public Health with Particular Reference to Cancer, Tuberculosis, and Poliomyelitis*, Washington University.

WILLIAMS, L. L. (1938), 'Economic importance of malaria control', *Proceedings of the Twenty-Fifth Annual Meeting of the New Jersey Mosquito Extermination Association*, Atlantic City, March 24th, pp. 148–51.

WHO (1957), 'Measurement of levels of health', Technical Report no. 137, WHO.

WOODS, E. A., and METZGER, C. B. (1927), *America's Human Wealth: The Money Value of Human Life*, Crofts.

World Health Organization and Pan American Sanitary Bureau (1961), Thirteenth Meeting of Directing Council, October.

# 5 Victor R. Fuchs

## The Output of the Health Industry

Victor R. Fuchs, 'The contribution of health services to the American economy', *Milbank Memorial Fund Quarterly*, vol. 44, 1966, pp. 65–101.

### Introduction

Good health is one of man's most precious assets. The desire to live, to be well, to maintain full command over one's faculties and to see one's loved ones free from disease, disability or premature death are among the most strongly rooted of all human desires. That is particularly true of Americans who, on the whole, eschew the fatalism or preoccupation with the hereafter that is characteristic of some other cultures.

These sentiments are widely held. Therefore, is not the question – what is 'the contribution of health services to the United States economy?' – presumptuous? Who can place a value on a life saved, on a body spared from pain or on a mind restored to sanity? If not presumptuous, is not the question a foolish one, and likely to evoke an equally foolish answer?

When an economist enters an area such as health – so tinged with emotion, so enveloped in an esoteric technology and vocabulary – he runs a high risk of being either irrelevant or wrong. What, then, is the justification for such an inquiry? The principal one is the fact that the question of the contribution of health services is being asked and answered every day. It is being asked and answered implicitly every time consumers, hospitals, universities, business firms, foundations, government agencies and legislative bodies make decisions concerning the volume and composition of health services, present and future. If economists can help to rationalize and make more explicit the decision-making process, can provide useful definitions, concepts and analytical tools, and can develop appropriate bodies of data and summary measures, they will be making their own contribution to health and to the economy.

### Plan of the paper

This paper has limited objectives. It does not pretend to offer a measure of the contribution of health services. Even partial completion of such a task would require a major effort by a research team over a period of several years. Statistics are presented, but for illustrative purposes only.

The primary purpose is to set out in nontechnical terms how the problem looks to an economist, to discuss definitions, concepts and methods of measurement, to indicate sources of information and to suggest promising research approaches. The paper offers a highly personal view of the problem rather than a synthesis of all points of view. Some discussion of relevant literature is included, but no attempt has been made to be exhaustive. Moreover, the paper is limited to the assigned topic and does not provide a general review of the health economics literature. An overall survey of the field, through 1964, is available in Klarman (1965). In addition, useful bibliographies may be found in Mushkin (1962), Wolf (1964), and the proceedings of a 1962 conference on the economics of health and medical care (University of Michigan, 1964).

First this paper will consider the meaning of 'contribution'. Then it will go on to discuss the inputs to health services (with special emphasis on health) and the contribution of health to the economy. The paper concludes with a brief summary and suggestions for research.

### The concept of contribution

One frequently reads discussions of the contribution of an industry couched in terms of the number of jobs the industry provides, the volume of capital investment of the industry, and the value of its purchases from suppliers. Such use of the term is ill-advised.

In economic terms the contribution of an industry to the economy should be measured in terms of its output (what does it provide for the economy?), not in terms of its input (what drains does it make on the available supply of resources?). The fundamental fact of economic life is that resources are scarce relative to human wants. Despite a good deal of loose talk about automation and cybernetics, the desires for goods and services in this country and the world exceed the available supplies. Indeed, if this were not the case, no reason could be found to study the economics of health or the economics of anything else. Additional resources would be devoted to health up to the point where no health want would be unmet. That this cannot be done at present is obvious. The reason should be equally obvious. To devote more resources to health services, the people must be willing to forego some other good or service. To the extent of the unused capacity in the economy, some increase could be obtained without diversion from other ends. The extent of this unused capacity, however, relative to the total economy, is very small at the present time.

What is the output of the health industry? No completely satisfactory answer is available. One possible way to think about the problem is to distinguish three different kinds of output that flow from health services. They are health, validation services and other consumer services.

Probably the most important of these, and certainly the one that has received the most attention, is the contribution of health services to health. However, to define the output of the health industry in terms of some ultimate utility, such as health rather than health services, runs counter to the general practice followed by economists in the study of other industries. For the most part, economists follow the dictum, 'whatever Lola gets, Lola wants'. They assume that consumers know what they want and know how to satisfy these wants. They further assume that goods and services produced under competitive conditions will be sold at a price which properly reflects (at the margin) the cost of production and the value to the consumer. The health industry, however, has certain characteristics, discussed by Arrow (Reading 1), Klarman (1965) and Mushkin (1962), which suggest that special treatment is required. In the present context, three important differences could be emphasized between the health industry and the 'typical' or 'average' industry.

*Consumer ignorance.* Although expenditures for health services account for more than 6 per cent of all personal consumption expenditures, consumers are, for the most part, terribly ignorant about what they are buying. Very few industries could be named where the consumer is so dependent upon the producer for information concerning the quality of the product. In the typical case he is even subject to the producer's recommendation concerning the quantity to be purchased. A recent report by the American Medical Association says flatly, 'The "quantity" of the hospital services consumed in 1962 was determined by physicians' (American Medical Association, 1963–4).

The question is even more complicated, as indicated in the following statement by J. Douglas Colman, president of the New York Blue Cross (Anon, 1965):

We must remember that most elements of hospital and medical care costs are generated by or based on professional medical judgment. These judgments include the decision to admit and discharge patients, the decision to order the various diagnostic or therapeutic procedures for patients, and the larger decision as to the types of facilities and services needed by an institution for proper patient care. For the most part, these professional judgments are rendered outside of any organizational structure that fixes accountability for the economic consequences of these judgments (pp. 45–9).

One reason for consumer ignorance is the inherent uncertainty of the effect of the service on any individual. How can the lay person be expected to know the value of a particular procedure or treatment, when in many cases the medical profession itself is far from agreed? Also, many medical services are infrequently purchased. The average consumer will buy many more automobiles during a lifetime than he will major operations. Therefore, he cannot develop the necessary expertise. Furthermore, the consumer is often not in a good position to make a cool, rational judgment at the time of purchase because he is ill, or because a close member of his family is ill. Finally, the profession does little to inform the consumer; in fact, it frequently takes positive action to keep him uninformed. This leads to the second important difference.

*Restrictions on competition.* In some other industries where the possibilities for consumer ignorance are considerable, the consumer obtains protection through the competitive behavior of producers. If the producers are engaged in vigorous competition with one another, some of them, at least, will go out of their way to inform the consumer about the merits of their product and those of the competition. Also, middle-men, such as retailers, are usually involved, one of whose main functions is to provide information and dispel consumer ignorance. In the case of physicians' services (and this is the keystone to health services because of the dominant role of the physician in the industry) the reverse is true. In the first place, severe restrictions on entry are assured through the medical profession's control of medical schools, licensing requirements and hospital appointments. Advertising is forbidden and price competition is severely frowned upon. Critical comment concerning the output of other physicians is also regarded as unethical.

A good example of the conflict and confusion on this point can be found in the report previously cited. An extensive discussion of medical care in America is presented, and an attempt is made to identify it with the competitive free enterprise system. The report then goes on to say, 'the Medical Care Industry has as its prime social goal the development and maintenance of optimum health levels' (American Medical Association, 1963–4, p. 9). The authors apparently fail to realize the inconsistency of this statement with their attempt to place the industry in the context of a market system. In such a system, industries do not have 'social goals'. The goal of the individual firm is maximum profit (or minimum loss); the achievement of social goals is a by-product of the profit-seeking activities of individual firms and industries.

Numerous arguments can be advanced in support of each of the restrictive practices followed by the medical profession. (Arrow's discussion of the role of uncertainty in health is particularly relevant.) In the present context, these restrictive practices mean that an appraisal of the industry's output and performance by economists cannot be pursued using the same assumptions that would be appropriate in appraising the output of a more competitive industry.

*The role of 'need'*. Health services are one of a small group of services which many people believe should be distributed according to need rather than demand (i.e. willingness and ability to pay). Other services in this category, such as education, police and fire protection, and sanitation are typically provided by government. For a time philanthropy and the generosity of physicians were relied upon to achieve this distribution for health services, but now increasing reliance is being placed on taxation or coverage in compulsory insurance schemes. If 'need' is to be criterion, however, a closer examination of the role of health services in filling that need seems in order.

If a person 'demands' an article of clothing or a haircut or some other good or service, in the sense of being willing and able to pay for it, usually no special cause for concern or inquiry arises on the part of anyone else regarding either the need underlying the demand or whether the purchase will satisfy the need. However, if a service, such as health, is to be provided to others on the basis of 'need', then those paying for it would seem to have some right to inquire into the actual presence of 'need', and an obligation to determine whether or how much the service actually satisfies the need. Because need is often the criterion for obtaining health services, much of the payment for these services is by a 'third party'. This means that the consumer has less incentive to make certain that the output (what he is getting) is truly worth the cost.

These characteristics of the health industry indicate why output cannot simply be equated with expenditures. However, that does not mean that economic analysis cannot be applied to this industry. On the contrary, precisely these special characteristics make the industry an interesting subject for economic analysis, both from the scientific and public policy points of view.

## Total versus marginal contribution

In studying the contribution of health services to health the *total* contribution must be distinguished from the *marginal* contribution. The total contribution can be appraised by asking what would happen if no health services at all were available. The results would almost surely be disastrous in terms of health and life expectancy. A reasonably safe conclusion seems to be that the total contribution is enormous. A modern economy could not continue to function without some health services.

The marginal contribution, on the other hand, refers to the effects on health of a small increase or decrease in the amount of health services provided. To expect a small change in services to have a large effect on the level of health is, of course, out of the question. But that is not what is being measured. Rather, the question is, what is the relative effect on health of a small relative change in health services?

The reason this question is crucial is that changes are usually being made at the margin. Most decisions are not of the 'all or nothing' variety, but involve 'a little more or a little less'. The goal of an economic system, in terms of maximum satisfaction, is to allocate resources in such a way that the last (marginal) inputs of resources used for each purpose make contributions that are proportionate to their costs.

## Health services

'Health services' can be defined as services rendered by:

1. Labor: personnel engaged in medical occupations, such as doctors, dentists and nurses, plus other personnel working directly under their supervision, such as practical nurses, orderlies and receptionists.

2. Physical capital: the plant and equipment used by this personnel, e.g. hospitals, x-ray machines.

3. Intermediate goods and services: i.e. drugs, bandages, purchased laundry services.

This definition corresponds roughly to what economists have in mind when they refer to the 'health industry'. Payment for this labor, capital and intermediate input is the basis for estimating 'health expenditure'.

This definition seems satisfactory for the purposes of this paper, but some classification problems are worth mentioning. First, some health-related resources might or might not be included in health services, such as the provision of a supply of sanitary water. A second problem arises because a portion of the personnel and facilities in hospitals is used to produce 'hotel services' rather than health. This paper will not exclude such inputs from health services, but will try to allow for them by showing that part of the output consists of other consumer services (see Figure 1).

One of the greatest problems concerns the unpaid health services that people perform for themselves and for members of their families. According to present practice in national income accounting, this labor input is not included in health services. Therefore, this 'home' production must be treated as part of the environmental factors that affect health.

Approximately two thirds of the value of health services in the United States represents labor input. Somewhat less than one sixth represents input of physical capital and the remainder represents goods and services purchased from other industries. These are all rough estimates. Information about the volume and composition of health services must be derived from a variety of official and unofficial sources. No census of the health industry compares to the census of manufacturing, trade or selected services. As the importance of the health industry grows, the government may wish to reconsider whether a periodic census of health should be undertaken.

Present sources of information are of two main types: those that give information about expenditures for health services, and those that report on one or more aspects of inputs of resources. A good example of the former is the material supplied by Reed and Rice (1964). A few problems arise when these data are used to measure inputs of health services. First, some of the items represent investment expenditures by the health industry rather than payment for current services. Expenditures for construction and medical research are the most important ones in this category. No particular economic justification may be found for treating these as inputs in the year that the investment takes place. On the other hand, current input of capital may be understated to the extent that hospital charges do not include an allowance for depreciation and interest.

The expenditures shown for drugs, eyeglasses, etc., do not all represent payment for intermediate goods purchased from other industries. A substantial portion (probably about one half) represents the labor services of pharmacists, opticians and the like and the services of the plant and equipment used by this personnel.

The net cost of health insurance represents output of the insurance industry. It may be thought of as an intermediate service purchased and resold by the health industry.

A final point concerns the failure of expenditures data to reflect contributed labor. This results in an underestimate of labor input, especially in hospitals.

Other sources of information on expenditures for health services include: the Office of Business Economics (1954, 1958), detailed annual data on personal consumption expenditures for health service; the Social Security Administration (Merriam, 1964, pp. 3–14), special emphasis on government spending for health services; the Public Health Service (1963, 1965), expenditures cross-classified with characteristics of the individual incurring the expense; the Health Information Foundation (Andersen and Anderson, 1965), and Bureau of Labor Statistics (1956, 1957).

The decennial population census is an excellent source of information about labor inputs to health services. In addition to providing a complete enumeration of the numbers employed and their geographical location, numerous economic and demographic characteristics are described in considerable detail. With the aid of the 1/1000 sample of the 1960 census (US Bureau of the Census, 1960a), comparisons may be made within the health industry and between health and other industries on such matters as education, earnings, age, sex, race and hours of work. The labor input to health services may be defined as all persons employed in the health and hospital industry, plus those persons in medical occupations employed in other industries. Health employment, so defined, amounted to almost three million in 1960. This represented almost 5 per cent of total employment.

Another good source of data on labor input is provided by the Public Health Service (1952–64). This source is particularly useful for those interested in such characteristics as physicians' type of practice, specialization, medical school and location of practice.

Information on capital inputs to health services is more difficult to obtain. The annual guide book issue of *Hospitals* reports the book value of hospital plant and equipment (American Hospital Association, 1964). This was given as 21·3 billion dollars in 1963. This figure is biased downward as a measure of present value, because of the rise in prices of construction in recent decades. It is biased upward to the extent that hospitals have failed to make deductions for depreciation. This same source also provides useful data on labor input by type and size of hospital.

Some information on the capital inputs associated with the labor input of physicians can be gleaned from the reports of the United States Internal Revenue Service (US Treasury Department, 1965). According to these reports, 163,000 returns were filed for unincorporated businesses under the heading of 'physicians, surgeons, and oculists' in 1962. These returns showed business receipts of six billion dollars. They showed net rent paid of 250 million dollars (most of this represents payment for capital services) as well as depreciation charges of 190 million dollars. Some information for other types of health services, such as those provided by dentists and dental surgeons, is also available from the same source.

One important source of information about inputs of equipment and intermediate goods that has not received much attention is the quinquennial Census of Manufacturers. The latest one (1963) provides considerable data on shipments by manufacturers of drugs, ophthalmic goods, dental equipment and supplies, ambulances, hospital beds and many other health items.

## Real versus money costs

One problem in measuring inputs that has already been alluded to in connection with volunteer labor is the need to distinguish between 'real' and 'money' costs. The person who is not an economist usually thinks of the cost of health services in money terms; when more money has to be spent, costs are said to be rising. This approach is readily understandable and for some purposes useful and proper. The analysis of many problems, however, requires a stripping away of the money veil and an examination of 'real' costs. The real cost to society of providing health services, or any other good or service, consists of the labor and capital used in the industry, plus the cost of producing the intermediate goods and services. For instance, if the workers employed in a given hospital are unionized, and they negotiate a large increase in wages, the money costs of that hospital clearly rise, other factors remaining unchanged. But the real cost of that hospital service has not changed at all.

In a perfectly competitive market economy, money costs usually provide a good measure of real costs. But in the health industry, with its curious mixture of philanthropy, government subsidies, imperfect labor markets and contributed labor time, concentration on money costs alone may frequently be misleading. Good decisions about the allocation of resources require information about the real costs involved.

One important element of real cost is often overlooked, namely, the time of the patient. When the patient is ill, the value of this time (measured by alternative opportunities) may be very low. But, in calculating the costs of periodic medical examinations and routine visits, omitting this cost would be a mistake (Becker, 1965, pp. 493–517).

## Health

Any attempt to analyse the relationship between health services and health runs headlong into two very difficult problems. The first concerns the definition and measurement of levels of health, or at least changes in levels. The second involves an attempt to estimate what portion of changes in health can be attributed to health services, as distinct from the genetic and environmental factors that also affect health. This section discusses the question of definition and measurement of levels of health.

### What is health?

Definitions of health abound. Agreement is hard to find. The oft-quoted statement of the World Health Organization (1958a) is framed in positive (some would say Utopian) terms – 'A state of complete physical and mental and social well-being.' Others, e.g. Ffrangcon Roberts (1952), simply stress the absence of, or the ability to resist, disease and death.

A few points seem clear. First, health has many dimensions – anatomical, physiological, mental and so on. Second, the relative importance of different disabilities varies considerably, depending upon the particular culture and the role of the particular individual in that culture. Third, most attempts at measurement take the negative approach. That is, they make inferences about health by measuring the degree of ill health, as indicated by mortality, morbidity, disability, etc. Finally, with respect to health, as in so many other cases, detecting changes in health is easier than defining or measuring absolute levels.

*Indexes of health*

The most widely used indicators of health levels are those based on mortality rates, either age-specific or age-adjusted. The great virtues of death rates are that they are determined objectively, are readily available in considerable detail for most countries, and are reasonably comparable for intertemporal and interspatial comparisons.

Health experts rely heavily on mortality comparisons for making judgments about the relative health levels of whites and non-whites in the United States, or of smokers versus non-smokers, and for other problems. A recent survey of health in Israel, for example, concluded:

> The success of the whole system of medicine in Israel is best judged, not by an individual inspection of buildings or asking the opinions of doctors and patients, but by an examination of the health statistics of the country. Infant mortality is about the same as in many European countries, and life expectancy is equal to, or better than, most (Johnson, 1965, pp. 842–45).

The tendency in recent years has been to dismiss mortality as a useful indicator of health levels in developed countries because very little intranational or international variation occurs. These reports of the demise of mortality indexes are premature.

Differences within the United States are still considerable. The most important differential is race, but even considering rates for whites only, the age-adjusted death rate (average 1959–61) in the highest state is 33 per cent greater than in the lowest; the highest infant mortality rate is 55 per cent above the lowest; and the death rate for males 45–54 in the worst state is 60 per cent higher than in the state with the lowest rate.

Comparing the United States with other developed countries, the differences are even more striking, as shown in Table 1. For males 45–54, (a critical age group from the point of view of production), the United States has the highest rate of any country in the Organization for Economic Cooperation and Development (OECD), and has a rate which is almost double that of some of

Table 1 **Death rates in OECD countries relative to the United States, average 1959–61**

| Country | Age-adjusted death rate * | Infant mortality | Mortality males 45–54 | Mortality females 45–54 |
|---|---|---|---|---|
| United States | 100 | 100 | 100 | 100 |
| White | 96 | 88 | 94 | 87 |
| Nonwhite | 138 | 164 | 155 | 220 |
| Iceland | 78 | 62** | 62 | 81 |
| Netherlands | 82 | 63 | 57 | 65 |
| Norway | 82 | 74** | 54 | 58 |
| Sweden | 86 | 63 | 52 | 69 |
| Greece | 86 | 155 | 56 | 64 |
| Denmark | 90 | 85** | 59 | 78 |
| Canada | 92 | 107 | 76 | 79 |
| Switzerland | 94 | 83 | 67 | 75 |
| France | 96 | 105 | 89 | 83 |
| Italy | 98 | 166 | 74 | 77 |
| Belgium | 102 | 113 | 82 | 79 |
| United Kingdom | 103 | 87 | 76 | 85 |
| Spain | 104† | 178 | 75† | 84† |
| West-Germany (excluding Berlin) | 107 | 129 | 77 | 84 |
| Luxembourg | 107 | 122 | 96 | 89 |
| Ireland | 109 | 118 | 74 | 105 |
| Austria | 110 | 142 | 87 | 87 |
| Japan | 115 | 127** | 83 | 102 |
| Portugal | 131 | 328 | 84 | 84 |

Sources: Age-Adjusted Death Rate, Mortality Males 45–54 and Mortality Females 45–54: United States Deaths: United States Public Health Service (1959, 1960, 1961). United States Population: United States Bureau of the Census (1960a). OECD Countries: Population and Deaths: World Health Organization (1959, 1960, 1961). Data for Luxembourg from United Nations (1960, 1961). Infant Mortality Rate: United Nations (1961, Table 17).

* Age-adjustment is by the 'indirect' method. For each country, United States age-specific death rates were applied to the actual population distribution and the result was divided into the actual number of deaths to obtain the mortality ratio, i.e. the age-adjusted death rate in index number form.

† 1957–9 average.

** 1958–60 average.

the other countries. Such gross differences surely present a sufficient challenge for scientific analysis and for public policy.

Another argument that seems to underly the objections to mortality indexes is that age-adjusted death rates (and average life expectancy) have been relatively stable in the United States for the past decade. The real costs of health services have increased over this period, and medical science has certainly made some progress; therefore, one may assume that some improvement in health levels occurred that was not captured by the mortality indexes.

This type of reasoning begs the question. Possibly the increase in health services has not resulted in improved health levels and the scientific advances of recent years have not had much effect on health. An alternative explanation is that changes in environmental factors in these years have had, on balance, a negative effect on health, thus offsetting the favorable effects of increases in services and medical knowledge. The latter explanation seems to be a very real possibility. Health services do not operate in a vacuum, nor can they be regarded as being matched against a 'health destroying nature' that remains constant over time. An apt aphorism attributed to Sigerist states that 'each civilization makes its own diseases' (Morris, 1964, p. 14).

Most of the suggestions for new and better indexes of health involve combining morbidity and mortality information. An excellent discussion of some of the problems to be encountered, and possible solutions, may be found in Sullivan (1966). One particularly intriguing approach, suggested by Sanders (1964, pp. 1063–70), consists of calculating years of 'effective' life expectancy, based on mortality and morbidity rates. Such an index would measure the number of years that a person could expect to live and be well enough to fulfill the role appropriate to his sex and age. This approach could be modified to take account of the fact that illness or disability is a matter of degree. The years deducted from life expectancy because of disability should be adjusted by some percentage factor that represents the degree of disability. The determination of these percentage weights is one of the most challenging research problems to be faced in calculating a health index.

### Health services and health

Writing this section would be more appropriate for a physician than for an economist since the relation between health services and health is a technical question best answered by those whose training is in that technology. All that is intended here is to record some impressions of an outsider who has reviewed a minute portion of the literature from a particular point of view.

The impact of health services on health depends upon two factors: 1. How effective are the best known techniques of diagnosis, therapy, etc.? 2. How wide is the gap between the best known techniques ('treatment of choice') and those actually used across the country? The latter question has been reviewed extensively in medical literature under the heading 'quality of care' (Anderson and Altman, 1962); it will not be discussed here. A useful introduction to the first question is provided in Terris (1963).

The belief that an important relationship exists between health services and health is of long standing. Reliable evidence to support this belief is of much more recent origin. For thousands of years sick people sought advice and treatment of physicians and surgeons, but many of the most popular remedies and courses of treatment of earlier centuries are now known to have been either harmful or irrelevant.

If this be true, how can one explain the demand for health services that existed in the past? Two possible explanations seem worth noting; they may even continue to have some relevance today. First, doctors probably received a great deal of credit that properly belonged to nature. The body itself has great healing powers, and most people who successfully consulted physicians would have recovered from or adjusted to their illness without medical intervention. Second, and probably more important, is the intensive need 'to do something' that most people have when faced with pain and the possibility of death.

In more recent times, the value of health services for certain illnesses has been established with considerable certainty; but broad areas of doubt and controversy still remain. The following discussion considers a few examples of each type.

Infectious disease is an area where medical services are demonstrably effective. Although the decline of some infectious diseases (e.g., tuberculosis) should be credited in part to environmental changes such as improved sanitation, the important role played by improvements in medical science cannot be downgraded. For many infectious diseases the health service is preventive rather than curative and 'one-shot' rather than continuous. Such preventive services do not occupy a large portion of total physician time, but the results should nevertheless be included in the output of the health industry.

Examples of the control of infectious disease through immunization are: diphtheria (Rosen, 1964, pp. 483–94), tetanus (Long, 1955; Long and Sartwell, 1947), poliomyelitis (American Medical Association, 1963, vol. 3, ch. 4); chemotherapy is effective in tuberculosis and pneumonia (American Medical Association, vol. 3, ch. 4 and 7). The decline in mortality from these causes has been dramatic and some correlation can be observed between changes in the rate of decline and the adoption of specific medical advances. For example, during the fifteen-year period, 1935 to 1950, which spanned the introduction and wide use of sulfonamides and penicillin, the United States death rate from influenza and pneumonia fell at a rate of more than 8 per cent per annum; the rate of decline was 2 per cent per annum from 1900 to 1935. In the case of tuberculosis, considerable progress was made throughout this century, but the relative rate of decline in the death rate accelerated appreciably after the adoption of penicillin, streptomycin and PAS (para-aminosalicylic acid) in the late 1940s, and of isoniazid in the early 1950s.

Even more dramatic examples are the death rate patterns of syphilis and poliomyelitis, where the introduction of new forms of treatment for the former and immunization for the latter were reflected very quickly in precipitous drops in mortality. To be sure, the diseases mentioned have not been eliminated. Partly for socio-cultural reasons, the incidence of syphilis has actually increased in recent years. In other cases, modern treatments of choice are losing their effectiveness because of the development of resistant strains of micro-organisms.

The situation with respect to the non-infectious diseases is more mixed. Some examples of demonstrable effectiveness are the following: replacement therapy has lessened the impact of diabetes (Marks, 1965, pp. 416–23), dental caries in children are reduced by fluoridation (World Health Organization, 1958; Schlesinger, 1965) and medical care has become increasingly successful in treating trauma (Farmer and Shandling, 1963). The diagnostic value of the Papanicolaou test for cervical cancer is established (Kaiser *et al.*, 1960; Dunn, 1956) and the incidence of invasive cancer of this site has been reduced in the 1960s, presumably due to medical treatment during the pre-invasive stage disclosed by the test. Also effective is the treatment of skin cancer (Krementz, 1961).

Less heartening are the reports on other cancer sites. The five-year survival rate for breast cancer (the most common single organ site of malignancy in either sex) is typically about 50 per cent. Moreover, a review of the breast cancer literature found such striking uniformity of results, despite widely differing therapeutic techniques, that the author was prompted to speculate whether such end results record therapeutic triumphs or merely the natural history of the disease (Lewison, 1963). Some writers stress the importance of prompt treatment for cancer; others question whether elimination of delay would dramatically alter survival rates. The problem of delay itself is complex, and not simply attributable to ignorance or lack of access to health services: 'Physicians with cancer are just as likely to delay as are laymen' (Sutherland, 1960).

Heart disease is another major cause of death where the contribution of health services to health leaves much to be desired. Despite the contributions of surgery in correcting congenital and rheumatic cardiac defects (Stout, *et al.*, 1964) and the decline in recurrence rates of rheumatic fever (Wilson *et al.*, 1958), apparently no curative treatment has been found for rheumatic fever (Rheumatic Fever Working Party, 1955; Kutner, 1965). The treatment of coronary heart disease is only partially effective (Brest, 1964). The value of anti-hypertensive drugs in preventing early death in case of malignant hypertension seems assured, but these drugs may be harmful in non-malignant hypertension (Combined Staff Clinic, 1965). The value of anticoagulants in reducing complications and mortality with acute myocardial infarction has been questioned by recent reports (Lindsay Jr and Spiekerman, 1964; Lockwood *et al.*, 1963).

Definitive therapy is still not available for widespread afflictions such as cerebral vascular disease (Cain *et al.*, 1963) and rehabilitation results indicate that only the more severely ill may benefit from formal therapy (the others seem to recover spontaneously) Lowenthal *et al.*, 1959). No cure is known for schizophrenia. The tranquilizing drugs and shock therapy have had a significant impact in shortening hospital stay, yet they do not seem to lower rehospitalization rates below those achieved with other methods (May and Tuma, 1965).

Health services have always been assumed to be very valuable in connection with pregnancy, but a recent study of prenatal care reveals little relation to prevention of pregnancy complications or prevention of early pregnancy termination, except in uncomplicated pregnancies of thirty weeks' gestation and over (Schwartz and Vinyard, 1965). The latter cases do not clarify whether the medical care component of prenatal care, as distinct from nutritional and other components, is due the credit.

Innovations in health services are not limited to improvements in drugs, surgical techniques or other technological changes. Research concerning the effects on health of group practice (Shapiro *et al.*, 1958, 1960), intensive care units (Lockwood *et al.*, 1963; US Public Health Service, 1964) and special arrangements for neo-natal surgery (Forshall and Rickham, 1960), has yielded encouraging results with respect to these organizational innovations. In other cases, results have been disappointing, e.g., multiple screening (Wylie, 1961), periodic medical examination of school children (Yankauer and Lawrence, 1955) and cancer control programs differing in duration, intensity and cost (McKinnon, 1960).

This very brief review indicates that no simple generalization is possible about the effect of health services on health. Although many health services definitely improve health, in other cases even the best known techniques may have no effect. This problem of relating input to output is one of the most difficult ones facing economists who try to do research on the health industry. They must gain the support and advice of doctors and public health specialists if they are to make progress in this area.

*Environmental factors and health*

One of the factors contributing to the difficulty in reaching firm conclusions about the relationship between health services and health is the importance of environmental factors. Some environmental changes are biological, involving the appearance and disappearance of bacteria, viruses and other sources of disease. Many environmental variables are related to economics in one way or another. Some are tied to the production process, e.g., the factors associated with occupation. Others are part of consumption, e.g., diet, recreation. Major attention has frequently been given to income, partly because many other environmental factors tend to be highly correlated with real income, both over time and cross-sectionally. Examples include housing, education, urbanization, drinking and the use of automobiles.

The prevailing assumption, in some cases with good evidence, has indicated that an increase in real *per capita* income has favorable implications for health, apart from the fact that it permits an increase in health services. This assumption for the United States at present, except for infant mortality, may reasonably be questioned. This country may have passed the peak with respect to the favorable impact of a rising level of living on health. This is not to say that some favorable elements are not still associated with a higher income, but the many unfavorable ones may outweigh them.

After a period of neglect of environmental factors by medical researchers, the tendency in recent years has been to over-emphasize the favorable aspects of rising income levels. For example, the American Medical Association recently stated, 'medical science does not seek major credit for the improvements in the health levels during the past twenty-five years. Certainly, our standards of living and higher educational levels have contributed substantially to the betterment of the health level in the United States (American Medical Association, 1963–4, vol. 3, p. 9). Although modesty is becoming, the Association provides no evidence to support this statement, and the chances are good that it is wrong.

Altenderfer (1947) was able to show some slight negative association between age-adjusted death rates and income across cities in the United States in 1940, but the adjustment for the effect of color was crude, and no allowance was made for the correlation between health services and income. The question at issue here is the relation between income and health, not of the fact that higher income permits a higher rate of utilization of health services.

Some preliminary work suggests that education is indeed favorable to health, but by far the largest share of the credit for improvement in health levels over the past twenty-five years probably should go to what economists call improvements in technology – better drugs, better medical knowledge, better diagnostic techniques, etc. Cross-sectional regressions across states, for instance, reveal a positive relation between income and mortality for whites, except in the case of infant mortality.

Death rate patterns in countries where the level of income is far below that of the United States, should also cause one to question the level of living argument. In Table 2, death rates for five European countries in 1960 are compared with rates for the United States in 1960 and 1925. The latter date was included because, in 1960, these five countries were at a level of real *per*

Table 2 **Comparison of death rates of United States in 1925 and 1960 with European countries 1960**

| | Age-adjusted death rate all causes* | Crude death rate all causes | Crude death rate tuberculosis (all forms) | Crude death rate influenza and pneumonia† |
|---|---|---|---|---|
| **1925** | | | | |
| United States | 1683·3 | 1170·0 | 84·8 | 121·7 |
| **1960** | | | | |
| United States | 945·7 | 945·7 | 5·9 | 32·9 |
| England and Wales | 926·8 | 1150·2 | 7·5 | 70·1 |
| France | 926·8 | 1136·2 | 22·1 | 48·1 |
| West Germany (excluding Berlin) | 983·5 | 1136·8 | 16·2 | 43·8 |
| Netherlands | 766·0 | 762·1 | 2·8 | 26·6 |
| Belgium | 1002·4 | 1244·7 | 17·1 | 36·5 |

Sources: United States in 1925; United States Bureau of the Census (1960). European countries 1960 population distribution, influenza and pneumonia deaths 1959–61, total populations 1959–61, and total deaths 1960 in West Germany and Belgium: World Health Organization (1959–61, Table 4). Other crude death rates in 1960: United Nations (1961, Table 17). United States age-specific death rates in 1960: United States Department of Health, Education and Welfare, Public Health Service, National Vital Statistics Division (1960, Vol. II, Part A, Table 1-C).

* Age-adjustment is by the 'indirect' method. For each country the United States age-specific death rates in 1960 were applied to the actual population distribution and the result was divided into the actual number of deaths to obtain the age-adjusted death rate index. This was multiplied by the United States crude death rate in 1960, to obtain the age-adjusted death rate.

† 1957–61 average used instead of 1960 rates because of influenza epidemic in 1960,

*capita* income roughly comparable to that of the United States in 1925 (Denison, unpublished).

The table shows that the overall age-adjusted death rates for the European countries are very similar to those for the United States, and far below the level of the United States in 1925. The European crude rates tend to be higher because of the larger proportion of older people in Europe. Despite this bias, the crude rates for tuberculosis and influenza and pneumonia (two causes where the rise in income levels has been alleged to be particularly important) are also much closer to the United States in 1960, than to the United States in 1925. One explanation worth investigating is that the European countries enjoy a medical technology that is similar to that of the United States in 1960, and that changes in medical technology have been the principal cause of the decrease in the United States death rate from 1925 to 1960.

One possible reason for the effect of income levels on health having been overestimated is that investigators often find a very high correlation between income and the health status of individuals. The tendency has been to assume that the latter was the result of the former, but some recent studies of schizophrenia (Morrison and Goldberg, 1963) and bronchitis (Meadows, 1961) suggest that the causal relationship may run the other way. Evidence shows that illness causes a deterioration in occupational status (from a skilled job to an unskilled job and from an unskilled job into unemployment). The evidence relates to the decline in occupational status from father to son (where the latter is a victim of the disease) and also within the patient's own history.

Even though research on the relation between health services and health would seem to be primarily the responsibility of those with training in medicine and public health, the long experience that economists have had with the environmental variables, such as income, education and urbanization, suggest that a multidisciplinary approach would be most fruitful.

## Other contributions of health services

The effect of health services on health probably represents their most important contribution. However, two other types of output are worth noting – validation services and other consumer services.

### Validation services

One type of output that is not directly related to improvements in health can be traced to the fact that only a physician can provide judgments concerning a person's health status that will be widely accepted by third parties. This type of output is designated 'validation services' in Figure 1. One familiar example is the life insurance examination. This examination may have some favorable impact on the health of the examinee, but it need not do so and is not undertaken primarily for that purpose. The insurance company simply wants to know about the health status of the person concerned. In obtaining and providing that information, the physician is producing something of value, but it is not health.

Other examples include a physician's testifying in court, providing information in a workmen's compensation case, or executing a death certificate.

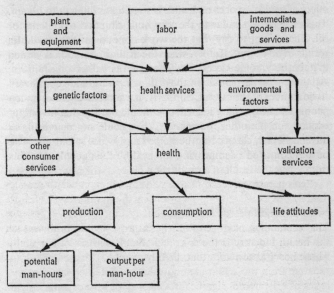

Figure 1  Schematic outline of the Paper

The validation role of physicians is probably much broader than in these sharply defined cases. Consider the following situation: a person feels ill; he has various aches, pains and other symptoms. He complains and looks for sympathy from family, friends, neighbors and co-workers. He may seek to be relieved from certain responsibilities or to be excused from certain tasks. Doubts may arise in the minds of persons around him. Questions may be asked. Is he really ill? Is he doing all that he can to get well? A visit, or a series of visits, to one or more doctors is indicated. The patient may not have the slightest hope that these visits will help his health, and, indeed, he may be correct. Nevertheless, the service rendered by the physician cannot be said to result in no output. The visit to the doctor is a socially or culturally necessary act. The examination, the diagnosis and the prognosis are desired by the patient to provide confirmation to those who have doubts about him. Only the professional judgment of a physician can still the doubts and answer the questions.

The validation service type of output should not be confused with another type of problem that arises in measuring the output of health services; namely, that advance knowledge about the effect of health services on health is sometimes difficult to obtain. This problem is similar to the 'dry hole' situation in drilling for oil. That is not to say that the work done in drilling dry holes results in no output. Rather, when the drilling operation is viewed in its entirety, some successes will be noted as well as some failures. All those who participate in the drilling operation are considered to be sources of the output. Similarly, if a surgeon operates on ten people and only six are helped, one should not say that no output occurred in the other four cases, if one could not determine in advance which cases could be helped and which could not. The output consisted of improving the health of six people, but this output was the result of a production process which encompassed the ten operations.

*Other consumer services*

The outstanding example of other consumer services produced by the health industry is the so-called 'hotel' services of hospitals. Those hospital activities that directly affect health are difficult to separate from those that are equivalent to hotel services, but the latter clearly are not significant. One way of getting some insight into this question would be to study the occupational distribution of health industry employment. A very significant fraction consists of cooks, chamber-maids, porters and others who are probably producing 'other consumer services' (Reed and Rice, 1964, pp. 11–21).

In mental hospitals and other hospitals providing long-term care a major proportion of all costs are probably associated with producing consumer services other than health. The fact that these other consumer services would have to be provided somehow, either publicly or privately, if the patients were not in the hospital, is often neglected in discussions of how total hospital costs are inflated by the presence of people who are not really ill. Possibly some of these consumer services are actually produced more inexpensively in a hospital than on the outside. This point comes to the fore in New York City, now grappling with the problem of housing and feeding patients who have been discharged from mental hospitals, not because they are cured, but because the new drugs mean they no longer need to be confined to an institution.

Some of the services rendered by nurses outside hospitals also bear little relation to health, but nevertheless they may have considerable value to consumers. This type of service is likely to grow in importance with the increase in the number of elderly people with income who are seeking companionship and help with their daily chores.

The failure of mortality indexes to decline with increased expenditures for health services in recent years has led some people to conclude that mortality no longer measures health levels properly. But if most of these increased expenditures have gone for health services that largely produce 'other consumer services' rather than health, a great deal of the mystery is removed.

### Health and the economy

An increase in health has two potential values for individuals – consumption and production. Good health is clearly something consumers desire for itself. (That they do not put an overriding value on health is also abundantly clear from the figures on smoking, drinking, over-eating, fast driving, etc.) To the extent that health services lead to better health, they make a contribution to the economy comparable to that of any industry producing a good or service wanted by consumers.

In addition, better health may contribute to the productive capacity of the economy. It may do this, first, by increasing the supply of potential man-hours through a reduction in mortality and decrease in time lost because of illness and disability. Second, better health may increase production by improving productivity, that is, increasing output per man-hour.

Beyond its potential direct contribution to production and consumption, better health probably has important indirect effects on the economy. These indirect effects occur through the changes in life attitudes which may accompany changes in health. When the average life expectancy in a country is only thirty or thirty-five years, attitudes toward work and saving, for instance, may be different from those in countries where life expectancy is fifty or seventy-five years. When infant mortality rates are very high, attitudes toward birth control are likely to be different from those in countries where mortality rates are low. Indeed, the idea of progress itself may be intimately bound up with the health levels of the population and the rate of change of these levels.

## Health and production

A substantial literature is now available which attempts to measure the impact of changes of health levels on the productive capacity of the economy (Klarman, 1965, pp. 162–72). The principal approach is to ask how many more people are available

Table 3 Age-value profile of United States males in 1960 estimated from discounted future earnings

| Age | Discount rate 4·0 per cent per annum (A) | 7·2 per cent per annum (B) | 10·0 per cent per annum (C) |
|---|---|---|---|
| 0 | $32,518 | $14,680 | $8114 |
| 10 | 43,133 | 29,361 | 21,047 |
| 20 | 68,363 | 52,717 | 45,023 |
| 30 | 81,300 | 70,515 | 64,697 |
| 40 | 73,057 | 67,365 | 64,012 |
| 50 | 54,132 | 52,406 | 51,363 |
| 60 | 30,285 | 29,853 | 29,570 |
| 70 | 9395 | 9395 | 9395 |
| 80 | 2465 | 2465 | 2465 |
| 90 | 0 | 0 | 0 |

Source: United States Bureau of the Census (1960a, Table 34).

*Note:* The indicated discount rates were applied to the following earnings:

| Age | Annual earnings |
|---|---|
| 0–14 | $ 0 |
| 15–24 | 1201 |
| 25–34 | 4582 |
| 35–44 | 5569 |
| 45–54 | 5327 |
| 55–64 | 4338 |
| 65–74 | 1386 |
| 75–84 | 493 |
| 85 and over | 0 |

No discounting was applied within ten-year age groups. No allowance was made for future increases in real earnings or for life expectancy.

No deduction was made for additional consumption attributable to decreased mortality. No earnings were imputed for males not in the labor force.

for work as a result of a decrease in death rates, and what potential or actual production can be attributed to this increased supply of manpower. The capitalized value of the increase at a given point in time can be obtained by summing the value of future potential production represented by the lives saved. Current earnings patterns are usually used with or without adjustment for future increases in earnings per man, and with future earnings discounted at some appropriate interest rate.

The details of calculating the value of lives saved vary greatly from one investigator to another, but one result is common to all: the value of a man (in terms of future production potential) is very different at different ages. Table 3 shows some calculated values for United States males at three different discount rates based on average patterns of earnings and labor force participation rates in 1960.

The principal implication of the age-value profile is that the economic return (in production terms) from saving a life is not the same at all ages. Different kinds of health programs and different kinds of medical research are likely to affect various age groups differently; therefore, wise planning should give some consideration to these matters. For example, accidents accounted for only 6·6 per cent of all male deaths in the United States in 1960, but accounted for 12·8 per cent of the economic cost of these deaths as measured by age-value profile B in Table 3. On the other hand, vascular lesions accounted for 9·5 per cent of all male deaths, but only 5·7 per cent of the economic cost of these deaths.

Table 4 shows how the age-value profile can be used to calculate the economic value (in production terms only) of the United States, using the 1960 death rate instead of the 1929 rate, or of lowering the United States rate in 1960 to the Swedish rate in 1960. In the former comparison, the greatest savings in number of lives were for infants and ages 75–84, but the greatest gain from a production point of view was from the reduction in the mortality rate for men 35–44. The United States–Swedish comparison highlights the current importance and potential of the 45–54 age group.

Most studies that attempt to place a value on a life saved (or on the cost of premature death) discuss the question of whether some deduction from discounted future earnings should be made for the future consumption of the individuals whose lives are saved. The arguments for and against are usually framed in terms of whether the value being measured is the value to society including

Table 4 **Lives saved and economic value of reduced United States death rate, 1929 and 1960 and of reduction of United States death rate to Swedish death rate, 1960**

*1960 United States rate compared with 1929 United States rate*

| Age | United States male population 1960 (thousands) | Death rate* 1929 | Death rate* 1960 | Number of deaths At 1929 rate (thousands) | Number of deaths At 1960 rate (thousands) | Number of lives saved (thousands) | Economic value of lives saved (millions) |
|---|---|---|---|---|---|---|---|
| Under 1 | 2090 | 79·8 | 30·1 | 166·8 | 62·9 | 103·9 | $1525 |
| 1–4 | 8240 | 6·5 | 1·2 | 53·6 | 9·9 | 43·7 | 834 |
| 5–14 | 18,029 | 2·0 | 0·6 | 36·1 | 10·8 | 25·3 | 743 |
| 15–24 | 11,906 | 3·7 | 1·5 | 44·1 | 17·9 | 26·2 | 1381 |
| 25–34 | 11,179 | 5·1 | 1·9 | 57·0 | 21·2 | 35·8 | 2524 |
| 35–44 | 11,755 | 7·8 | 3·7 | 91·7 | 43·5 | 48·2 | 3247 |
| 45–54 | 10,093 | 13·9 | 9·7 | 140·3 | 97·9 | 42·4 | 2222 |
| 55–64 | 7537 | 26·7 | 22·7 | 201·2 | 171·1 | 30·1 | 899 |
| 65–74 | 5116 | 57·6 | 48·3 | 294·7 | 247·1 | 47·6 | 447 |
| 75–84 | 2025 | 126·8 | 99·6 | 256·8 | 201·7 | 55·1 | 136 |
| 85 and over | 362 | 256·0 | 208·4 | 92·7 | 75·4 | 17·3 | 0 |
| Total | 88,331 | 16·2 | 10·8 | 1435·0 | 959·4 | 475·6 | 13,958 |

*Swedish death rate compared with United States death rate*

| Age | Death rate* Sweden 1960 | Number of deaths at Swedish rate (thousands) | Lives saved if US rate lowered to Swedish rate (thousands) | Economic value of lives saved (millions) |
|---|---|---|---|---|
| Under 1 | 19·1 | 39·9 | 23·6 | $ 347 |
| 1–4 | 1·0 | 7·8 | 2·1 | 39 |
| 5–14 | 0·5 | 9·0 | 1·8 | 53 |
| 15–24 | 1·0 | 11·9 | 5·9 | 314 |
| 25–34 | 1·2 | 13·4 | 7·8 | 552 |
| 35–44 | 2·0 | 23·5 | 19·9 | 1346 |
| 45–54 | 5·1 | 51·5 | 46·4 | 2433 |
| 55–64 | 14·1 | 106·3 | 65·6 | 1958 |
| 65–74 | 38·2 | 195·4 | 51·2 | 481 |
| 75–84 | 98·2 | 198·9 | 4·5 | 11 |
| 85 and over | 236·0 | 85·4 | −9·3 | 0 |
| Total | 8·4 | 743·1 | 219·5 | 7533 |

Sources: United States Death Rates: 1929. United States Bureau of the Census (1960b). United States Public Health Service (1960–1, Table 1C). United States Population: United States Bureau of the Census (1960a, Tables 45, 46). Swedish death rates: (World Health Organization, 1959–61, Table 4).

* Three-year average centered on year indicated.

the individual or excluding him. A slightly different way of looking at this problem could be suggested. Consider someone contemplating whether a certain expenditure for health services is worthwhile for him in terms of its expected benefits. He is highly

unlikely to think that his own future consumption must be subtracted to calculate the benefits. Many collective decisions might
be listed concerning the allocation of resources to health in the
same way. Who will be the beneficiary of these additional services
is not known. Each person, therefore, will tend to evaluate the
potential benefits in much the same way that he would a decision
concerning his own expenditures for health; i.e., he will see no
reason for deducting consumption, since he may be the one who
will benefit from the expenditure. *Ex post* he may reason that
saving someone else's life did not do him any good, but in advance
of the event and in the absence of knowledge concerning who the
beneficiary will be, the full value of the discounted earnings seems
the appropriate basis for valuation.

Better health can increase the number of potential man-hours
for production by reducing morbidity and disability, as well as by
reducing mortality. Some estimate of the potential gains to the
economy from this source can be obtained from data collected
periodically as part of the National Health Survey. In 1964,
approximately 5·5 workdays per person were lost for health
reasons by those currently employed (United States National
Health Survey, 1965, p. 16). Additional loss was contributed by
those persons who would have been employed except for reasons
of health.

*Health and productivity*

Common sense suggests that better health should result in more
production per man, as well as more men available for work.
Unfortunately, very little research has been done to provide a
basis for estimating the magnitude of this effect. Company
sponsored health programs would seem to offer an excellent
opportunity for the study of this question, but not much has been
done. In one investigation of what executives *thought* were the
results of their company's health program, 'less absenteeism'
was mentioned by 55 per cent of the respondents, 'improved
employee health' was mentioned by 50 per cent, but 'improved
productivity on the job' was mentioned by only 12 per cent of the
respondents (National Industrial Conference Board, 1959).

A number of studies have examined company health programs
(Grant, 1960; National Health Forum, 1960; Cipolla, 1963;
Blankenship, 1963), but their emphasis is on turnover rates,
accident rates, absenteeism and Workmen's Compensation insurance premiums, rather than on output per man-hour. Whether

this is because the latter effect is small, or because it is difficult to measure, is not clear. Many of the studies suffer from failure to consider other relevant variables along with the presence or absence of a company health program. Also, these studies do not clarify whether the benefits of company health programs should be attributed to improvements in health. For example, absenteeism and medical expenses may be lowered because of better controls rather than because of any change in health.

One special aspect of company health programs is the periodic health examination, much favored by those interested in preventive medicine. The basic notion is that if diseases or other injurious conditions are discovered early enough the chances for arrest or cure are greatly enhanced. An extensive literature exists on this subject, reviewed by Roberts (1959, pp. 95–116), but, unfortunately, the studies do not clearly establish the economic value of such examinations. Roberts lists several values served by such examinations but concludes that both public health service activities and personal health practices have much more effect on health than do periodic examinations.

A thorough economic analysis of the costs and benefits of company health programs and periodic health examinations is needed. Such an analysis should pay special attention to all the real costs of these programs including, for example, the time demanded of the examinees. It should attempt also to distinguish between those benefits which are realized through improvements in health and those which are unrelated to health.

## Health and consumption

In contrast to the substantial number of studies that look at the economic value of health in terms of production, very little information is available concerning its value as an end in itself (consumption). Klarman has suggested that one way of approaching the problem would be to observe the expenditures that people are willing to incur for the elimination of non-disabling diseases or the expenditures incurred by those not in the labor force (Klarman, 1965, p. 64).

Many people in the public health field greatly overestimate the value that the consumer places on health. The health literature frequently seems to read as if no price is too great to pay for good health, but the behavior of consumers indicates that they are often unwilling to pay even a small price. For example, surveys have shown that many people do not brush their teeth regularly, even when they believe that brushing would significantly reduce tooth decay and gum trouble (Kirscht, 1965; Haefner *et al.*, 1965). Smokers who acknowledge the harmful effects of smoking refuse to stop (Swinehart and Kirscht, 1965), and a group of executives whose obesity was called to their attention by their physicians took no action to correct a condition which is acknowledged to be injurious to health (Wade *et al.*, 1962). Some cases (mostly communicable diseases) may be noted where the social consumption value of health is greater than the private consumption value because of important external effects. The examples cited, however, do not fall into this category.

One of the problems that should be squarely faced in framing a social policy for health services is that people differ in the relative value that they place on health, just as they differ in the relative value that they place on other goods and services. Any system which attempts to force all people to buy the same amount of health services is likely to result in a significant misallocation of resources.

## Health and life attitudes

This is another area where one can do little more than say that research would be desirable. Many people have speculated about the effect of changes in health levels on attitudes toward work, saving, birth control and other aspects of behavior, but not much evidence has been accumulated. One interesting question concerns the ability of various populations to perceive changes in health levels. A study of low income Negroes in Chicago revealed very little awareness that a significant decline in infant mortality had actually occurred (Bogue, 1965). This suggests that changes in life attitudes, if they are related to changes in health levels, probably occur only after a lag.

## Conclusion

The principal line of argument in this paper may be stated briefly: health services represent the combined inputs of labor, capital and intermediate goods and services used by the health industry. Their contribution to the economy must be measured by the output of this industry, which takes three forms: health, validation services and other consumer services. Of the three, health is probably the most important. The problem of measuring changes in health levels was examined and followed by a discussion of the relationship between health services and health. Measure of the latter is greatly complicated by the fact that health depends upon environmental factors as well as health services. Most of the studies treat rising income as favorable to health, but some reasons are presented for questioning the validity of this assumption for the United States at present. The economic importance of changes in health levels flows first, from the importance of health as a consumption goal in itself and, second, from the effect of health on production. This effect can take two forms – changes in potential man-hours and changes in output per man-hour. Changes in life attitudes attributable to changes in health levels also may indirectly affect the economy.

Throughout the paper the need for additional research on each of these concepts and relationships has been stressed. Many of the studies cited have also dealt at length with the question of needed research. The best stimulus to good research is a good example; exhortation is a poor substitute. Nevertheless, this paper will conclude with a few comments on possible points of departure for research.

One promising line of inquiry would be to capitalize on the fact that health services in this country and abroad are produced and financed under a bewildering array of institutional arrangements. Important differences may be found with respect to the ownership and control of facilities, the organization of medical practice, the pricing of health services, the remuneration of health personnel and many other aspects of industrial organization. A basic question to be asked in each case is, 'What are the implications of these differences for health and for the economy?'

Another potentially fruitful area of work concerns the advances in medical technology which are the principal source of productivity gain for this industry. The American Medical Association has compiled a list of 'significant advances and technological developments' for the period 1936–62, by specialty, based on the response of knowledgeable physicians to a mail survey (American Medical Association, 1963–4, vol. 3, pp. 4–12). The same source presents a list of thirty important therapeutic agents now in use that have been introduced since 1934 (vol. 3, pp. 13–14). Both could provide a useful departure for research on the costs and benefits of medical research as well as for studies of innovation and diffusion similar to those that Mansfield (1961) and Griliches (1957) have developed for other parts of the economy.

The introduction to this paper argued that one of the principal reasons for wanting to know something about the contribution of health services to the economy is to be able to make better decisions concerning the allocation of resources to health. These decisions are increasingly made by government and are implemented in the form of subsidies for hospital construction, medical education and even medical care. This suggests that one line of fruitful research might be developed as follows:

1. First, the question of health versus other goals must be considered. Although lip service is often paid to the notion that health is a goal to be desired above all else, the most casual inspection of human behavior provides ample refutation of this proposition. Viewed as a source of consumer satisfaction, good health is often shunted aside in favor of the pleasure to be derived from other objects of expenditure and other patterns of behavior. Although the path to better health is frequently portrayed in terms of more hospitals, more doctors and more drugs, most people have the potential of improving their own health by their own actions. Ignorance may be cited to explain the failure of people to take these actions, but this is manifestly untrue in many cases (e.g., doctors continue to smoke). Furthermore, 'ignorance' frequently means nothing more than that people have not taken the time or trouble to obtain readily available information about health.

Health also contributes to the economy through production, but alternative ways of increasing output are available. To cite two important ones, resources allocated to increasing health could be allocated to increasing the stock of physical capital, or to increasing the rate of technological change through research and development. Anyone arguing for greater investment in health to increase production should be prepared to show that the return to investment in health is greater than the return to alternative forms of investment.

2. Once a decision has been made regarding the allocation of resources for health relative to other consumer goals and alternative forms of investment, a second allocation decision is required to divide resources among health services and alternative routes to better health. For instance, expectant mothers may benefit from frequent visits to a board-certified obstetrician, but they may also benefit from a better diet, or from not having to work during the last months of pregnancy, or from having someone to help them with their other children.

One can think of health problems where the environmental factors are of negligible importance and health services can make the difference between life and death. However, many situations also exist where both the environment and health services have a role to play and, given a fixed amount of resources to be used for health purposes, knowing the relative contributions (at the margin) of each is important so that resources may be allocated efficiently.

3. The third and most detailed level of decision-making concerns the allocation of resources among various types of health services. More doctors, more nurses, more hospitals, more dentists – in short, more of everything – is needed. Given the decision about resources available for health and the allocation of these resources among health services and other health factors, however, one must have some notion about the contribution (again at the margin), of various types of health services. The absence of such knowledge probably means that public decisions concerning increases in these services can be made on only an arbitrary basis. The argument that the various health resources must be increased in fixed proportion is refuted by the evidence from other countries where health systems are successfully using doctors, nurses, hospital facilities and other health inputs in proportions that differ strikingly from those used in the United States, as well as differing among themselves.

One final note of caution seems to be in order. Whatever research approach is pursued, and whatever questions are attacked, economists must become familiar with health institutions and technology. The practice of medicine is still more an art than a science. The intimate nature of the relationship between patient and doctor, the vital character of the service rendered, and the heavy responsibilities assumed by medical personnel suggest the dangers inherent in reducing health care to matters of balance sheets, or supply and demand curves. Economics has something to contribute to health problems, but it should proceed as the servant of health, not its master.

*References*

ALTENDERFER, M. (1947), 'Relationship between per capita income and mortality in the cities of 100,000 or more population', *Public Health Reports*, vol. 62, pp. 1681–91.

AMERICAN HOSPITAL ASSOCIATION (1964), *Hospitals*, Guide Issue, part 2, vol. 38, August 1st.

AMERICAN MEDICAL ASSOCIATION (1963–64), *Commission on the Cost of Medical Care Report*, vol. 1, p. 19, vol. 3, chs. 4, 7.

ANDERSEN, R., and ANDERSON, O. (1965), 'Trends in personal health spending', *Progress in Health Services*, vol. 14, November–December.

ANDERSON, A., and ALTMAN, I. (1962), *Methodology in Evaluating the Quality of Medical Care, An Annotated Selected Bibliography 1955–61*, University of Pittsburgh Press.

ANONYMOUS (1965), 'An interview with J. Douglas Colman', *Hospitals*, vol. 39, pp. 45–9.

BECKER, G. S. (1965), 'A theory of the allocation of time', *The Econ. J.*, vol. 75, pp. 493–517.

BLANKENSHIP, M. (1963), 'Influenza immunization and industrial absenteeism – A seven month study', in *Proceedings of the Fourteenth International Congress on Occupational Health*, vol. 2, pp. 291–5.

BOGUE, D. (1965), 'Inventory explanation and evaluation by interview of family planning: motives – attitudes – knowledge – behaviour: fertility measurement?', document prepared for discussion at International Conference on Family Planning Programs, Geneva, Switzerland, August 23–27.

BREST, A. N. (1964), 'Treatment of coronary occlusive disease: critical review', *Diseases of the Chest*, vol. 15, pp. 40–45.

CAIN, H. D., *et al.* (1963), 'Current therapy of cardiovascular disease', *Geriatrics*, vol. 18, pp. 507–18.

CIPOLLA, J. A. (1963), 'The occupational health experiences of two American hotels for 1955 and 1956', *Proceedings of Fourteenth International Congress on Occupational Health*, vol. 2, pp. 290–1, Madrid, Spain.

COMBINED STAFF CLINIC (1965), 'Recent advances in hypertension', *Amer. J. of Medicine*, vol. 39, pp. 634–8.

DENISON, E. F. (n.d.), 'Study of European economic growth', The Brookings Institution, (unpublished).

DUNN, J. E. Jr (1956), 'Cancer of the cervix – and results report', National Cancer Institute and American Cancer Society, *Fifth National Cancer Conference Proceedings*, J. B. Lippincott Company, pp. 253–7.

FARMER, A. W., and SHANDLING, B. S. (1963), 'Review of burn admissions, 1956–1960 – the hospital for sick children', *J. of Trauma*, vol. 3, pp. 425–32.

FORSHALL, I., and RICKHAM, P. P. (1960), 'Experience of a neonatal surgical unit – the first six years', *The Lancet*, vol. 1, pp. 751–4.

GRANT, E. S. (1960), 'The US concept of and experience in small-plant health services', *Proceedings of Thirteenth International Congress on Occupational Health*, pp. 113–20.

GRILICHES, Z. (1957), 'Hybrid corn: an exploration in the economics of technological change', *Econometrica*, vol. 25, pp. 501–22.

HAEFNER, D. P., *et al.* (1965), 'Preventive actions concerning dental disease, tuberculosis and cancer', paper delivered at the 22nd Annual Meeting of the Association of Teachers of Preventive Medicine, Chicago, October 17th.

JOHNSON, R. H. (1965), 'The health of Israel', *The Lancet*, no. 7417, pp. 842–5.

KAISER, R. F., *et al.* (1960), 'Uterine cytology', *Pub. Health Reports*, vol. 75, pp. 423–7.

KIRSCHT, J. P. (1965), *A National Study of Health Beliefs*, University of Michigan, manuscript.

KLARMAN, H. E. (1965), *The Economics of Health*, Columbia University Press.

KREMENTZ, E. T. (1961), 'End results in skin cancer', in National Cancer Institute and American Cancer Society, *Fourth National Cancer Conference Proceedings*, J. B. Lippincott Co.

KUTNER, A. G. (1965), 'Current status of steroid therapy in rheumatic fever', *Amer. Heart J.*, vol. 70, pp. 147–9.

LERNER, M., and ANDERSON, O. W. (1963), *Health Progress in the United States 1900–1960: A Report of the Health Information Foundation*, University of Chicago Press.

LEWISON, E. F. (1963), 'An appraisal of long-term results in surgical treatment of breast cancer', *J. of Amer. Medical Assoc.*, vol. 186, pp. 975–8.

LINDSAY, M. I. Jr, and SPIEKERMAN, R. E. (1964), 'Re-evaluation of therapy of acute myocardial infarction', *Amer. Heart J.*, vol. 67, pp. 559–64.

LOCKWOOD, H. J., *et al.* (1963), 'Effects of intensive care on the mortality rate of patients with myocardial infarctions', *Pub. Health Reports*, vol. 78, pp. 655–61.

LONG, A. P. (1955), 'Immunization to tetanus', in Army Medical Services Graduate School, *Recent Advances in Medicine and Surgery*, Walter Reed Army Institute of Research, pp. 311–13.

LONG, A. P., and SARTWELL, P. E. (1947), 'Tetanus in the US army in World War II, *Bull. of the US Army Medical Department*, vol. 7, pp. 371–85.

LOWENTHAL, M., *et al.* (1959), 'An analysis of the rehabilitation needs and prognoses of 232 cases of cerebral vascular accident', *Archives of Physical Medicine*, vol. 40, pp. 183–6.

McKINNON, N. E. (1960), 'The effects of control programs on cancer mortality', *Canadian Medical Assoc. J.*, vol. 82, pp. 1308–12.

MANSFIELD, F. (1961), 'The diffusion of technological change', National Science Foundation Reviews of Data on Research and Development.

MARKS, H.H. (1965), 'Longevity and mortality of diabetics', *Amer. J. of Pub. Health*, vol. 55, pp. 416–23.

MAY, D. R. A., and TUMA, A. H. (1965), 'Schizophrenia – an experimental study of five treatment methods', *British J. of Psychiatry*, vol. 111, pp. 503–10.

MEADOWS, S. H. (1961), 'Social class migration and chronic bronchitis: a study of male hospital patients in the London area', *British J. of Preventive and Social Medicine*, vol. 15, pp. 171–5.

MERRIAM, I. C. (1964), 'Social and welfare expenditures, 1963–64', *Social Security Bull.*, vol. 27, pp. 3–14.

MORRIS, J. N. (1964), *Uses of Epidemiology*, second edition, The Williams & Wilkins Co.

MORRISON, S. L., and GOLDBERG, E. M. (1963), 'Schizophrenia and social class', *J. of Mental Sci.*, vol. 109, pp. 785–802.

MUSHKIN, S. J. (1962), 'Health as an investment', *J, of Pol. Econ.*, supplement, vol. 70, pp. 129–57.

MUSHKIN, S. J. (1964), 'Why health economics?', in *The Economics of Health and Medical Care*, pp. 3–13, University of Michigan Press.

NATIONAL HEALTH FORUM (1960), Are occupational health programs worthwhile?', in A. Q. Maisel (ed.), *Health of People Who Work*, National Health Council.

NATIONAL INDUSTRIAL CONFERENCE BOARD (1959), *Company Medical and Health Programs*, Studies in Personnel Policy, no. 171, National Industrial Conference Board.

OFFICE of BUSINESS ECONOMICS (1954), *National Income, 1954 Edition, A Supplement to the Survey of Current Business*, United States Government Printing Office.

OFFICE of BUSINESS ECONOMICS (1958), *US Income and Output, A Supplement to the Survey of Current Business*, United States Government Printing Office.

PUBLIC HEALTH SERVICE (1963), *Measurement of Personal Health Expenditures*, series 2, United States Government Printing Office.

PUBLIC HEALTH SERVICE (1965), *Personal Health Expenses: Distribution of Pensions by Amount and Type of Expense, United States, July-December 1962*, series 10, United States Government Printing Office.

REED, L. S., and RICE, D. P. (1964), 'National Health expenditures: object of expenditures and source of funds,' 1962, *Social Security Bull.*, vol. 27, pp. 11–21.

RHEUMATIC FEVER WORKING PARTY (1955), 'Treatment of acute rheumatic fever in children: a co-operative clinical trial of ACTH, cortisone and aspirin', *British Medical J.*, vol. 1, pp. 555–74.

ROBERTS, F. (1952), *The Cost of Health*, Turnstile Press.

ROBERTS, N. J. (1959), 'The values and limitations of periodic health examinations', *J. of Chronic Diseases*, vol. 9, pp. 95–116.

ROSEN, G. (1964), 'The bacteriological immunologic and chemotherapeutic period 1875–1950', *Bull. of the New York Academy of Medicine*, vol. 10, pp. 483–94.

SANDERS, B. S. (1964), 'Measuring community health levels', *Amer. J. of Pub. Health*, vol. 54, pp. 1053–70.

SCHLESINGER, E. R. (1965), 'Dietary fluoride and caries prevention', *Amer. J. of Public Health*, vol. 55, pp. 1123–29.

SCHWARTZ, S., and VINYARD, J. H. (1965), 'Prenatal care and prematurity', *Public Health Reports*, vol. 80, pp. 237–48.

SHAPIRO, S., *et al.* (1958), 'Comparison of prematurity and prenatal mortality in a general population and in a population of a prepaid group practice', *Amer. J. of Pub. Health*, vol. 48, pp. 170–87.

SHAPIRO, S., *et al.* (1960), 'Further observations on prematurity and prenatal mortality in a general population and in the population of a prepaid group practice medical plan', *Amer. J. of Pub. Health*, vol. 50, pp. 1304–17.

STOUT, J., *et al.* (1964), 'Status of congenital heart disease patients ten to fifteen years after surgery', *Pub. Health Reports.*, vol. 79, pp. 377–82.

SULLIVAN, D. F. (1966), 'Conceptual problems in developing an index of health', *Vital and Health Statistics Data Evaluation and Methods Research*, Public Health Service Publication No. 1000, series 2, no. 17, United States Government Printing Office.

SUTHERLAND, R. (1960), *Cancer: The Significance of Delay*, Butterworth.

SWINEHART, J. W., and KIRSCHT, J. P. (1965), 'Smoking: a panel study of beliefs and behavior following the PHS Report', paper delivered at the Annual Meeting of the American Psychological Association, Chicago.

TERRIS, M. (1963), 'The relevance of medical care to the public health', paper delivered before American Public Health Association, November 13th.

UNITED NATIONS (1961), *Demographic Yearbook*, UN.

UNITED STATES BUREAU of LABOR STATISTICS (1956), *Study of Consumer Expenditures, Incomes and Savings, Volume VIII, Summary of Family Expenditures for Medical Care and Personal Care*, University of Pennsylvania Press.

UNITED STATES BUREAU of LABOR STATISTICS (1957), *Study of Consumer Expenditures, Income and Savings, Volume XVIII, Summary of Family Income, Expenditure and Savings, All Urban Areas Combined*, University of Pennsylvania Press.

UNITED STATES NATIONAL HEALTH SURVEY (1965), *Disability Days: United States July 1963–June 1964*, series 10, United States Government Printing Office.

UNITED STATES PUBLIC HEALTH SERVICE (1952–64), *Health Manpower Source Book*, sections 1–19, United States Government Printing Office.

UNITED STATES PUBLIC HEALTH SERVICE (1959–61), *Vital Statistics of the United States*, United States Government Printing Office.

UNITED STATES PUBLIC HEALTH SERVICE (1964), *Coronary Care Units: Specialized Intensive Care Units for Acute Myocardial Infarction Patients*, United States Government Printing Office.

UNIVERSITY of MICHIGAN DEPARTMENT of ECONOMICS and BUREAU of PUBLIC HEALTH ECONOMICS (1964), *The Economics of Health and Medical Care*, The University of Michigan Press.

US BUREAU of the CENSUS (1960a), *Census of Population*, volume 1, Government Printing Office.

US BUREAU of the CENSUS (1960b), *Historical Statistics of the United States, from Colonial Times to 1957*, Government Printing Office.

UNITED STATES TREASURY DEPARTMENT (1965), *Statistics of Income . . . 1962: US Business Tax Returns*, United States Government Printing Office.

WADE, L., *et al.* (1962), 'Are periodic health examinations worthwhile?', *Annals of Internal Medicine*, vol. 56, pp. 81–93.

WILSON, M. G; *et al.* (1958), 'The decline of rheumatic fever – recurrence rates of rheumatic fever among 782 children for twenty-one consecutive calendar years', *J. of Chronic Diseases*, vol. 7, pp. 183–97.

WOLF, B. M. (1964), *The Economics of Medical Research and Medical Care From the Point of View of Economic Growth*, Public Health Service, manuscript.

WORLD HEALTH ORGANIZATION (1958a), 'Constitution of the world health organization annexe 1', in World Health Organization, *The First Ten Years of the World Health Organization*, WHO.

WORLD HEALTH ORGANIZATION (1958b), *Expert Committee on Water Fluoridation, First Report*, Technical Report Series, number 146, The World Health Organization.

WORLD HEALTH ORGANIZATION (1959–61), *Annual Epidemiological and Vital Statistics*, WHO.

WYLIE, C. M. (1961), 'Participation in a multiple streaming clinic with five year follow-up', *Public Health Reports*, vol. 76, pp. 596–602.

YANKAUER, A., and LAWRENCE, R. A. (1955), 'A study of periodic school medical examinations', *Amer. J. of Pub. Health*, vol. 45, pp. 71–8.

# 6 Donald E. Yett

## The Nursing Shortage

Donald E. Yett, 'The chronic "shortage" of nurses: a public policy dilemma', in H. E. Klarman (ed.), *Empirical Studies in Health Economics*, The Johns Hopkins Press, 1970, pp. 357–89.

For thirty years there have been complaints of a shortage of professional nurses. Hundreds of articles concerning the problem have been published in scholarly journals and popular magazines. Although much attention has been given this issue, surprisingly few attempts have been made to specify what the term nurse 'shortage' means. The few authorities who have attempted to do so usually have defined it as the number of 'active' nurses relative to the number 'required' to provide the desired level of patient care.

A chronological review of the attempts to estimate the size of the shortage in this sense indicates the following trend: before the Second World War, nurse employment levels were considered adequate; during the war a shortage developed, estimated at approximately 75,000 in 1943 and 110,000 by the end of the war; despite predictions to the contrary, the shortage declined dramatically until 1949, when it was approximately 50,000, a level which was maintained throughout the Korean War; by the mid-1950s the shortage numbered 70,000, and subsequent estimates climbed to a new high of 125,000 in 1966; by 1970, according to a 1963 forecast, the shortage will be between 170,000 and 200,000.

Despite some discussion of whether there has been a misuse of professional nursing skills rather than an actual shortage, most experts remain convinced that the situation has deteriorated since the 1950s. They agree that there has been a large increase in the *supply* of nurses but emphasize that there has been a greater increase in the nation's *need* for nurses. This is the sense in which we must take the statements of hospital and nursing leaders that we have had a chronic nurse shortage for almost thirty years. And it is in this same sense that the existence of the 'shortage' has become part of the 'conventional wisdom'.

## Definitions of economic shortage

To an economist, a labor shortage does not generally mean that additional manpower is 'needed' to satisfy a certain public policy goal. Simply described, an economic shortage exists when the amount of something demanded by the public exceeds the amount supplied at the existing market price. Demand is negatively related to price, whereas need is generally construed to be independent of price; thus there is no necessary relationship between an economic and a 'need' shortage. However, if both types of shortage exist, the market adjustment process would normally lead to an increase in nurse employment, which, *ceteris paribus*, would reduce each type of shortage simultaneously. Thus it should be interesting to compare the available evidence concerning the probable size of any economic shortage(s) of nurses that may have existed in recent years with the figures based upon 'need' given above. To do so, it will first be necessary to specify more rigorously what is meant by an economic shortage.

Few economists have expressed opinions on market conditions in nursing. Although certain occupations said to be experiencing serious 'shortages' have been analysed, no general model has been developed which is directly applicable to the market for nurses. In fact, the literature reveals several disconcerting instances in which 'shortage' studies based on virtually identical data resulted in different conclusions. Two economic analyses of the 'shortage of engineers' illustrate how opposite conclusions can be reached by applying different models to the same facts. A critical summary of both is given in sections following, and their applications to relevant nurse data are discussed.

### The Blank–Stigler model of a shortage

David M. Blank and George J. Stigler (1957) specify that a shortage 'exists when the number of workers available (the supply) increases less rapidly than the number demanded *at the salaries paid in the recent past*. Then salaries will rise [relative to those for other occupations] and activities which once were performed by (say) engineers must now be performed by a class of workers who are less well trained and less expensive' (1957, p. 24).

Figure 1 illustrates their definition. Functions $D_1$ and $S_1$ are initially in equilibrium at relative wage $W_1$ and employment $L_1$. If demand and supply shift to $D_2$ and $S_2$, a shortage of $X_1$ is indicated. Subsequent shifts to $D_3 S_3$ and $D_4 S_4$ would produce shortages of $X_2$ and $X_4$. However, since theirs is a comparative

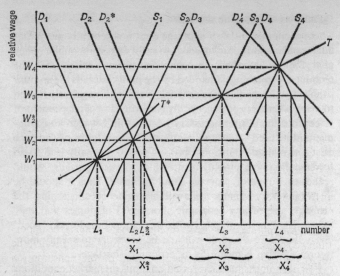

Figure 1 The Blank–Stigler shortage model

equilibrium approach, they do not expect to observe any $X_i$, but must rely on relative wage trends to indicate *ex post* whether a shortage exists. Thus the upward-sloping $T$ line indicates the existence of a 'shortage'.[1]

1. Blank and Stigler implicitly assumed that, in the absence of disequilibrium, wages for the occupation would rise at the same rate as those of the reference group; that is, in the absence of a disturbance all workers will benefit equally from productivity gains and/or product price increases. However, if the reference group selected were all workers, it is entirely possible that no occupation would have the same wage trend as the deflator, so that a strict application of their definition would imply that about half of all occupations had experienced a 'shortage' and the other half a 'surplus'. Even if their approach is accepted as an adequate approximation to *ceteris paribus*, the most that could be inferred from a relative wage increase is a 'relative shortage' in comparison to other occupations. In times of widespread unemployment such a finding would clearly be meaningless, but even in prosperous times this might be the case. For example, assume that there are shortages in both the general and specific labor markets, that 'excess demand' is proportionally larger in the general market, and that the demand and supply curves are steeper in the specific than in the general labor market. As both markets adjust toward equilibrium, the wage for the specific occupation may rise relative to the average of all wages. This would clearly represent a definitional contradiction, as a larger wage increase would have been required to regain equilibrium in the specific than in the general market – even though the specific 'shortage' was smaller than the general 'shortage'.

Data on median nurse salaries relative to those for other workers suggest, in Blank–Stigler terms, a shortage of nurses during the Second World War [2] but no postwar shortage until after 1962; in fact, there appears to have been a 'surplus' relative to teachers.[3] Between 1962 and 1966 the situation changed, with evidence of an economic shortage according to the relative wage increase criterion.

The expected rate of return on an investment in training was also studied as an alternative measure of remuneration (Yett, 1968). Specifically, the following equation was solved for the internal rate of return $r$.[4]

$$\int_0^T [R_i(t) - O_i(t) - C_i(t)]e^{-rt}dt = 0 , \qquad\qquad 1$$

where, for option $i$, $R_i(t)$ is the receipts stream, $O_i(t)$ is the opportunity cost stream, and $C_i(t)$ is the direct cost stream. Ideally, the returns stream should include the value of the consumption aspects of education, options to increase training, non-monetary rewards, etc., with adjustments at the margin for individual ability differences, motivation, family status, on-the-job training, prior experience, market discrimination, the 'quality' of the training, and amount spent on 'human capital' improvement (e.g. health care). In practice, such factors are assumed to average out.

It was assumed that the receipts streams for nurses and female college graduates are best estimated by their average survivor-adjusted, after-tax earnings (including expected values for

2. This trend may not be reliable in view of the existence and differential administration of wartime wage controls.

3. Another possibility is, of course, that there were shortages in both fields, but that the 'shortage' of teachers was more severe.

To test the sensitivity of these results to the measure of remuneration employed, estimates were made of overtime pay and of the cash value of maintenance provided nurses, plus salary supplements received by all earners, as well as annual hours worked. Switching from wages and salaries to total compensation, and from monthly to hourly data, gave nurses an absolute advantage over workers in general, but relative trends were little affected.

4. In view of the well-known conceptual deficiencies of the internal rate of return as a criterion for investment decisions (Hirshleifer, 1958, pp. 350–52), estimates were also made of the present values and the rates of return over cost ('crossover points') associated with each training option. The results were not substantially different from those obtained on the basis of internal rates of return.

**Table 1 Professional nurse salaries relative to earnings of all workers, all female workers, and teachers**

| Year | All workers | All female workers | Teachers |
|------|-------------|--------------------|----------|
| 1939 | 0·83 | 1·18 | 0·72 |
| 1946 | 0·89 | 1·25 | 0·99 |
| 1949 | 0·89 | | 0·86 |
| 1959 | 0·85 | 1·21 | 0·77 |
| 1962 | 0·86 | 1·28 | 0·76 |
| 1966 | 0·91 | 1·37 | 0·79 |

**Table 2 Internal rates of return for nurses compared with all females with four or more years of college**

| Year | Nurses | Female college graduates | Ratio |
|------|--------|--------------------------|-------|
| *100 per cent labor force participation rates applied* | | | |
| 1939 | negative | 10·2 | negative |
| 1946 | 8·5 | 9·4 | 0·90 |
| 1949 | 9·8 | 9·3 | 1·05 |
| 1959 | 2·9 | 9·0 | 0·32 |
| 1966 | 7·6 | 8·6 | 0·88 |
| *Occupational education-specific labor force participation rates applied* | | | |
| 1939 | 18·1 | 15·2 | 1·19 |
| 1946 | 10·2 | 14·3 | 0·71 |
| 1949 | 18·4 | 14·0 | 1·31 |
| 1959 | 13·5 | 14·4 | 0·94 |
| 1966 | 12·7 | 12·6 | 1·01 |

scholarships, stipends and maintenance during training), from the beginning of training (age eighteen) to retirement. Opportunity costs are taken to be the similarly weighted earnings of female high school graduates. Costs of both forms of training include fees and other educational expenses but not living expenses unrelated to training. The first set of estimates assumes 100 per cent employment from graduation to age sixty-five; the second is actuarial, in that the age-specific labor force participation rates for nurses and for female college and high school graduates are applied to their receipts streams up to age eighty.

The estimates based upon 100 per cent labor force force participation yield essentially the same results, in Blank–Stigler terms, as did relative wages. The estimates based upon group-specific labor force participation rates diverge from this pattern only with respect to the wartime period, during which they indicate that there may have been a surplus rather than a shortage.[5] Thus, it would appear that there was an economic shortage of nurses during and shortly after the Second World War, a surplus during the 1950s, but a shortage again in the 1960s.

However, this interpretation disregards the second component of the Blank–Stigler definition – that activities formerly performed by professionals would then be performed by cheaper and less experienced workers. Surprisingly few data exist on the substitution of non-professional for professional nurses, and those that are available pertain exclusively to hospitals. What is known is that there has been a fairly steady increase in the ratios of practical nurses and non-professional nursing personnel to hospital-employed registered nurses and, even more dramatically, to general duty nurses.

In Blank–Stigler terms, the conclusions concerning personnel substitution indicate a shortage during the 1950s, whereas the data on relative remuneration imply a surplus. This apparent inconsistency is easily explained. The substitution of non-professionals for registered nurses should be based on their relative costs and productivities. If registered nurse salaries declined compared with those of all workers yet increased relative to those of non-professionals,[6] the first relative salary decline

5. There is a reasonable explanation for this difference. Prior to the war, nursing was one of the few areas open to career-oriented women, and, since most training was in hospitals which typically provided maintenance and small stipends, it represented one of the most highly skilled careers open to women unable to finance a college education. The war brought expanded job opportunities, rising wages, and an increase in employment rates for all women. However, employment rates for nurses somewhat declined, and came to resemble more closely those for other females. The higher employment rates for high school graduates meant higher opportunity costs for all post-high school training. The lower group-specific rates of return for nurses were a consequence of both shifts. Concomitantly, the group-specific rates of return for college graduates declined only slightly, owing to the rise in their employment rates. A strict application of the Blank–Stigler definition would seem to imply a wartime surplus of nurses. Such an interpretation not only lacks intuitive appeal but also ignores the second element of their definition, namely, the substitution of less skilled personnel for those in short supply.

6. This occurred between 1946 and 1959, when the ratios of general duty nurse starting salaries to those of practical nurses and untrained female and male hospital workers were, respectively, 1·37, 1·69, and 1·47 in 1946 and 1·39, 1·79, and 1·59 in 1959.

Table 3 **Ratio of non-professional to professional nurses in hospitals, 1946–66.**

| Year | Ratio to registered nurses of | | Ratio to general duty nurses of | |
|---|---|---|---|---|
| | Non-professional nurses | Practical nurses | Non-professional nurses | Practical nurses |
| 1946 | 0·997 | | 1·723 | |
| 1949 | 1·178 | 0·167 | 1·878 | 0·266 |
| 1959 | 1·449 | 0·314 | 2·426 | 0·527 |
| 1962 | 1·467 | 0·336 | 2·401 | 0·551 |
| 1966 | 1·677 | 0·372 | 3·152 | 0·590 |

would still indicate a surplus, although the second would encourage substitution, indicating a shortage.

The evidence thus supports the initial application of the Blank–Stigler definition. The size of the shortages during the 1940s and 1960s still must be determined. Unfortunately, since Blank and Stigler found no shortage (of engineers), they did not explain how to measure one, but certain inferences can be drawn from their model. Given an upward-sloping $T$ curve, three factors will determine, *ceteris paribus*, the size of the shortage.

1. The larger the increase in demand relative to supply, the steeper will be the slope and, hence, the greater the indicated shortage. Thus, if demand shifts from $D_1$ to $D^*_2$ (instead of $D_2$), the steeper curve $T^*$ (not $T$) and the larger shortage $X^*_1$ (rather than $X_1$) are indicated (see Figure 1).

2. Moving along a single linear $T$ curve, the larger the absolute shifts in demand and supply, the greater will be the implied shortage. If, for example, demand and supply shift in one year from $D_1S_1$, to $D_3S_3$, (rather than $D_2S_2$), a larger shortage $X_3$ (not $X_2$) will ensue.

3. Changes in demand and supply slopes can also affect the size of the shortage after a shift. The flatter the curves, the larger will be the implied shortage (e.g., a movement from $D_3S_3$, to $D'_4S_4$, rather than $D_4S_4$, results in a shortage of $X'_4$ rather than $X_4$).

Since their approach precludes our observing $X_i$, the 'size' of a Blank–Stigler shortage can be measured only by its effect on relative remuneration. This would not be difficult if one could estimate the initial equilibrium and the slopes of the relevant demand and supply curves. Some crude estimates of the short-run supply curve are given below, but it has not yet been possible to make the other required estimates. One may conclude only that, given the elasticities of the demand and supply curves, the larger the relative wage increase the bigger the shortage. But if the curves are steep, a large relative wage increase might indicate a trivial Blank–Stigler 'shortage'.

Although Blank and Stigler admitted that the situation depicted by their definition 'is not necessarily objectionable from a social viewpoint', they nevertheless maintained that it 'is a well-defined and significant meaning of the word "shortage"' (Blank and Stigler, 1957, p. 24). If, in fact, this is so, then any relative wage increase in a freely adjusting market must be evidence of a 'shortage'. Likewise, if a 'significant' definition is one which calls attention to a 'problem' that warrants policy consideration, then all relative wage increases should be a source of public concern.

Wartime experience proved that a conclusion based on relative rates of return may be the opposite of one based on relative wage trends if an increase occurs in training costs (including foregone earnings) for an occupation relative to the reference group. This implies that 'short-run' and 'long-run' market conditions differed for that occupation (Yett, 1965, p. 29). By basing their analysis on salary trends, Blank and Stigler appear to be concerned mainly with testing a 'shortage' in the short-run sense. However, they claim that the study of long-run determinants of supply and demand is their real subject (1957, p. 33). It is surprising that they paid so little attention to relative training costs[7] especially because, as W. Lee Hansen demonstrated, these effects can be easily incorporated into their model.

Figure 2 summarizes Hansen's reformulation of the Blank–Stigler model. Starting from equilibrium at $W_1 L_1$, demand shifts from $D_1$ to $D_2$. As employers bid against one another for the existing supply of labor, the average wage rises to $W_2$. The rate of return on training increases, attracting entrants, the short-run supply curve shifts from $S^*_1$ to $S^*_2$, and wages fall to $W_3$. The flow of entrants stabilizes at $W_3$, since the relative wage advantage and training costs are now equal at the new equilibrium rate of return (Hansen, 1964, p. 80).

7. All they say on the subject is that 'since the differentials of engineers' earnings above those of the academically untrained labor force are still in excess of the costs of obtaining an engineering degree, we may expect this trend to continue in the future: (1957, p. 31).

In this situation, Blank and Stigler expected to observe only $W_1$ and $W_3$, from which they would have inferred the 'shortage' $X_1$. Yet Hansen argues that a movement from $W_1$ to $W_2$ to $W_3$ might occur,[8] and with no shortage at $W_1$ he would consider this sequence to mean the development of a shortage and its elimination. If Blank and Stigler encountered $W_2$, they would interpret the wage decline to $W_3$ as indicating a surplus rather than a correction of a shortage.[9]

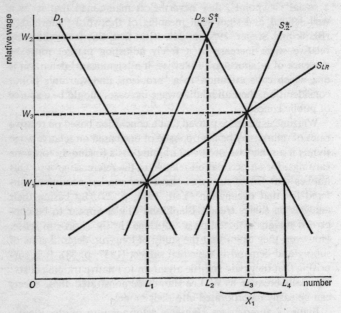

Figure 2 Lee Hansen's reformulation of the Blank–Stigler model

Extending Hansen's analysis, assume that as the wage approaches $W_3$ there is another increase in demand. The $T$ curve will then rise again, and, if this process is repeated, a virtually uninterpretable cyclic $T$ curve will be traced out, indicating, in

8. In order to simplify the argument, it was assumed that $D_1$ and $D_2$ represent long-run demand curves. If, in moving between the long-run equilibrium points $W_1 L_1$ and $W_3 L_3$, the short-run demand curves always increase much faster that the short-run supply curves, beyond some point the market wage must decline to the new long-run supply price ($W_3$).

9. Since Blank and Stigler assumed that all historically observed combinations of wages and employment were equilibrium levels, they must have had in mind short-run conditions.

Blank–Stigler terms, alternating periods of shortage and surplus. However, before the $T$ curve can be interpreted unambiguously in Hansen's terms, additional evidence is needed about equilibrium somewhere along the $T$ curve;[10] otherwise, an upward movement could mean either a declining surplus or a developing shortage. Since the reverse is true of a downward movement along a cyclic $T$ curve, no $T$ curve which does not continuously rise or fall from a known equilibrium can be unambiguously interpreted.

In the nurse market, rates of return based on continuous employment after graduation could be interpreted as indicating a developing shortage or adjustment to a previous surplus between 1939 and 1949 and recovery from a shortage or a developing surplus during 1949–59. Yet the group-specific rate of return estimates indicate recovery from a shortage or a developing surplus during the war, a developing shortage or recovery from a postwar surplus, and an adjustment to the shortage or a developing surplus during the 1950s. (Both sets of estimates indicate either recovery from a surplus or a developing shortage in the mid-1960s.) Measured in these terms, a change in relative remuneration proves neither a shortage nor a surplus in the Blank–Stigler sense.

If relative wage increases do indicate a shortage, is it significant for policy? Blank and Stigler considered all wage–employment combinations to be short-run equilibria; thus no 'excess demand' would occur unless wages were prevented from rising. If relative wage increases do not provide evidence of excess demand, what type of shortage do they indicate? Although Blank and Stigler never directly answered this question, two possibilities can be inferred from their analysis.[11]

1. Even if observed wage-employment combinations indicate short-run equilibria, they may not represent long-run equilibria. Thus short-run wages may exceed long-run supply prices, which

10. As Hansen explained, 'the choice of one base date over another for comparison can give quite different results; there is no logical basis for determining the beginning of a shortage' (1964, p. 80).

11. Still another possibility has been suggested. During the Second World War alternative opportunities for employment developed for those who had previously been servants; the higher wages in alternative lines of employment lured many to these occupations, so that '*at the price they had been paying for household help*, many families found they could no longer find such people. Rather than admit that they could not pay the higher wages necessary to keep help, many individuals found it more felicitous to speak of a "shortage".' (Arrow and Capron, 1959, p. 307).

certainly is true if the short-run supply curve is steeper than the long-run curve. Under these conditions increased demand might indicate a shortage in the sense that the short-run employment level would be less than the long-run level. If this is their meaning, it may serve to reconcile the fact that Blank and Stigler expressed their model in short-run terms with their claim of primary interest in the study of long-run factors, but it still does not represent a *significant* shortage, in the sense of a manpower problem worthy of serious policy consideration.

2. It is more likely that they considered a 'shortage' as a measure of unfulfilled employer expectations, i.e., the difference between *ex ante* and *ex post* hiring decisions. When an employer's demand for labor increases, he expects to hire additional workers at the prevailing wage, but if many employers have demand increases at the same time, the prevailing wage must rise. Each employer discovers that market conditions have changed when he is unsuccessful in expanding employment at the 'going wage'. Before raising his wage offers, the typical employer will complain of job 'vacancies' and of the fact that he is losing some of his older workers. As the new market wage is gradually accepted, hiring expectations will be revised. Whether there will be a 'significant' shortage will depend upon the difference between supply and demand at the previous wage and upon the speed at which employer expectations are brought into line with changed market realities. Although Blank and Stigler could not have assumed instant market adjustments and still maintained that theirs was a 'significant' definition, they did not incorporate into their model the determinants of a market's adjustment speed. Fortunately, Arrow and Capron included this refinement in their subsequent analysis of the engineer 'shortage'.

*The Arrow–Capron model of a 'dynamic' shortage*

In contrast to Blank and Stigler, Arrow and Capron sought to explain 'not only the direction of price adjustment (i.e., toward equilibrium) but [also] the rate of adjustment in the face of continued shifts in the short-run functions' (1959, pp. 293–4). Their model is dynamic. It recognizes time lags in responses to demand or supply shifts and applies to situations in which demand for an occupation is continuously increasing. They define a 'shortage' as the excess of demand over supply at the prevailing market wage. Further, they specify the 'market reaction speed' as the ratio of the rate of increase in the market wage to the excess demand. This ratio depends upon 'the time it takes the firm to recognize the existence of a shortage at the current salary level, the time it takes to decide upon the need for higher salaries, and either the time it takes employees to recognize the salary alternatives available and to act upon this information or the time it takes the firm to equalize salaries without outside offers' (1959, p. 299). The slower the market reaction speed and the more inelastic short-run demand and supply, the longer it will take the market to adjust. If demand continuously increases, and the reaction speed is finite, wages will increase without ever becoming high enough to clear the market. The shortage will continue to grow, but it will approach a limit which 'is greater the greater the rate of increase of demand and the slower the speed of adjustment' (1959, p. 300).

Arrow and Capron's unusual definitions of supply and demand pose a problem which must be resolved before their model can be applied to the market for nurses. To them, 'demand' (supply) means the amount of labor which would be hired (offered) in a particular labor market, in equilibrium at the prevailing wage, *after complete rational calculation* of the alternatives. In this sense few firms are likely to know, immediately following an increase in demand, what their demand is. Moreover, an increase in perfect-knowledge demand is not automatically equivalent to an increase in effective demand, which occurs when management suspects a change in product demand or labor productivity. In the presence of such a change, a typical firm will decide to increase employment but, in trying to do so at the going rate, will find little or no labor available. Realizing that it must pay more, the firm eventually will do so, but ordinarily this process takes time, and must be repeated.

Even when the firm has hired the desired number of workers at the new salary, the market will not be in equilibrium, since some firms now pay lower salaries to old employees than to the new ones. Established workers notice they are no longer in equilibrium situations; some change jobs, and management comes to realize that higher starting salaries eventually mean higher salaries for all. Equilibrium is restored only when each firm's effective demand is consistent with its perfect information demand, and when *ex ante* and *ex post* employment levels are equal at the existing market wage.

Blank and Stigler's definition implies that observed wage-employment combinations represent equilibria, but Arrow and

Capron's leads to the opposite conclusion. It is almost impossible for the market to return to an Arrow–Capron equilibrium immediately following a general increase in demand because to do so requires *all firms* to be in equilibrium. Since each firm must discover the new market wage and its own true demand individually whenever market demand increases, it follows that every firm 'will not, *by definition*, be on its demand . . . curve'.[12] This disequilibrium is what Arrow and Capron call a 'shortage'. Its existence is indicated by job 'vacancies', but because vacancy statistics do not measure the difference between perfect-information demand and supply, they cannot reliably measure the shortage.

Thus the Arrow–Capron definition is no better than Blank and Stigler's in two critical respects: it fails to measure the size of the shortage, and the 'problem' it identifies is the difference between behavior under conditions of imperfect and of perfect knowledge. Arrow and Capron also fail to explain why wages will approach equilibrium in their sense if firms are able to hire the amount of labor desired, utilizing only imperfect information.

One may eliminate the latter problem by adding an equation specifying the relation between the firm's actual and its perfect-information demand curves.[13] This approach is not operational, however, because identification of the latter curve requires perfect information. Alternatively, one might redefine demand and supply in a manner more consistent with traditional economic theory. If 'demand' is redefined as each firm's best *estimate* of the labor it wants at the existing rate, then market demand would represent the sum of their desired employment goals. Such an 'effective' demand curve would lie to the left of the Arrow–Capron curve. When effective demand increases, the resulting adjustment will be the same as that described by Arrow and Capron, except that each firm will know how many workers it

12. The analytical problem suggested by this quotation is further compounded if it is explicitly recognized that there is not a single market wage during the adjustment process and that observed wage-employment combinations are not necessarily points on the perfect-information market supply curve (Arrow and Capron, 1959, p. 293).

13. As shown above, Arrow and Capron define the market reaction speed ($k$) as the rate of change in wages relative to the difference between perfect information demand and supply. Obviously, $k$ could be allowed to vary in relation to the difference between the two types of demand. The form of the function would depend, of course, upon the institutional arrangements which determine costs of search, information, etc.

wants at a given wage – but will not know the relation between its demand and overall market conditions (which can be discovered only by trial and error). In summary, a 'dynamic shortage' can be measured at any time by reported job vacancies, which depend upon the rate of increase in demand, the slopes of the short-run market supply and demand curves, and the market reaction speed.

In recent years, 10 to 20 per cent of all budgeted positions for hospital registered nurses, but only 4 to 8 per cent of public health nurse and 1 to 2 per cent of school nurse positions, have been reported vacant. Although there are no data on openings in the industrial and office nurse fields, there is indirect evidence that such vacancies are extremely low.[14] Further, it appears that there are half again as many unfilled jobs in private duty as in hospitals. The figures for the early 1950s indicate an average 'frictional' vacancy rate of approximately 30 per cent in this field.[15] The slight upward trend since the mid-1950s suggests an increase in either 'frictional' vacancies or demand.

Reported hospital vacancies were higher for general duty nurses than for directors, supervisors and head nurses; vacancy rates for general duty nurses also exceeded those for public health nurses and nurse educators. This seems to conflict with the opinion of many experts that the 'shortage' is greatest in the most highly skilled areas of nursing (US Department of Health, Education and Welfare, 1963). However, the experts have never claimed merely a shortage of bodies but rather a lack of qualified nurses to fill high-level positions. Nursing and hospital leaders agree that teaching and supervisory positions should be filled by college-trained nurses, but the existing supply is not sufficient.[16] Conse-

14. In industrial and office nursing the typical firm employs only a few nurses. Since there are few opportunities to 'stretch out' existing staff the urgency in filling a vacancy is pronounced. Therefore, the fact that less than 0·1 per cent of the calls received by professional nurse registries are for even temporary placements in these fields suggests that such vacancies do not constitute a serious problem.

15. The transitory nature of private duty employment implies a high frictional vacancy rate even in the absence of a 'shortage'. Moreover, the reported figures are biased upward because they include canceled as well as unfilled calls.

16. There have, however, been sharp differences of opinion as to the relative importance of master's and bachelor's degrees and as to whether the position of head nurse should be included as one of the supervisory levels requiring advanced training. In 1963 it was reported that one fourth of nurse educators, two thirds of public health nurses, and nine tenths of

quently, many of these positions have been filled by nurses who otherwise would have been assigned to general duty, an area in which, as a result, the shortage appears to be concentrated.

The foregoing analysis assumes, of course, that reliable comparisons can be made among the vacancy series, which is unlikely, except in broad terms. Interpreting the year-to-year pattern for a given field is even more difficult.[17] The most consistent data are provided by seven American Nurses' Association surveys of hospitals. They suggest that vacancies rose during the 1950s, then declined between 1962 and 1968.[18] Although the 1958 and 1966 US Public Health Service figures imply a continuously increasing shortage, the absence of an observation for an early year in the 1960s prevents a meaningful comparison with the trend in the ANA data. (The figures are, however, consistently higher in the former than in the latter series.)

While no definitive statement can be made concerning vacancy trends, it is apparent that hospitals have long been reporting relatively high rates. These figures indicate a 'shortage' in the Arrow–Capron sense during the 1950s, when the Blank–Stigler approach suggested the opposite. The probable decline in vacancies between 1962 and 1968 implies a declining shortage at the very time when the Blank–Stigler approach suggests a developing shortage. In view of this conflict, it must be determined whether

nurses in hospitals and other fields lack degrees. By contrast, almost 30 per cent of hospital nurses have administrative or supervisory responsibilities (1963, p. 9).

17. In 1966, for example, the US Employment Service reported approximately thirty-five thousand nursing vacancies, which is about 5 per cent of total or 7 per cent of hospital registered nursing positions. In the same year an American Hospital Association survey reported a vacancy rate of 13·5 per cent for all hospital nurses. Both figures represent a tremendous decline from the 1962 figure of 20·7 per cent reported by the American Nurses' Association. In turn, the latter figure suggests a large increase in hospital vacancies at the end of the 1950s. Conceptual differences, as well as differences in definitions, survey design, non-response rates, and possibly even seasonal factors are largely responsible for the size of the fluctuations observed. A detailed analysis of these differences will be given in my forthcoming book, *An Economic Analysis of the Nurse Shortage*, chap. 3.

18. Even this pattern is suspect. The 1967 and 1968 ANA samples included only large, non-federal general hospitals (which tend to report above average vacancy rates), and positions were quoted in 'full-time equivalent' terms. While the selection of hospitals undoubtedly contributed an upward bias and the definition of positions a downward bias, their net effect is uncertain. The present author implicitly assumes that they cancel each other out.

Table 4 Vacancy rates by nursing field and hospital position, 1951–1968

| Field and position | 1951 | 1953 | 1954 | 1956 | 1958 | 1959 | 1961 | 1962 | 1963 | 1964 | 1965 | 1966 | 1967 | 1968 |
|---|---|---|---|---|---|---|---|---|---|---|---|---|---|---|
| **Hospitals** | | | | | | | | | | | | | | |
| All RNs | 11·9 | 13·6 | 11·1 | 12·9 | 9·3 | — | 20·1 | 20·7 | — | — | — | 13·5 | — | — |
| General duty | — | 14·6 | 13·0 | 14·5 | 10·0 | — | 23·2 | 23·0 | — | — | — | — | 18·1 | 15·0 |
| Directors | — | — | — | 6·0 | 7·3 | — | 12·0 | 13·4 | — | — | — | — | — | — |
| Supervisors | — | — | — | 7·5 | 5·3 | — | 13·1 | 15·3 | — | — | — | — | — | — |
| Head nurses | — | — | — | 10·0 | 9·3 | — | 14·0 | 17·0 | — | — | — | — | — | — |
| **Other** | | | | | | | | | | | | | | |
| Private duty | 28·7 | 31·8 | 27·6 | 34·2 | 31·6 | 34·2 | 32·9 | 37·3 | 38·3 | 37·8 | 40·0 | 40·5 | 41·1 | — |
| Public health | | | | | | | | | | | | | | |
| Total | — | — | — | — | — | 3·7 | 4·9 | — | 5·5 | — | 5·6 | 7·2 | 8·0 | — |
| Schools | — | — | — | — | — | 0·9 | 0·8 | — | — | — | 1·8 | 1·4 | 2·6 | — |
| Nurse educators | — | — | — | 7·3 | — | — | — | 10·1 | — | 7·8 | — | 9·4 | — | 6·8 |

the other Arrow–Capron criteria are met. According to their model, a 'dynamic shortage' will occur whenever '(1) there has been a rapid and steady increase in demand, (2) the elasticity of supply [or demand] is low, especially for short periods, and (3) the reaction speed . . . may, for several reasons, be expected to be slow' (Arrow and Capron, 1959, p. 302).

Throughout the period 1930 to 1960 census data provide evidence of a strong upward trend in the demand for nurses. The number of employed registered nurses consistently rose faster than the size of the population or the total labor force. However, during the depression decade of 1930 to 1940 the 'stock' of living graduate nurses increased faster than the number employed – 55 per cent compared with 33 per cent (Folk and Yett, 1968, p. 300). Hospital nurse salaries declined in relation to the overall average and in absolute terms. Nevertheless, serious unemployment was reported during the Depression and was probably still widespread in 1940.

Between 1940 and 1950 the total stock of nurses increased by almost 50 per cent, but the number of active nurses by only one third. The implication that supply increased relative to demand during and following the Second World War is unlikely, especially with rising wages and the alleged wartime shortage. This apparent paradox is easily resolved by noting that only employed nurses were counted as 'active' in the 1930 and 1950 figures. However, the 1940 'active' figure included all nurses in the labor force, including a substantial number of unemployed. The 1940–50 trend in active nurses thus understates the growth in demand because the unemployed were included in the 1940 figure for active nurses.

The evidence concerning the 1950–60 period is more difficult to explain. On the one hand, the slower increase in the stock than in the number of 'active' registered nurses (30 versus 40 per cent) and the steady increase in hospital nurse vacancies would seem to imply that demand grew faster than supply. However, as we have seen, the relative decline in nurse remuneration would lead Blank and Stigler to the opposite conclusion.

Like the census figures, my estimates of postwar employment by field of nursing are generally indicative of a strong upward demand trend. Total nurse employment grew by 129 per cent from 1946 to 1966. However, the rate of increase appears to have diminished since the late 1940s, possibly because in twenty years the stock expanded by only 72 per cent. (Again, the widening gap between the increase in employment and the stock is indirect evidence that the vacancy data shown in Table 4 might have resulted from the type of market behavior posited by Arrow and Capron.) Over three fourths of the increase in total active registered nurses is attributable to the 178 per cent growth in hospital nurse employment during this period, as a result of which the proportion of hospital to total active registered nurses rose from 55 to 67 per cent.

Although it accounted for only about 8 per cent of the increase in all active registered nurses, employment grew even more rapidly in the nurse educator and school nurse than in the hospital field. The increase in school nurses paralleled the postwar expansion of the school-age population. The situation with respect to nurse educators is more complex and reflects the shift from diploma to baccalaureate and associate degree programs, with their typically higher faculty-student ratios.

Of the remaining fields, the fastest-growing was office nursing (140 per cent), followed by industrial nursing (94 per cent), and public health nursing (63 per cent). Private duty nursing, the second largest field, showed the lowest postwar growth (5 per cent) and actually declined after 1954.

It is interesting to compare the foregoing employment trends with the salaries paid in different fields of nursing. Although salaries were quite similar for all fields in 1946, their postwar growth trends have exhibited a marked dichotomy. One group, composed of school nurses, nurse educators, public health and industrial nurses, gained substantial wage increases of about 60 to 90 per cent from 1946 to 1966. The other group, which constitutes over 85 per cent of all active nurses and is composed of office, hospital and private duty nurses, had salary increases of less than 50 per cent. Moreover, the latter group displayed much less dispersion than the former. Surprisingly, all but one of the low-paid fields was among the faster-growing in terms of employment. Taken together, these facts raise two significant questions: what common factor links the three fields with the lowest salaries, and why have their salaries increased so slowly?

Differences in educational preparation are not sufficient to explain the observed groupings. For example, most school and industrial nurses are diploma-school graduates, and lack of a baccalaureate degree does not automatically preclude employment of a registered nurse in public health, or even as a nurse educator. With its high salary scale, the nurse educator field has

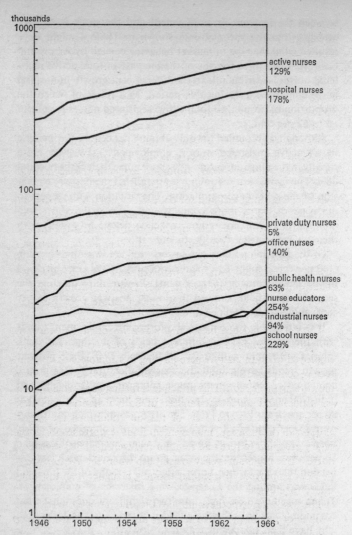

Figure 3 Estimated number of professional nurses, by field of practice

expanded over 300 per cent without a marked rise in its low vacancies. The school, public health, and industrial nursing fields also expanded rapidly without experiencing vacancy increases. According to the Arrow–Capron model, these areas would appear to have relatively elastic supply and demand curves and/or rapid market reaction speeds. To test both hypotheses, the salary-setting process for these markets should be examined.

Given the trend in hospital salaries, the rapid gains by nurse educators are surprising in view of the large proportion of them employed in hospital-affiliated schools. The pressure for higher salaries undoubtedly stems from the expanding baccalaureate programs and reflects the general salary rise of other academicians. The growing demand for college degrees may also explain the belief that there is a more acute 'shortage' of nurse educators than of hospital nurses, although reported vacancies for the former are lower. Requirements that teachers in baccalaureate programs have terminal degrees have intensified the sense of urgency associated with this problem and have boosted the salaries of nurses holding such degrees. Doubtless competition in this market has also resulted in higher salaries for hospital-affiliated faculty.

The correspondence between the salaries of nurse educators and other academic salaries illustrates a general rule: that nurses employed in an industry where nursing is a minority occupation receive compensation more representative of that industry than of the nursing profession. This principle is further supported by data on school and industrial nurses. In both instances personnel policies are set on the basis of market conditions for typical workers in the industry; management finds it worth a substantial salary premium to hire and retain a few well-qualified registered nurses. This premium is easy to establish where the average salary of other employees with similar training is higher than the going salary for nurses.

The foregoing hypothesis implies that the ratios of the average salaries of school nurses to teachers and of industrial nurses to manufacturing workers should tend toward unity. As a test, both ratios were calculated, and it was found that the former fluctuated from 0·98 to 1·11 and the latter from 0·98 to 1·07. Moreover, since the policy of paying a premium for not having to worry about nursing services would not be continued if it were unsuccessful, low turnover rates for these fields would be expected. No figure for industrial nurses in available, but a 1956 study of New Jersey school nurses disclosed that only 11 per cent were newly appointed that year (compared with turnover rates of 66·9 and 57·5 per cent for general duty nurses and female manufacturing workers, respectively) (Johnson, 1957, p. 465; Levine, 1957, p. 52; US Bureau of Labor Statistics, May 1955, p. 27; August 1955, p. 31; November 1955, p. 31; February 1956, p. 31).

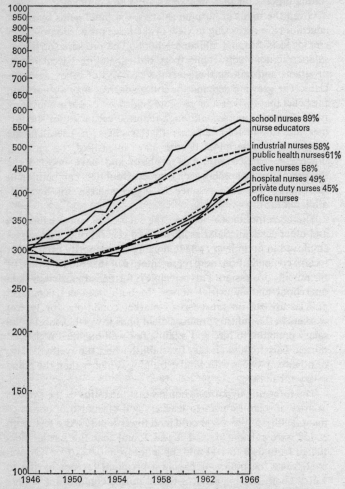

Figure 4 Monthly salaries of professional nurses, by field of practice (1966 dollars)

Market conditions in the public health field also support the above hypothesis. Salaries are commonly regulated by civil service and tend to be based upon years of training and seniority. However, unlike school nurses, public health nurses have not received higher salaries because of the rapid expansion of their 'parent' industry. This may partly explain why the vacancy rates for public health nurses are higher than those of school nurses even though employment in the former field rose more slowly than in the latter.

It is significant that the high-salaried fields account for under 15 per cent of total active registered nurses and that this employment level is determined by demand. At the prevailing salaries, employers in these fields face a virtually horizontal supply curve. They could pay lower wages without losing their recruiting advantage but choose not to do so because the convenience outweighs the cost. In Arrow–Capron terms, the market reaction speed is inconsequential.

Nurses who cannot find jobs in the top-paying fields must choose among hospitals, private duty and doctors' offices. It is tempting to ascribe the clustering of the salaries paid in these fields to competition, but in reality the pay scales for both private duty and office nurses are largely determined by salaries of hospital nurses. The basic eight-hour fees for private duty nurses hired through registries (which place most of them) are generally set in conformity with local hospital salary levels.[19] It is therefore unlikely that private duty earnings would diverge from general duty salaries except in areas where individual bargaining is common or where there is a deliberate attempt by the state nurses' association to upset the traditional pattern. For their part, physicians commonly recruit office staff from among the nurses who make the best impression in the hospital. Moreover, since many physicians have some hospital affiliation, they are undoubtedly familiar with hospital salary scales. By offering shorter hours and better working conditions, doctors are able to recruit nurses from the hospitals without open salary competition.

Clearly, hospital employment conditions set the scale for private duty and office nurses, and these three fields employ almost all nurses with salaries not administratively set above the 'going wage'. If hospitals can be shown to have inelastic demand

19. I am indebted to Elizabeth C. Carroll, State Section Advisor of the California Nurses' Association, for explaining the process by which basic eight-hour fees are determined.

and supply curves and/or slow market reaction speeds, it would appear that the Arrow–Capron model provides a reasonable economic explanation of the nurse 'shortage'. Superficially, the small salary rise accompanying the large expansion of hospital employment might seem to indicate a high short-run supply elasticity. The data necessary to test this proposition directly are unavailable, but rough calculations were made of the average short-run supply of elasticity for all nurses, which suggest the opposite. In 'real' wage terms, the average supply elasticity was low, between 0·25 and 0·34 (or from 0·11 to 0·17 in money wage terms) (Yett, 1965, p. 99). Since those fields paying 'above scale' do not represent a large source of additional nurses, the figures indicate that the short-run supply elasticities are indeed low in hospital-related fields.

Less is known about the average short-run elasticity of demand. The demand for nurses is a derived demand, determined by the demand for different medical services and by all the factors affecting the productivity of nurses in each of the health fields. It would be necessary to know both the demand and production functions for each health service (in addition to achieving econometric identification) before nurse demand elasticities could be estimated. The notion that short-run demand is inelastic is implicit in the views of the experts who have established nurse-patient ratios as 'requirements' for adequate care.[20] On the other hand, it appears that non-professional personnel are often substituted for registered nurses (albeit reluctantly), suggesting that the typical market demand curve for hospital nurses may not be as inelastic as the supply.[21]

20. Actually, the 'typical' hospital's demand for nurses depends not only upon its demand and production functions but also upon the supply-price relationships of the other factors it employs. The hypothesis that demand is relatively elastic depends upon the production function implications of the observed substitution of non-professional for professional nurses and the conviction of hospital administrators that while the nurse supply curve is upward-sloping, the supply of non-professionals is essentially horizontal. The implication of the latter is that the ratio of professional to non-professional wages will increase if the hospital attempts to hire more of both.

21. On the other hand, it is known that the elasticity of demand for a factor is positively related to the elasticity of the product demand, as well as to the proportion of total cost attributable to the factor. The results of several studies show that the demand for hospital services is quite inelastic (Feldstein and Sevorson, 1964, pp. 67–8; Rosenthal, 1964, pp. 26, 35). It was estimated that compensation to registered nurses amounted to approxi-

Although the probability that vacancies evidence a 'dynamic shortage' is reduced if demand is elastic, it must be noted that such a shortage depends upon the net effect of the interaction between relative demand increases, the slopes of the supply and demand curves, and the market reaction speed. Given a stable and inelastic supply curve, there is a good possibility that the increased demand for nurses may have caused such a shortage if the market reaction speed was slow.

Arrow and Capron gave three reasons to expect the reaction in a market for professional personnel to be 'slower than that in the markets for other commodities, such as manufactured goods, or even in other labor markets. They are the prevalence of long-term contracts, the influence of the heterogeneity of the market in slowing the diffusion of information, and the dominance of a relatively small number of firms' (Arrow and Capron, 1959, p. 303). Long-term hospital employment contracts still are the exception[22] and, aside from administrative and supervisory staff, few hospital registered nurses accumulate the type of seniority or tenure-related benefits that would slow the market adjustment mechanism. However, most hospitals are non-profit institutions constrained by annually fixed budgets, which would have the same effect as long-term contracts on the market reaction speed.

Although not all registered nurses are 'eligible' to be administrators or supervisors, the qualifications for such positions are not independent of the availability of applicants – i.e., lacking 'qualified' applicants, management will reluctantly hire less skilled personnel. Since hospitals do not publicize such practices, information on these job opportunities may be limited, and in Arrow and Capron's terms this factor would slow the market reaction speed. Dispersion of local markets may also hinder spread of information about opportunities elsewhere. However, this fact may not be too important, as over 60 per cent of the nurses are married and are constrained by their husbands' locations. Unmarried nurses may be in a better position to move

mately 14 per cent of total hospital expenses in 1963. Both factors will reduce the elasticity, but their net effect is uncertain.

22. The only collective bargaining contracts which cover registered nurses are those negotiated by unions in enterprises employing few nurses (e.g., industrial nurses) or by the ANA's Economic Security Program. As of January 1, 1967, the various state nurses' associations had obtained only 121 contracts, covering 245 employers and approximately 16,850 nurses. In all, less than 5 per cent of active nurses are covered by collective bargaining agreements.

elsewhere in response to higher wage offers, but it appears that their mobility is not great,[23] whether due to lack of information or of incentive is not known. Nevertheless, the nature of the market probably creates information breakdowns.

At first glance it seems improbable that the market reaction speed would be slowed by 'the dominance of a relatively small number of firms' in the nurse market. Nationally, there are thousands of employers as well as employees in each field of nursing. However, an evaluation of the extent of competition in this market must be tempered by the evidence of the concentration of employment in hospitals and the low geographical mobility of registered nurses. The latter fact implies that the relevant market is local rather than national, and the former indicates that hospitals are likely to be the dominant nurse employers in most localities. Moreover, in most cases, hospitals are either monopsonists or oligopsonists. According to separate surveys of general hospitals in 1949 and in 1960–62, more than 10 per cent of the hospitals were the only ones in their Hill–Burton Service Area, about 30 per cent were located in areas with one or two hospitals, 45 per cent were in areas with less than four hospitals, and over 60 per cent were in areas with less than six hospitals (Reed and Rice, 1949, pp. 88–156).

Even in metropolitan areas the market for nurses in less competitive than might be expected. In a survey of the thirty-one largest metropolitan hospital associations, all but one association of the fifteen replying reported having established successful 'wage-standardization' programs (Yett, 1965, p. 100). (The association that did not already have such a program asked for information on how to establish one.) The incentive to engage in such practices is quite strong, as unilateral wage changes are likely to evoke retaliation which will result in higher labor costs with little, if any, change in registered nurse employment. Because Arrow and Capron found no comparable situation for engineers, they did not explore its implications. They simply noted that the fear of precipitating a 'wage war' tends to slow the market reaction speed. Since hospitals must be aware of their ability to influence

23. One study found that 25 per cent of all married nurses made a geographical move when they changed jobs (probably because of a family move) but that only 5 per cent of the job changes of unmarried nurses involved a geographical move. Moreover, the same study disclosed that only 4 to 8 per cent of the nurses surveyed changed jobs because they were dissatisfied with their pay and only 10 to 15 per cent because they had found a better job (Smith, 1962, pp. 8, 11).

local nurse salary scales, the typical nurse market undoubtedly has a slow reaction speed.

Although nearly all the evidence available favors the 'dynamic shortage' hypothesis, not even its aggregate magnitude can be measured by the vacancy statistics in Table 4. In addition to the problems of measurement described above, a more fundamental difficulty exists at the theoretical level. Since monopsonistic and oligopsonistic employers will express the desire to hire more workers at the equilibrium wage, vacancies will be reported even though there is no 'dynamic shortage'. If one does exist, its severity will be overstated by vacancy data. Thus, before one can test for a 'dynamic shortage', the 'equilibrium vacancy' level of the market must be determined. The first step is to specify theoretical models describing the equilibrium positions of such markets.

## Model of an imperfectly competitive labor market

Under conditions of monopsony and oligopsony, firms face an upward-sloping factor supply curve. Consequently, since 'the marginal cost of labour exceeds its average cost an employer who is maximizing his profits at the existing marginal cost will . . . offer no more, although he may report vacancies (Archibald, 1954, pp. 188-9).

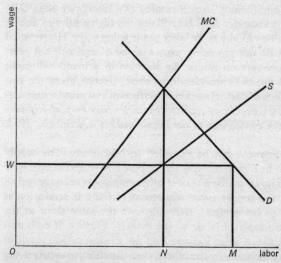

Figure 5  Model of a monopsonistic market

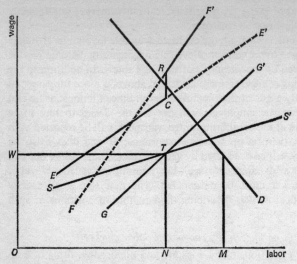

Figure 6 Model of an oligopsonistic market

Figure 5 shows a rising supply curve, $S$, and a corresponding marginal factor cost curve, $MC$, that is above $S$ for all employment levels. An employer in this situation will hire workers until the value of their marginal product equals their marginal cost. Thus, in equilibrium, he will employ $ON$ labor, pay wage $OW$, and report vacancies $NM$. He will not pay higher salaries, but he will be willing to hire more labor at the going wage. His reported vacancies do not represent 'excess demand' and will not exert upward pressure on wages. An increase in demand will cause wages to rise and vacancies to increase. 'Hence, given the two assumptions of [factor] market imperfection and profit maximization, *a large number of reported vacancies may be perfectly consistent with equilibrium in the labour market*' (Archibald, 1954, p. 189).

This argument can be extended to oligopsony. The supply curve $SS'$ in Figure 6 shows the response to wage changes by a single employer acting alone. If other employers are expected to retaliate, the supply curve will resemble $GG'$. If retaliation is expected to be 'perfect', $GG'$ will have the same slope as the aggregate supply of labor to the market. Further, if each employer expects a wage increase (but not a wage cut) to result in retaliatory increases by the others, then the effective supply is the kinked curve $STG'$. The marginal cost curve $FF'$ corresponds to the supply curve $GG'$, and the marginal cost curve $EE'$ corresponds to $SS'$. Thus the marginal cost curve for the kinked supply curve $STG'$ is the discontinuous curve $ECRF'$. In order for equilibrium to exist, the demand curve D must pass through the vertical section $CR$ of the marginal cost curve, yielding an equilibrium wage of $OW$ and vacancies of $NM$.

Since vacancies $NM$ do not represent 'excess demand', they do not affect the equilibrium wage, and their size is determined by the demand curve slope and the point at which it passes through $CR$. Any increase in demand within $CR$ will cause increased vacancies. No wage increase will occur until the demand curve cuts the marginal cost curve at a point above $R$. Below $R$ employers know that they will not gain by raising wages, but they will continue to report vacancies in the hope that their efforts will cause a shift in the supply curve. Under these conditions, wage increases will probably come in 'rounds', each being initiated by an employer who is temporarily strong enough (or hard-pressed enough) to act as the 'leader'. Other employers must follow suit. When the adjustment is over, relative stability will obtain until another employer is tempted to raise wages.

According to G. C. Archibald (1954), 'we will find oligopsony in the labour market whenever there are few employers of a given type of labour in an area and the cost of mobility is positive'. This would explain 'the apparent stickiness of the wages of many of the skilled and comparatively rare craftsmen. . . . The employer of skilled men who are limited in number will fear retaliation if he attempts to increase his share; the employer of casual labour will not'. Thus excess demand may often 'squeeze' the margin for skill'. Moreover, if 'solidarity' among employers exists and leads to collusion, it will 'help to deter employers from making increased wage offers which . . . will, *in any case*, look doubtful and risky' (1954, pp. 193–95).

Archibald, like Arrow and Capron, assumed that all employers are profit maximizers. Only a few employers of nurses are even profit seekers, much less maximizers. However, this strong assumption is not necessary. All that is required is that employers try to produce the output they desire as efficiently as possible, utilizing factors of production (including nurses) in the least-cost combination (Yett, 1970, p. 91). As a first approximation, it is not unreasonable to assume that hospitals – the major employers of nurses – behave in this fashion (Carr and Feldstein, 1967, pp. 50–51; Mann and Yett, 1968, p. 197).

Given the evidence that hospitals are monopsonistic or oligopsonistic nurse employers, the 'shortage' might be explained by the increasing number of registered nurses concentrated in hospitals.[24] 'Equilibrium' nurse vacancies may represent a misallocation of resources, but they are not likely to be 'corrected' by normal market forces. This should not be interpreted as implying that there has been no 'dynamic shortage' of nurses. The problem is that the vacancy statistics (Table 4), taken alone, measure neither 'dynamic shortage' nor 'equilibrium' vacancies. The author is currently engaged in research which, it is hoped, will lead to numerical estimates of both types of vacancies. To guide this effort, a model of the nurse market was developed which includes the dynamic factors brought out by Arrow and Capron as well as the effects of monopsony and oligopsony.

## Summary and eclectic model of the nurse market

Since most nursing statistics are national in scope, it is tempting to think of the market in such terms. Actually, the data should be viewed as weighted averages of behavior in local markets that possess a high degree of autonomy because of low wage-induced geographical mobility and the site-specific nature of nurse services. Most local nurse markets are variants of two basic prototypes in the hospital sector. Conditions in the other fields of nursing exert little influence on salaries because hospitals are the dominant employers, and two thirds of the nurses employed outside them have salaries directly tied to hospital scales, while the remainder work for employers who pay 'above-scale'. The more nurses in the latter category, or the greater the differential, the higher the average local wage will be. The same effect obtains with respect to the size of the hospital-related fields because, in the short run, they can increase only at the expense of the hospital supply, which would, of course, mean higher hospital salaries.

The ratio of hospital to all active nurses grew during the post-war period by almost the same amount (15 percentage points) as the drop in the proportion in private duty. This shift in the hospital supply curve undoubtedly contributed to the widening of the salary differentials between hospital-related and other nursing fields but in itself cannot explain the low level or slow rate of

24. It will be recalled that in 1946 salaries in all fields were more nearly uniform than at present. The dichotomous nurse salary pattern did not appear until hospitals became the dominant employers in local nurse markets.

increase of the hospital nurse salaries. This trend is explained by the hospital's position in the structure of local markets. Since the Depression, hospitals have become either monopsonistic or oligopsonistic[25] and in recent years have tended toward collusion on employment policies. Nurses demonstrate little wage-induced geographical mobility and, since positions in the highest paid non-hospital fields are scarce, they must often choose between hospitals and jobs outside of nursing. Few other occupations for which nurse training provides any advantage pay competitive salaries. In two studies, done in 1955 and in 1964, only 2 per cent of the nurses surveyed reported being employed in non-nursing positions (Deutscher et al., 1956, p. 56).[26] It might be expected that the growth in the proportion of registered nurses holding baccalaureate degrees would increase this percentage.[27] Fragmentary evidence suggests that this has not been the case. The 1955 survey included both diploma-holding and degree-holding registered nurses, while the 1964 figure was for diploma graduates only. The fact that the two figures are the same would seem to indicate that nurses with baccalaureates do not have a significantly greater propensity toward non-nursing employment than others, perhaps because they hold a disproportionate number of positions in the highest-paid nursing fields.[28] Thus, interoccupational mobility is not likely to diminish monopsony or oligopsony in local markets.

As monopsonists and oligopsonists, hospitals normally report registered nurse vacancies at the going wage, indicating a 'short-

25. During the 1920s and 1930s hospitals employed few graduate nurses, relying instead on students to provide most patient care. Offering free room, board and small stipends, hospital nursing schools attracted girls in financial need. The steady stream of poorly trained graduates produced by this system was not absorbed into hospital employment. Those who could not find jobs in other fields went into private duty or became unemployed (often indistinguishable states).

26. The 1964 Income was obtained from Margaret D. West and represents one of the findings of her survey of Hagerstown Hospital Nursing School during 1909–63.

27. Between 1956 and 1966 the percentage of active registered nurses holding baccalaureate degrees increased from 7·0 to 10·4 (American Nurses Association, 1967, p. 11).

28. In 1966, for example, 10·4 per cent of total nurses employed were baccalaureate graduates. By comparison, 33·8, 41·5, 30·4, and 18·7 per cent, respectively, of public health nurses, nurse educators, hospital nursing service directors, and hospital nursing supervisors held baccalaureates (1967, p. 10).

age' only in welfare theory terms (i.e., fewer nurses employed than at the competitive optimum). This situation could persist indefinitely because the market is in equilibrium, and no endogenous adjustment will 'correct' the problem. However, this misallocation of resources is not what nursing authorities mean when they complain about the 'shortage'. They refer to a deficit of demand relative to 'needs'. The elimination of monopsony and oligopsony would undoubtedly result in higher registered nurse employment, but there is no reason to suppose that this increase would fully satisfy their criteria.

Monopsony or oligopsony increases the probability of a 'dynamic shortage'. When demand increases rapidly, salaries do not rise as much as they do in a competitive market. The smaller the increase in registered nurse salaries, the less the increase in the rate of return on training will be. Thus, to the extent that short-run supply shifts depend upon the number of new recruits, the lower salaries attributable to monopsony and oligopsony will work against increases in the supply of nurses. Monopsony and oligopsony also affect the other two factors responsible for dynamic shortages. The market reaction speed depends partly upon the availability of job information, the paucity of which accentuates the effects attributable to isolated local markets. Moreover, since monopsonists and oligopsonists 'set' (rather than react to) the market wage, administrative delays will slow the market reaction speed even when job information is abundant. Monopsony and oligopsony further increase the probability of a 'dynamic shortage', since it is inversely related to the elasticity of the marginal cost curve, and the latter is more inelastic than the average cost curve representing supply in a competitive market. Unfortunately, data on local nurse markets are insufficient to test this model. The national figures which are available must be interpreted as weighted averages of local statistics. This procedure presents no conceptual difficulties, but estimates of true 'weights' would require considerably more knowledge of local markets than is now available.

From a policy standpoint, it is essential to distinguish between the two types of vacancies in the model. In equilibrium, all observed vacancies can be attributed to monopsony or oligopsony. Otherwise, some fraction will represent 'excess demand'. If the demand (or supply) function is continually shifting, it is extremely difficult to estimate the number of vacancies which would exist in equilibrium. However, such an estimate must be made before the size of the dynamic shortage can be measured.[29]

Although the relative numbers of each type of vacancy have not yet been estimated, their relationship to nurse demand and and supply elasticities should be considered. *Ceteris paribus*, the lower the elasticity of demand, the higher the number of dynamic relative to equilibrium vacancies. Similarly, the lower the elasticity of supply, the greater the number of both types of vacancies. Thus if the initial distribution of the two types of vacancies were known, the effect of a change in either demand or supply elasticity could be predicted.

The fact that the separate sizes of the two types of shortage cannot currently be estimated would seem to preclude implementing remedial policies. This fact would not matter if only one type of shortage were 'significant' or if the same remedies were invariably applicable to both. However, both types of shortage involve resource misallocation and, therefore, in the absence of quantitative information to the contrary, are equally worthy of policy consideration. The critical question is whether they respond to the same or to different policy measures.

## Some policy implications

Table 5 summarizes the effect on vacancies of policy measures which would change the elasticity or the position of nurse demand and supply curves. The effects of alternative policies on both economic and 'needs' shortages are given. Any measure which increases nurse employment (relative to 'requirements') would reduce the size of the nurse 'needs' shortage.

The only policy which will reduce all vacancies simultaneously is one which will increase the elasticity of supply. Although decreasing the elasticity of demand reduces 'equilibrium' and 'needs' vacancies, it will increase 'dynamic' vacancies. Any policy to decrease demand reduces all except 'needs' vacancies. This is usually done by substituting less-skilled personnel for registered nurses, which, unfortunately, could have adverse effects on the quality of patient care. Nursing leaders have long advocated policies which would have the effect of increasing the short-run supply elasticity and to some extent shift the curve itself (e.g.

29. As wages rise in response to disequilibrium, the number of dynamic vacancies will decline, but the number of equilibrium vacancies will rise. As a result of this process of transforming dynamic into monopsony vacancies, the difference between the ultimate level of equilibrium vacancies and the total number of current vacancies will underestimate the true magnitude of the dynamic shortage.

Table 5 Implications for number of vacancies of alternative policy approaches to alleviate various types of nurse 'shortage'

| Type of vacancy | Effects of policies designed to result in | | | | | | | |
|---|---|---|---|---|---|---|---|---|
| | Increase in supply elasticity[a] | Decrease in supply elasticity[a] | Increase in demand elasticity[a] | Decrease in demand elasticity[a] | Increase in supply | Decrease in supply | Increase in demand | Decrease in demand |
| 'Equilibrium' | Decrease | Increase | Increase | Decrease | Increase | Decrease | Increase | Decrease |
| 'Dynamic' | Decrease | Increase | Decrease | Increase | Decrease | Increase | Increase | Decrease |
| Total economic | Decrease[b] | Increase | Indeterminate | Indeterminate | Indeterminate | Indeterminate | Increase | Decrease |
| Relative to specified 'needs'[c] | Decrease | Increase | Increase | Decrease | Decrease | Increase | Decrease | Increase |

[a] The assumption is made that the elasticities are evaluated at the point of intersection between supply (average factor cost) and demand.

[b] If the elasticity of supply increase is due to collective bargaining, the introduction of long-term contracts may make the result indeterminate.

[c] The current employment level is assumed to be below the specified 'needs'.

flexible hours, more part-time personnel positions, child-care centers, refresher courses, non-discriminatory hiring, etc.). Except for the expansion of part-time employment (which I estimate was responsible for a 12 per cent increase in full-time-equivalent registered nurse employment between 1946 and 1964), hospitals have done little to implement any proposals which might involve higher costs. This behavior is, of course, not unexpected, as monopsonists will not incur higher costs to reduce 'equilibrium' vacancies, but will institute 'costless' measures to do so.

On the 'seller's' side, collective bargaining is frequently espoused. Although the establishment of standard pay scales through such bargaining would reduce the *effects* of monopsony or oligopsony, it would not ensure their *elimination*, which would occur only if the negotiated wage were equal to the competitive wage.[30] Collective bargaining could even replace monopsony with monopoly resource misallocation, but experience indicates that this result is unlikely in the near future.[31] Its effect on dynamic vacancies is indeterminate because the introduction of a long-term contract decreases the market reaction speed at the same time that the reduction in monopsony power increases it. Moreover, collective bargaining may have a greater impact on hospital salaries than is indicated by the number of nurses directly involved. A negotiated settlement may cause other hospitals to offer higher salaries to forestall the spread of collective bargaining or as a response to the publicity which usually accompanies it (Moses, 1967; Stelluto, 1967). This effect could be viewed as an increase in the market reaction speed, which, of course, decreases dynamic vacancies.

Professional registries offer an untried but potentially effective instrument for raising nurse salaries. Private duty fees are tied to general duty salaries and appear to be below market clearing rates. In an open market private duty earnings would rise, and, to

30. The same could be said with respect to a special minimum wage for nurses, with the additional complication that a standard rate sufficient to eliminate all local market shortages would probably reduce registered nurse employment in some areas, thereby aggravating existing non-economic shortages.

31. Between 1965 and 1967 the number of bargaining agreements in force as part of the ANA's Economic Security Program increased from 92 to 121. The number of nurses covered went from approximately 9,000 to 16,850. Some observers feel, however, that this rate of increase presages a bigger role for such bargaining in the future – especially if *bona fide* unions are formed and/or nurses are given the legally protected 'right' to organize (Kleingartner, 1967, p. 238; Hawley, 1967, p. 149; Kruger, 1961, p. 704).

the extent that hospital nurses were attracted by these higher earnings, hospital salaries would also rise and equilibrium vacancies would fall. (There would, however, be a temporary increase in dynamic vacancies.) The higher the proportion of private duty to hospital employment, the greater would be the increase in the hospital supply elasticity and the consequent decrease in both equilibrium and dynamic vacancies.[32]

At the national level, the establishment of a nationwide nurse registry would greatly improve the flow of information, which in turn would increase both the elasticities of supply and reaction speeds in local markets, simultaneously reducing equilibrium and dynamic vacancies.[33] 'Moving cost' subsidies for the 35 per cent of all nurses who are primary wage earners would have the same type of effect.

Still another way to offset monopsony or oligopsony would be to pay subsidies to hospitals as an incentive for them to hire enough nurses to eliminate equilibrium vacancies. The size of the subsidy to a specific hospital would be the amount necessary to lower its marginal cost of nurses curve until it coincided with the pre-subsidy supply curve. Such a program would be difficult to implement and would have to be continued indefinitely, since, by itself, it would generate no forces which would continue to offset monopsony power if the subsidy were cut off. Moreover, the subsidy would have to be increased whenever the hospital experienced an increase in demand relative to supply.

It is most unlikely that Congress would pass legislation giving different subsidies to equivalent facilities facing different nurse market conditions. Experience suggests that legislators are more inclined to support demand for particular services. Medicare is a good example. By making it possible for hospitals to shift part of the burden of higher costs, the program had the same effect as would an increase in the elasticity of the supply of nurses. On the

32. If registries became the standard source of placement in all nursing fields, it might be possible to eliminate equilibrium vacancies by breaking down the existing market segmentation. This would require, however, that three unlikely preconditions be met: each nurse would have to be willing to accept employment in any field at the market wage for her skill level; hospitals would no longer be able to identify their individual influences on supply; and registries would have to set salaries at market-clearing levels. By increasing the availability of job information, this plan might also increase the market reaction speed and thereby reduce dynamic vacancies as well.

33. Although the ANA operates a 'clearinghouse', its scale is too small to have much influence (American Nurses Association, 1967, p. 241).

other hand, the resulting rise in demand for hospital services (approximately 5 per cent) meant some increase in relative demand for nurses as well (Ball, 1967, p. 60). The former would tend to decrease both equilibrium and dynamic vacancies, while the latter would have the opposite effect; thus nothing definite can be said at this time about the net result of Medicare.

The Nurse Training Act of 1964 (amended and continued in the Health Manpower Act of 1968) represents the major federal attempt to reduce the postwar nurse shortage. Not concerned with demand *per se*, the Act was an attempt to expand the supply of nurses, a policy which, if successful, would reduce both dynamic and 'needs' shortages while increasing equilibrium vacancies. When the NTA was enacted, I criticized it on the grounds that any serious attempt to eliminate the nurse 'shortage' would have to be addressed to its demand as well as its supply side. Moreover, within the bounds of its limited goals, I correctly predicted that student loans would not cause the increase in nursing school enrollments to be greater than was expected without them (Yett, 1966, p. 200). Therefore, the funds allocated for new building were excessive, although they did help to improve obsolete facilities and to build college-based programs to offset the decline in hospital schools.

In 1967 the NTA Program Review Committee recommended continuation of the same approach for another five years. As a dissenting member, I endorsed efforts 'to improve the *quality* of both the existing and future supplies of nurses'. However, in company with Frank Furstenberg, M.D., I took 'exception to those aspects of the program designed to bring about a substantial increase in the *quantity* of professional nurses by 1975'.

We expressed our belief that 'without a program to translate the nation's "needs" into *effective* demand, the proposal to greatly increase the *supply* of nurses could cause large relative salary declines. Under such circumstances, nursing will become an even less attractive career than at present; and we will soon be faced with still another ... "shortage". ... If the determination of the supply of nurses is an appropriate Federal responsibility, so too is the assurance that effective demand will be sufficiently high to create employment opportunities at salaries attractive enough to eventually eliminate the discrepancy between the number of nurses "needed" and those "demanded" (US Department of Health, Education, and Welfare, 1967, p. 3).

Given the structure of the nurse market and the continuing increases in demand relative to supply, both equilibrium and dynamic vacancies are probably permanent phenomena, but it is doubtful that even economists would pay much attention to them if there were no longer a 'shortage' of nurses, in the popular sense of the word.

## References

AMERICAN NURSES ASSOCIATION (1967), *Facts about Nursing*, ANA.

ARCHIBALD, G. C. (1954), 'The factor gap and the level of wages', *Econ. Record*, vol. 30, pp. 188–9.

ARROW, K. J., and CAPRON, W. M. (1959), 'Dynamic shortages and price rises: the engineer-scientist case', *Q.J. of Econ.*, vol. 73, p. 307.

BALL, R. M. (1967), 'Problems of cost – as experienced in medicare', in US Department of Health, Education and Welfare, *Report of the National Conference on Medical Costs*, Government Printing Office.

BLANK, D. M. and STIGLER, G. J. (1957), *The Demand and Supply of Scientific Personel*, NBER.

CARR, W. J., and FELDSTEIN, P. J. (1967), 'The relationship of cost to hospital size', *Inquiry*, vol. 4, pp. 50–51.

CARR, W. J., and YETT, D. E. (1967), 'The relationship of cost to hospital size', *Inquiry*, vol. 4, pp. 50–51.

DEUTSCHER, I. *et al.* (1956), 'A survey of the social and occupational characteristics of a metropolitan nursing complement', mimeograph.

FELDSTEIN, P. J., and SEVERSON, R. (1964), 'The demand for medical care', in American Medical Association *Report of the Commission on the Cost of Medical Care*, vol. 1, pp. 67–8, AMA.

FOLK, H., and YETT, D. E. (1968), 'Methods of estimating occupational attrition', *Western Econ. J.*, vol. 6, p. 300.

HANSEN, W. L. (1964), ' "Shortages" and investment in health manpower', in S. J. Axelrod (ed.), *The Economics of Health and Medical Care*, University of Michigan.

HAWLEY, K. S. (1967), *Economics of Collective Bargaining by Nurses*, Iowa State Industrial Relations Center.

HIRSHLEIFER, J. (1958), 'On the theory of optimal investment decision', *J. of Pol. Econ.*, vol. 66, pp. 350–52.

JOHNSON, W. J. (1957), 'Public health nursing turnover', *Amer. J. of Nursing*, vol. 57, p. 465.

KLEINGARTNER, A. (1967), 'Nurses, collective bargaining and labor legislation', *Labor Law J.*, vol. 18, p. 238.

KRUGER, D. H. (1961), 'Bargaining and the nursing profession', *Monthly Lab. Rev.*, vol. 84, p. 704.

LEVINE, E. (1957), 'Turnover among nursing personnel in general hospitals', *Hospitals*, vol. 31, p. 52.

MANN, J. K., and YETT, D. E. (1968), 'The analysis of hospital costs: a review article', *J. of Bus.*, vol. 41, p. 197.

MOSES, E. B. (1967), Memorandum to Executive Directors of State Nurses Association, July 13th.

REED, L. S., and RICE, D. P. (1949), 'The nation's needs for hospitals and health centers, a summary of data from plans submitted by the states under the hospital survey and construction act', US Public Health Service Division of Hospital Facilities, pp. 88–156, mimeograph.

ROSENTHAL, G. D. (1964), *The Demand for General Hospital Facilities*, American Hospital Association mineograph 14, AMA.

SMITH, P. L. (1962), *Influence of Wage Rates on Nurse Mobility*, University of Chicago Graduate Program in Hospital Administration.

STELLUTO, G. L. (1967), 'Earnings of hospital nurses, July 13th, 1966', *Monthly Lab. Rev.*, vol. 90, pp. 57–8.

US BUREAU of LABOR STATISTICS (1955–6), *Employment and Earnings*, vol. 1, (May 1955), p. 27, vol. 2, (August 1955), p. 31, vol. 2, (November 1955), p. 31, vol. 2, (February 1956) p. 31.

US DEPARTMENT of HEALTH, EDUCATION and WELFARE (1963), *Toward Quality in Nursing: Needs and Goals, Report of the Surgeon General's Consultant Group on Nursing*, Public Health Service Publication 992, pp. 15–17, Government Printing Office.

US DEPARTMENT of HEALTH, EDUCATION and WELFARE (1967), *Nurse Training Act of 1964*, Public Health Service Publication no. 1740, Government Printing Office.

YETT, D. E. (1965), 'The supply of nurses: an economist's view', *Hospital Progress*, vol. 46, p. 29.

YETT, D. E. (1966), 'The nursing shortage and the nurse training act of 1964', *Ind. and Labor Rels. Rev.*, vol. 19, p. 200.

YETT, D. E. (1968), 'Lifetime earnings for nurses in comparison with college-trained women', *Inquiry*, vol. 5, pp. 35–70.

YETT, D. E. (1970), 'The causes and consequences of salary differentials in nursing', *Inquiry*, vol. 7, p. 91.

# 7 M. S. Feldstein

## Planning Health Care

Martin S. Feldstein, 'An aggregate planning model of the health care sector', *Medical Care*, vol. 5, 1967, pp. 369–81.

The growing interest in policy in the health care sector reflects both an inherent concern with the nation's health and an awareness that the price mechanism is an inadequate regulator of resource allocation in this area.[1] A prerequisite of appropriate government policy is an understanding of the aggregate behavioral relations of the millions of independent producers and consumers whose decisions determine the supply and use of health care services. The purpose of this paper is to show how this information could be estimated and analysed in the framework of an econometric model of the health care sector.[2]

### The uses of a health sector model

Federal government policy in the health care field currently concentrates on subsidizing the construction of hospital facilities and, through the Medicare and Medicaid programs, providing health insurance for the aged and medically indigent. Future developments may involve the government more directly in the supply of nursing home facilities, the training of medical personnel, and the care of individual patients. Through each of these

1. A recent discussion of the reasons why the market mechanism does not yield even a Pareto-optimal allocation in the health care sector is given by Arrow (Reading 1). For a survey of previous writing on this subject, see Klarman (1965).

2. The presentation in this paper recognizes that readers generally will not be familiar with the current use of econometric models in macroeconomic forecasting and policy. The concepts and methods are therefore explained as they are required; for further discussion, readers may consult the excellent expository paper by Suits (1962, p. 104) as well as fuller treatments in Marschak (1953), Tinbergen (1952), Theil (1964), and Goldberger (1959, 1964).

Although technical discussion is kept to a minimum, care has been taken to provide information about the statistical estimation procedure which will be of interest to those familiar with the problems of econometric model estimation.

activities, the government influences, both directly and indirectly, all aspects of the provision and use of health care services. For example, providing additional support for hospital building in one state would not only influence its pattern of hospital admissions but would also affect the building of private nursing homes, the attraction of doctors to the state, the wages of nurses and paramedical personnel, etc. All of these effects are relevant to determining the optimal level of such support for hospital construction.

More generally, associated with each possible government health sector policy are:

1. A set of *available* facilities – both those directly influenced by the government (e.g. hospital beds) and those indirectly influenced (e.g. private nursing homes);

2. The *costs* incurred by the government and by others;

3. The pattern of *utilization* of facilities (e.g. hospital admission and duration of stay by diagnosis);

4. The ultimate effect of this care on the *health* of the nation.

In principle, the government should select that policy which maximizes a 'welfare function' (the variables of which are measures of the nation's health, the costs incurred by the government, and other costs) subject to the constraints imposed by the behavioral and technological relations between government policy variables, total availabilities, costs, utilization and health. In practice, this approach to health sector policy-making is far from attainable. The behavioral relations linking government policy to the overall availability and use of services are almost completely unexplored. Technological relations between the use of health services and the resulting improvements in community health are known only for a quite limited range of activities. Because of the extreme difficulties in estimating these technological relations, a less demanding approach to health sector policy must be sought.

It is nevertheless important to preserve, as much as possible, the idea of choosing among policies in terms of their effects. If the ultimate impact which a government action will have on the nation's health cannot be assessed, it is at least possible to use estimated behavioral relations to predict its overall effects on the pattern of availability and use of health care services. The making of such conditional predictions would be the primary use of an econometric model of the health care sector.

Although such conditional prediction planning requires using the entire model, each individual equation can by itself provide information which could aid policy makers. It is helpful to distinguish two types of information, which may be called monitoring information and explanatory information.[3]

Monitoring information permits assessing individual aspects of the current operation of the health care system. More specifically, it answers the question: How do differences in variable $x$ affect some other variable(s) in the health care system? An example will clarify this. It is known that areas differ in the number of hospital beds available per thousand population. National officials should know what effects this has on the types of cases treated, the mean duration of stay per case, etc. Because clinicians serve in single areas, they will not be aware of these differences between areas in the patterns of admission and treatment. Similarly, a crude statistical comparison of admission rates or mean durations of stay in different areas would not distinguish the effects of bed availability differences from other factors which vary among areas. In contrast, the equations of an econometric model can indicate conveniently how the health care system responds to differences in bed availability, demographic characteristics, income, etc.

Explanatory information relates to specific suspected problems and to the causal relations which must be understood as a prerequisite of a general appraisal of health sector operations. It answers questions of the form: What are the reasons for the differences between areas and through time in variable $y$? Do these imply any malfunctioning of the health care sector? For example, officials might start with the observation that hospital admission rates differ substantially between states and then ask whether this is due to differences in population age-sex structure and medical characteristics or whether it also reflects differences in income, insurance coverage, hospital availability, etc.

### Estimates of a preliminary specification

A fully-developed model of the health care sector would show how hospitals and other institutions, doctors and paramedical personnel, governments at all levels, insurance agencies, and patients interact to determine: the pattern of services provided;

3. Both structural and reduced form equations are relevant here. The distinctions between these two forms of equations and between the types of information they contain will be made later in this paper.

resources used in their production; patients who consume the services; payments received by institutions and individuals; and prices paid by consumers. It would moreover be dynamic, indicating the reaction lags and time paths along which variables respond to each other. The model developed in the current paper is far less ambitious. It is small and its dynamic properties are limited severely. But it does provide a preliminary core for a larger model and permits exploring a problem of substantial importance, the supply and demand for hospital inpatient care.

Before looking at the specification and estimates of the model, it will be useful to review the general concepts and terminology of complete-system econometric models.[4] An econometric model is a set of interdependent statistically-estimated equations. The model as a whole explains the values taken by one set of variables (known as *endogenous* variables) in terms of the values taken by the remaining variables (*predetermined* variables). The number of equations in the model is equal to the number of endogenous variables. Some equations may be merely definitional, i.e., true as an identity, and therefore need not be statistically estimated. Each non-definitional equation describes some behavioral or technological relationship. The dependent ('left-hand side') variable of such an equation is one of the endogenous variables; some of the explanatory ('right-hand side') variables may also be endogenous. The estimated coefficients of the explanatory variables in a particular equation indicate the *direct effects* of each such variable on the dependent variable of that equation. The set of behavioral, technological and definitional equations together constitute the *structural form* of the model.

If the equations are all linear, it is easy to solve the set of equations for the endogenous variables, i.e., to express each endogenous variable as a linear function of all of the predetermined variables. This new set of equations is known as the *reduced* form of the model. Each coefficient in a reduced form equation indicates the total effect that a predetermined variable has on an endogenous variable. An example will clarify the distinction between the *direct* effect coefficients of the structural form equations and the *total* effect coefficients of the reduced form equations. Assume that the structural equation with the number of private nursing home admissions as dependent variable has among its explanatory variables the number of beds in federal government hospitals (a predetermined variable) and the number of beds in private

4. See footnote 2 for references to further discussion.

hospitals (an endogenous variable). Both variables would have negative coefficients, indicating that an increase in the availability of either type of hospital bed would decrease the number of persons admitted to nursing homes. Now consider the effects of an increase in the number of federal hospital beds. The *direct* effect is to decrease the number of nursing home admissions by the amount indicated by the coefficient of the federal beds variable in the structural equation for nursing home admissions. But the increased number of federal hospital beds would decrease the building of private hospitals; and the existence of fewer private hospitals beds would increase the demand for nursing home admissions. The total effect on nursing home admissions of the change in the number of federal hospital beds, reflecting both its direct effect and its indirect effects (such as that through the availability of private hospital beds), would be indicated by the coefficient of the federal hospital bed variable in the reduced form equation for nursing home admissions.

The structural form coefficients are important both for monitoring and explanatory information and as raw material from which the reduced form coefficients are calculated. The reduced form coefficients are also useful for monitoring and explanation as well as in the calculation of conditional predictions.

The six-equation model presented below was originally constructed to study the relation between supply and demand for hospital inpatient care on the basis of cross-sectional information for individual states for 1960.

## The specification

The endogenous variables of the model are: number of persons with health insurance (*INS*); number of general practitioners (*GP*); number of medical specialists (*SPEC*); number of available short-term general hospital beds (*BA*); number of admissions (*ADM*), and mean duration of stay per case (*MS*). All variables except the last are expressed as rates per thousand population. The predetermined variables are of two types. The first consists of past (1950) values of the endogenous variables.[5] The second group is the exogenous variables, i.e., those which are 'causally prior' to the variables determined within the health sector; population age structure as measured by the percentage of persons aged 65

5. The lagged value of the proportional utilization of hospital capacity, $P = (ADM) \times (MS)/365 \, (BA)$, is included among the lagged endogenous variables.

and above ($AGE$); income distribution as measured by the percentage of families with incomes below $2000 ($INC$); the percentage of persons living in communities designated as urban by the census ($URB$); and the percentage of married females in the population ($MAR$).

The selection of variables and the specification of the individual equations is based on previous work by others, [6] on the author's study of the British health care sector (Feldstein, 1967), and on experiments with the current data. It would be wrong to claim that the specification finally selected is a 'correct' picture of the health sector or even a resonably accurate one. The model is too small; too many variables are omitted; the measurement of the exogenous variables is too crude. It is proffered only as a rough first approximation.

All equations in the model were assumed to be linear in the logarithms of the variables. This has two advantages. First, the coefficients are estimates of constant elasticity [7] responses. Second, certain identities linking the variables are linear in logarithms, e.g. log. (proportional utilization of hospital capacity) = log. $MS+$ log $ADM-$log $BA-$log 365 .

*Variables*

The current (1960) value of the proportion of persons with health insurance ($INS$) was posited to depend on the population's age and income distributions, urbanization, and the previous (1950) proportion of persons with health insurance ($INS_{-10}$). Including the variable $INS_{-10}$ implies that changes in the exogenous variables do not have their full direct effect on $INS$ immediately, but rather that the current value of $INS$ reflects a gradual adjustment from previous values. This is a very plausible assumption for a variable which measures a type of behavior (being insured) which once acquired is very likely to be maintained. This lagged response process can be easily formalized. Using each variable symbol (e.g. $INS$) to stand for the logarithm of the value of that variable, the structural insurance equation may be written:

6. A summary of research published before 1965 is given by Klarman (1965). Other useful sources include: Anderson (1956), Auter (1966), Axelrod (1964), McNerney (1962), Roemer (1959), Rosenthal (1964, 1965), Somers (1961), Stageman (1962), Weisbrod (1961) and US Dept of Health, Education and Welfare (1962).

7. 'Elasticity' is the economist's term for percentage responsiveness; e.g. if a 1 per cent increase in $x$ leads to a 2 per cent increase in $y$, then the elasticity of $y$ with respect to $x$ is two.

$$INS = b_0 + b_1 \ AGE + b_2 \ INC + b_3 \ URB + b_4 \ INS_{-10}. \qquad \textbf{1}$$

If there were no delay in the response of $INS$ to changes in the exogenous variables, the equation of the (fully-adjusted) insurance variable ($INS^*$) could be written:

$$INS^* = \beta_0 + \beta_1 \ AGE + \beta_2 \ INC + \beta_3 \ URB, \qquad \textbf{2}$$

where $\beta_1$, $\beta_2$ and $\beta_3$ are the 'long-run' elasticities. Instead of assuming an immediate response, we posit

$$INS - INS_{-10} = \lambda(INS^* - INS_{-10}); \qquad \textbf{3}$$

i.e., the decade change in (the logarithm of) the insurance variable is proportional to the difference between the new fully-adjusted value ($INS^*$) and the past actual value ($INS_{-10}$). The value of the response elasticity ($0 \leqslant \lambda \leqslant 1$) measures the reaction speed. Substituting equation **2** into equation **3** yields:

$$INS = \lambda\beta_0 + \lambda\beta_1 \ AGE + \lambda\beta_2 \ INC + \lambda\beta_3 \ URB + (1 - \lambda) \ INS_{-10}. \qquad \textbf{4}$$

This provides an interpretation of the coefficients of equation **1**. The value of $b_4$ equals $1 - \lambda$ or, $\lambda = 1 - b_4$. The higher the value of $b_4$, the slower the response of $INS$ to changes in the other variables. Moreover, the values of $b_1$, $b_2$ and $b_3$ are first-decade ('short-run' or 'impact') elasticities; to obtain the corresponding long-run elasticities ($\beta$'s), each $b$ value must be divided by $1 - b_4$.

A similar dynamic specification was also used for the numbers of general practitioners ($GP$) and specialists ($SPEC$) and for the availability of hospital beds ($BA$). The number of general practitioners in the state was related in the model to insurance, income, and the previous number of general practitioners. The number of specialists was assumed to depend directly on insurance, bed availability, age, income and the previous number of specialists. The bed availability equation included insurance, the number of general practitioners and specialists, income, urbanization, the previous stock of beds, and the previous utilization of available beds ($P_{-10}$). The two hospital-use variables ($ADM$ and $MS$) were not related to their own lagged values on the assumption that, since these did not represent stocks, they would not be influenced by their own distant past. Admissions were assumed to depend upon bed availability, age, urbanization and the number of married women. The mean duration of stay per case was assumed to be influenced by insurance and the number of general practitioners, as well as by urbanization and the number of married women.

## The estimated structural equation

Using ordinary least squares to estimate equations with current endogenous as well as predetermined explanatory variables produces coefficients which are biased even in large samples.[8] The model was therefore estimated by a modified form of two-stage squares.[9, 10]

Table 1 presents the estimated structural equations. Although the coefficients generally have reasonable signs and relatively small standard errors, there are several exceptions. Each equation will not be considered in detail. Instead, the *INS* equation will be examined to show the general method of interpretation; then several coefficients elsewhere in the model will be discussed.

The coefficients of the three exogenous variables in the *INS* equation indicate that the proportion of the population with health insurance increases with the proportion over age 65 and decreases with the proportion of low-income and urban families. The values of the coefficients are estimates of the impact elasticities, i.e., effects within ten years of a change in the exogenous variable. The low value of the coefficient of $INS_{-10}$ indicates a relatively high speed of response of *INS* to changes in the other explanatory variables; the estimated value of $\lambda$ is 0·717. This implies that the long-run elasticities are only $(1/0·717) = 1·39$ times the size of the impact elasticities.

8. This bias is due to the lack of independence between the endogenous explanatory variables and the stochastic disturbances in the equations. For introductory discussions of this problem see: Klein (1962), Hood and Koopmans (1953), Johnston (1963) or Goldberger (1964).

9. All predetermined variables were treated as uncorrelated with the current stochastic errors, a common but theoretically unsound procedure. If the lagged endogenous variables are correlated with the current errors, the estimates will not be consistent. Using only exogenous (including lagged exogenous) variables as instruments would increase the confidence with which consistency could be asserted but would probably increase the mean square error of the estimates. In a more complete model with additional exogenous variables and more than two periods of observation, the use of only exogenous variables as instruments might well be more desirable. See Fisher (1966) and Nerlove (1965).

10. Expositions of the two-stage least squares procedure may be found in Johnston (1963) or Goldberger (1964). The modification used in this paper recognizes the block-recursive structure of the model (Fisher, 1965) without making any assumption about the correlation between the residuals in different equations. Because *INS* depends only on predetermined variables, it was estimated by ordinary least squares. Whenever *INS* subsequently appeared as an explanatory variable, it was 'replaced' (for the second stage of two-stage least squares) by the predicted value derived in the

## Table 1 Health sector model: estimated structural form parameters *

| Dependent variable | INS | GP | SPEC | BA | ADM | MS | AGE | INC |
|---|---|---|---|---|---|---|---|---|
| INS | −1 | | | | | | 0·322 (0·090) | −0·209 (0·093) |
| GP | 0·258 (0·128) | −1 | | | | | | 0·225 (0·089) |
| SPEC | −0·288 (0·159) | | −1 | −0·157 (0·113) | | | 0·159 (0·118) | −0·327 (0·097) |
| BA | 0·249 (0·128) | 0·127 (0·115) | −0·187 (0·091) | −1 | | | | 0·081 (0·102) |
| ADM | | | | 0·641 (0·085) | −1 | | −0·053 (0·073) | |
| MS | 0·186 (0·109) | 0·026 (0·116) | | 0·229 (0·132) | | −1 | | |

* Standard errors shown in parentheses.
A −1 indicates the dependent variable of the equation.

It is interesting to compare the response speeds of general practitioners, specialists and hospital beds. All three respond much more slowly than *INS* to changes in the determining factors. As might be expected, specialists respond more quickly than general practitioners and the availability of beds more quickly than either type of doctor. Also interesting is the relation between income and the availability of general practitioners and specialists. The signs of the *INC* coefficients in the *GP* and *SPEC* equation indicate that general practitioners become relatively more abundant than (are 'substituted for') specialists in states in which low-income families are more common. Moreover, the values of the elasticities (both impact and long-run) suggest that the total number of doctors actually increases with the proportion of low-

---

structural equation for *INS* rather than by a regression of *INS* on *all* the predetermined variables. Similarly, once the coefficients of the *GP* equation were obtained, the corresponding predicted value of *GP* was used in subsequent 'second-stage' equations. The model is not fully recursive since *SPEC* and *BA* depend on each other; in estimating the *SPEC* equation, the variable *BA* was therefore replaced by the value predicted by a regression on all the predetermined variables. Because this modified estimation procedure is essentially a method of choosing the instruments for instrumental variable estimation, the parameters' estimates will have the same desirable consistency properties as two-stage least squares (subject to the inconsistency which may be introduced by using lagged endogenous variables as instruments, discussed in the previous footnote). Moreover, the modified procedure incorporates more information (i.e., the zero restrictions on the reduced form) and is therefore more efficient.

| URB | MAR | $P_{-10}$ | $INS_{-10}$ | $GP_{-10}$ | $SPEC_{-10}$ | $BA_{-10}$ | Constant | $\bar{R}^2$ |
|---|---|---|---|---|---|---|---|---|
| −0·224 | | | 0·283 | | | | 5·715 | 0·711 |
| (0·090) | | | (0·048) | | | | | |
| | | | | 0·972 | | | −1·882 | 0·776 |
| | | | | (0·102) | | | | |
| | | | | | 0·712) | | 2·934 | 0·905 |
| | | | | | (0·052) | | | |
| −0·112 | | 0·159 | | | | 0·616 | −1·397 | 0·742 |
| (0·099) | | (0·210) | | | | (0·084) | | |
| −0·118 | 0·561 | | | | | | 2·249 | 0·639 |
| (0·040) | (0·337) | | | | | | | |
| 0·190 | −1·559 | | | | | | 5·955 | 0·600 |
| (0·079) | (0·440) | | | | | | | |

income families;[11] this surprising result warrants further study in the next section.

## The reduced form equations

Table 2 presents the coefficients of the reduced form equations which express each endogenous variable as a linear function of the predetermined variables. As explained above, these coefficients measure the total effects (both direct and indirect) of the predetermined variables and thus complement the monitoring and explanatory information of the structural equations. Although the reduced form coefficients differ from those of the structural equations (except the coefficients of the $INS$ equation and of certain lagged dependent variables), the signs and magnitudes are approximately the same. Of course, some predetermined variables have indirect but not direct effects on given endogenous variables; in such cases, the structural coefficient is zero and the reduced form coefficient nonzero.

This estimated reduced form can be used to predict the values which the endogenous variables would take in each state in 1970 if the structural parameters of the health care sector remained unchanged. A prerequisite of such a predicition is a forecast of the 1970 values of the exogenous variables: $AGE, INC, URB$ and $MAR$. The lagged endogenous variables (e.g., $INS_{-10}$) are merely the 1960 values and therefore are known already.

11. This statement reflects not only the coefficient values but also the fact that there are on the average nearly twice as many general practitioners as specialists.

**Table 2 Health sector model: reduced form parameters**

| Dependent variable | Predetermined variable | | | | | | | | | |
|---|---|---|---|---|---|---|---|---|---|---|
| | $AGE$ | $INC$ | $URB$ | $MAR$ | $P_{-10}$ | $INS_{-10}$ | $GP_{-10}$ | $SPEC_{-10}$ | $BA_{-10}$ | $Constant$ |
| $INS$ | 0·322 | −0·209 | −0·224 | | | 0·283 | | | | 5·715 |
| $GP$ | 0·083 | 0·171 | −0·058 | | | 0·073 | 0·972 | | | −1·001 |
| $SPEC$ | 0·054 | −0·283 | 0·095 | | −0·026 | −0·097 | −0·020 | 0·734 | −0·100 | 1·792 |
| $BA$ | 0·081 | 0·104 | −0·193 | | 0·164 | 0·098 | 0·127 | −0·137 | 0·635 | 0·186 |
| $ADM$ | −0·001 | 0·066 | −0·242 | 0·561 | 0·105 | 0·063 | 0·082 | −0·088 | 0·407 | 2·427 |
| $MS$ | 0·081 | −0·107 | 0·103 | −1·559 | 0·038 | 0·077 | 0·054 | −0·031 | 0·145 | 7·253 |

**Table 3 Health sector model: policy reduced form**

| Dependent variable | Predetermined variable | | | | | | | | |
|---|---|---|---|---|---|---|---|---|---|
| | $BA$ | $AGE$ | $INC$ | $URB$ | $MAR$ | $INS_{-10}$ | $GP_{-10}$ | $SPEC_{-10}$ | $Constant$ |
| $INS$ | | 0·322 | −0·209 | −0·224 | | 0·283 | | | 5·715 |
| $GP$ | | 0·083 | 0·171 | −0·058 | | 0·073 | 0·972 | | −1·001 |
| $SPEC$ | −0·157 | 0·066 | −0·267 | 0·065 | | −0·082 | | 0·071 | 1·591 |
| $ADM$ | 0·641 | −0·053 | | −0·118 | 0·561 | 0·055 | | | 2·306 |
| $MS$ | 0·229 | −0·062 | −0·034 | 0·147 | −1·559 | 0·025 | | | 7·585 |

Substituting the exogenous and lagged endogenous variables into each equation yields estimates of (the logarithms of) the 1970 variables.[12] The process can be repeated to predict the endogenous variables for 1980 by using the 1970 predictions as forecasts of the lagged endogenous variables.

The structural and reduced form equations together can also be used to predict the effects of a federal government policy which causes a once-for-all change in the value of one of the endogenous variables. To be more specific, assume that in 1960 the government causes an increase in the proportion of the population with health insurance in one state. This also affects the values of the other endogenous variables in 1960. To calculate these effects, the government policy can be represented as an increase in the constant term of the *INS* structural equation and the modified system solved for the reduced form equations. The new reduced form coefficients, which would be the same as those of Table 2 except for the constant terms, permit calculating the revised values of all of the endogenous variables. Of course, a once-for-all government policy in 1960 will continue to have effects in the future. If the revised 1960 endogenous values are used as the lagged variables for predicting the 1970 values, a revised set of 1970 predictions will be obtained. The government can therefore associate with any single current action a time path of effects on all variables.

A different type of conditional prediction problem is raised by a government policy that changes the structural relations of the health care sector. For example, if the supply of all hospital beds were made an instrument of federal government policy, the *BA* structural equation would become irrelevant and incorrect. Nevertheless, the other structural equations (estimated with *BA* treated

12. More accurate predictions for each state could probably be obtained by recognizing that the expected value of the error term for each state is not zero, i.e., by adding to each predicted value a systematic 'state effect' that differs among states but is assumed to remain constant through time. The best available estimates of these state effects would be the differences between the 1960 observed endogenous variables and the values 'predicted' for 1960 for that state by the reduced form equations. Unfortunately, this procedure implies that the structural form disturbances also contain systematic 'state' components and therefore that each lagged endogenous variable is correlated with the current disturbance for that state. This would make the use of lagged endogenous variables as instruments inappropriate; see preceding footnote 9. The pooling of several cross-sections in a more elaborate health sector model would avoid this problem as well as providing more accurate estimates of the state effects in the structural equations.

as endogenous, for the period before the policy change) still could provide the basis for conditional predictions of the effects of different government bed-supply policies. These five remaining structural equations would be solved for the corresponding endogenous variables as functions of the old predetermined variables and the now exogenous $BA$. Table 3 presents the coefficients of such reduced form equations.

Because the new bed-supply policy changes the structure of the health sector (and not merely the value of one variable), the reduced form coefficients of the predetermined variables are also changed. For example, in the original structure a higher value of $URB$ caused both a higher $MS$ and a lower $BA$. The lower $BA$ in turn caused a lower $MS$. Thus, the total effect of $URB$ on $MS$ ($0 \cdot 10$) was less than its direct effect ($0 \cdot 19$). The substitution of a government bed-supply policy stops the indirect effect of $URB$ on $MS$ through $BA$ and thus causes the new total effect ($0 \cdot 15$) to be higher than the old.

The equations of Table 3 could be used to make conditional predictions of the effects in 1960 and future years of different supply policies, i.e. different time paths of $BA$.

### The supply and demand for hospital care

Before considering the implication of the model for planning the supply of hospital facilities, we shall examine the use of the model to yield monitoring information about the effects of current interstate differences in the availability of hospital beds.

#### Effects of availability on use

The *per capita* availability of short-term hospital beds varies widely among the states. In 1960, when the average was $36 \cdot 3$ beds per 10,000 population, the distribution had a standard deviation of $6 \cdot 4$. The structural and reduced form equations for $BA$, both indicate that this current interstate variation largely reflects inherited stocks. Although supply changes in response to demographic and economic factors, the response is slow; the coefficients of $BA_{-10}$ in the structural and reduced form equations indicate that less than 40 per cent of any ultimate change occurs in the first decade.[13] Examining the effects of these bed availability differences on the way in which beds are used is an important

13. Because the model is estimated in the logarithms of the variables, the coefficient of a lagged dependent variable does not exactly express the proportion of total response that occurs in the first period. But for small changes the approximation is sufficiently close.

form of the monitoring information that a health sector model provides.

The most basic classification of bed use is into the number of cases treated and the mean stay per case. One would probably expect and hope to find that in areas of greater bed scarcity the mean stay per case declines relatively more than the admission rate. In this way, fewer cases would be untreated because of local bed scarcity. But the evidence of both the structural and reduced form equations points in the opposite direction. The structural equations indicate that the 'direct' elasticity of the admission rate with respect to bed availability (0·641) is more than twice the mean stay elasticity (0·229)[14] As the specification of the model implies, the reduced form equation shows the same relative 'total' effects of the lagged supply of beds on the current admissions rate (0·407) and on the mean stay (0·145).[15]

Although the reasons for this apparently undesirable performance of the health care sector are uncertain, the assumption that admission and duration-of-stay patterns reflect primarily the decisions of doctors rather than patients suggests several hypotheses. The hospital physician focuses his attention on the patients in his own direct care, i.e. those currently in hospital. Medical training and medical ethics urge him to give 'the best possible care' to these patients. The decision to discharge a patient is influenced little, if at all, by the thought that other persons in the community might make better use of the scarce beds.[16] The resulting tendency to treat fewer cases where beds are more scarce rather than reduce duration of stay is reinforced by the doctors' aversion to risk. By not reducing durations of stay, doctors protect their patients and therefore themselves from the dangers of insufficient care or facilities. The risks incurred by those patients who are not admitted to hospital need not affect doctors' decisions.[17]

14. Note that the sum of these elasticities (0·870) is the elasticity of the number of beds used with respect to the number of beds available. Thus percentage utilization of capacity falls, but only slightly, as availability increases.

15. A similar pattern of high admission rate elasticity and low mean stay elasticity was also found in a study of the health care sector in England and Wales (cf. Feldstein, 1965, 1967). When hospital service regions were used as the unit of observation, the elasticities were 0·58 and 0·37.

16. Indeed, the doctors' insensitivity to opportunity costs is one of the basic reasons why an unregulated health care sector will not achieve an optimal allocation of resources.

17. For a discussion of other manifestations of doctors' risk-avoiding behavior, see Scheff (1964).

Finally, durations of stay may be less sensitive to bed availability simply because duration-of-stay norms are easier to state and therefore to follow than standards of admission. Although doctors cannot easily learn the admission criteria used in other parts of the country, durations of stay can readily be compared and 'standards maintained.'[18]

Whatever the correct explanations for the observed relative elasticities, the evidence does indicate that substantial numbers of patients are not hospitalized because of local bed scarcities. It would be useful to investigate this in greater detail by estimating admission rate and mean stay elasticities for individual diagnostic categories, surgical procedures, and patient age groups (Feldstein, 1967). Monitoring information of this type could serve two purposes. The first follows from the suggestions in the preceding paragraph that the doctors in areas of greater bed scarcity may not recognize the opportunity costs of longer durations of stay and may not know that doctors in other areas are hospitalizing relatively more patients. By making doctors more aware of the influence of scarcity on their patterns of care, monitoring information might change their behaviour. Second, the information could help government officials and others responsible for health care policy. An understanding of the effects of hospital bed scarcity is a first step in planning the appropriate provision of nursing homes, outpatient departments, visiting nurse services, diagnostic campaigns, etc. Of course, knowing the way in which increasing the number of beds is likely to affect individual admission rates and durations of stay is the basis of conditional prediction planning of the supply of hospital facilities.

## Planning the supply of hospital facilities

The current stock of hospital beds and its annual growth reflect the decisions of governments at all levels, of charitable organizations, and of the profit-oriented builders of proprietary hospitals. Since 1946, the federal government has subsidized the construction of non-profit hospitals under the Hill-Burton program. This is done not only to increase the availability of hospital facilities

18. These hypotheses make no reference to doctors' incomes. The effect of this on the balance between more patients and longer stays is unclear. Because the doctor's fee is often (especially in surgery) a fixed amount for the case plus a variable amount per day, doctors might be inclined to cut duration of stay rather than number of cases.

but also to introduce planning and co-ordination into hospital building.[19]

The Hill-Burton act provides that support is available only for hospital construction that is part of a wider hospital plan and in an area that is deemed to have an insufficient supply. The Hill-Burton criterion of the adequacy of supply is very crude: 4·5 beds per thousand population in states with more than twelve persons per square mile, 5·0 beds in states with six to twelve persons per square mile, and 5·5 beds in states with fewer than six persons per square mile.[20]

A number of writers have criticized the planning of supply on the basis of such uniform bed:population ratios and have proposed alternative criteria designed to reflect local conditions more appropriately. These methods seek to determine the number of beds required to satisfy a local demand which is assumed to be independent of supply. One approach, originated in England (Bailey, 1956, 1962) but subsequently advocated in continental Europe (World Health Organization, 1965) and the United States (Blumberg, 1961), would measure local demand for hospital admission by the number of cases currently admitted to hospital plus additions to the waiting list. A 'critical number' of beds is then defined as the number required to treat these admissions with the average duration of stay desired by local clinicians. The 'correct' supply is the critical number plus two standard deviations (based on the assumption that the demand for admission is a Poisson process) to allow for fluctuation in demand. The second approach would use cross-sectional data and a multiple regression equation to find the relation between current demand (admissions and total patient days) and population demographic and economic characteristics (Rosenthal, 1964, 1965). Beds would then be built to satisfy the future demand predicted by this equation for forecast values of the population characteristics, again with extra capacity to allow for random fluctuation.

Both methods make the implicit conceptual error of assuming that the observed demand for hospital care is not influenced by supply. The model examined in this paper clearly indicates that although percentage utilization of capacity does decrease as the

19. For discussion of some of the economic issues in the supply of hospital facilities, see Reder (1965), Rosenthal (1964), and Somers (1961). The Hill-Burton program is described in Palmer (1956).

20. Palmer (1956) reviews the history of opinions about 'correct' bed: population ratios.

number of available beds rises, the decrease is small. The number of persons demanding admission and, to a lesser extent, the mean stay per case, are both sensitive to local supply.[21, 22] Several writers have criticized the proposed methods for disregarding the effects of supply (Reder, 1965; Roemer and Shain, 1959; Somers and Somers, 1961). Probably the primary reason why these methods have not been more widely accepted by those responsible for planning hospital supply is that they too recognize this inadequacy.

The search for a formula to identify the 'correct' number of beds, whether in terms of a simple bed:population ratio or a multiple regression prediction of demand, is understandable. Finding a formula relieves the responsible officials of the difficult task of choosing on the basis of their preferences. Choice in public expenditure is always arduous; it is especially so in the emotion-laden health field. More important, officials are very unlikely to have preferences about numbers of beds as such. Their preferences will be in terms of patterns of care and, ultimately, of measures of community health.

The importance of supply as a determinant of demand and the nature of policy-makers' preferences together imply that the planning of hospital facilities should be done with the aid of an econometric model of the health care sector. The reduced form of such a model would indicate that total effects of different bed-supply levels on the overall pattern of care. Conditional predictions of this type could then be the basis for choosing among alternative supply policies. Moreover, such an approach would emphasize that hospital construction is only one of an interrelated set of policy instruments.

### Conclusions

During the past twenty years, economy-wide econometric models have been developed as important tools of research and policy.

21. The argument (Rosenthal, 1964) that the effect of supply need not be taken into account because the utilization of capacity is lower in areas of greater availability, is incorrect. Supply has an important effect on demand even though additional supply does not induce an *equal* increase in demand.

22. The results of a study of the effects on observed demand of regional supply differences in Britain supports these conclusions. Demand (both admissions and total patient days) was found to increase with supply in a way which implied no upper limit beyond which demand would not rise. This British evidence is particularly useful because, since supply has remained essentially unchanged since the 1930s, there is no difficulty in interpreting supply as the exogenous variable (Feldstein, 1964, 1967).

Complete models should be able to play a similar role in individual sectors of the economy where public policy influences, but does not fully control, the sector's behavior. In addition to health, obvious examples include transportation, power, education and housing.

The current paper has indicated the ways in which an econometric model of the health-care sector could be used to provide monitoring and explanatory information and to make conditional predictions of the effects of alternative policies. These ideas were illustrated by a study of the demand and supply of hospital inpatient care.

The model presented is obviously too crude to be of practical use. A more detailed specification must be developed on the basis of careful studies of individual behavioral relations. Additional variables should be included to extend the model to other institutions and personnel, to out-of-hospital care, and to costs and prices. Currently included variables such as hospital admission and duration of stay should be disaggregated. The measurement of variables such as income distribution or age composition should be improved. Time-series information for each variable and state should be used to estimate the time patterns of lagged responses and the characteristics of individual states.

Although the state-by-state data on utilization expenditures and prices which would be required in order to develop such an operationally useful model are not currently available, the growing recognition of the urgent need for information to use in health-sector planning should soon lead to a correction of this deficiency. When such data become available, an econometric health sector model could provide a useful framework for conditional prediction planning.

### References

ANDERSON, O. W., and FELDMAN, J. J. (1956), *Family Medical Costs and Voluntary Health Insurance: A Nationwide Survey*, McGraw-Hill.

ANDERSON, O. W., COLLETTE, P., and FELDMAN, J. J. (1963), *Changes in Family Medical Care Expenditures and Voluntary Health Insurance: A Five-Year Resurvey*, Harvard University Press.

ARROW, K. J. (1963), 'Uncertainty and the welfare economics of medical care', *Amer. Econ. Rev.*, vol. 53, p. 941.

AUTER, R., LEVESON, I., and SARACHECK, D. (1966), *The Production of Health, An Exploratory Study*, National Bureau of Economic Research, mimeographed.

AXELROD, S. J., (ed.) (1964), *The Economics of Health and Medical Care*, University of Michigan.

BAILEY, N. T. J. (1956), 'Statistics in hospital planning and design', *Applied Statistics*, vol. 5, p. 146.

BAILEY, N. T. J. (1962), 'Calculating the scale of inpatient accommodation', in J. O. F. Davies *et al.*, *Toward a Measure of Medical Care*, Oxford University Press.

BLUMBERG, M. (1961), 'DPF concept helps determine bed needs', *Mod. Hosp.*, vol. 75.

FELDSTEIN, M. S. (1964), 'Hospital planning and the demand for care', *Bull. Oxford Univ. Inst. Econ. and Stats*, vol. 26, p. 361.

FELDSTEIN, M. S. (1965), 'Hospital bed scarcity: an analysis of the effects of interregional differences', *Economica*, vol. 32, p. 393.

FELDSTEIN, M. S. (1967), *Economic Analysis for Health Service Efficiency: Econometric Studies of the British National Health Service*, North-Holland Publishing Company.

FISHER, F. M. (1965), 'Dynamic structure and estimation in economy-wide econometric models', in J. S. Duesenberry *et al.* (eds.), *The Brookings Quarterly Econometric Model of the United States*, Rand-McNally.

FISHER, F. M. (1966), *The Identification Problem in Econometrics*, McGraw-Hill.

GOLDBERGER, A. S. (1959), *Impact Multipliers and Dynamic Properties of the Klein-Goldberger Model*, North-Holland Publishing Company.

GOLDBERGER, A. S. (1964), *Econometric Theory*, John Wiley.

HOOD, W. C., and KOOPMANS, T. C. (eds) (1953), *Studies in Econometric Method*, John Wiley.

JOHNSTON, J. (1963), *Econometric Methods*, McGraw-Hill.

KLARMAN, H. E. (1965), *The Economics of Health*, Columbia University Press.

KLEIN, L. R. (1962), *An Introduction to Econometrics*, Prentice-Hall International.

MARSCHAK, J. (1953), 'Economic measurement for policy and prediction', in W. C. Hood, and T. C. Koopmans (eds), *Studies in Econometric Method*, John Wiley.

MCNERNEY, W. J., *et al.* (1962), *Hospital and Medical Economics*, Hospital Research and Education Trust.

NERLOVE, M. (1965), *Estimation and Identification of Cobb-Douglas Production Functions*, Rand-McNally.

PALMER, J. (1956), *Measuring Bed Needs for General Hospitals: Historical Review of Opinions with Annotated Bibliography*, GPO.

REDER, M. W. (1965), 'Some problems in the economics of hospitals', *Amer. Econ. Rev. Proc.*, vol. 55, p. 472.

ROEMER, M. I., and SHAIN, M. (1959), *Hospital Utilization Under Insurance*, American Hospital Association.

ROSENTHAL, G. D. (1964), *The Demand for General Hospital Facilities*, American Hospital Association.

ROSENTHAL, G. D. (1965), 'Factors affecting the utilization of short-term general hospitals', *Amer. J. Public Health*, vol. 11, p. 1734.

SCHEFF, T. J. (1964), 'Preferred errors in diagnosis', *Medical Care*, vol. 2, p. 166.

SOMERS, H. M., and SOMERS, A. R. (1961), *Doctors, Patients and Health Insurance*, The Brookings Institution.

STAGEMAN, A., and BARREY, A. M. (1962), *Hospital Utilization Studies: Selected References Annotated*, GPO.

SUITS, D. B. (1962), '*Forecasting and analysis with an econometric model*', *Amer. Econ. Rev.*, vol. 52, p. 104.

THEIL, H. (1964), *Optimal Decision Rules for Government and Industry*, North-Holland Publishing Company.

TINBERGEN, J. (1952), *On the Theory of Economic Policy*, North-Holland Publishing Company.

US DEPARTMENT of HEALTH, EDUCATION and WELFARE (1962), *Research in Hospital Use: Progress and Problems*, GPO.

US DEPARTMENT of HEALTH, EDUCATION and WELFARE (1964), *Conference on Research in Hospital Use*, GPO.

WEISBROD, B. A. (1961), 'Hospitalization insurance and hospital utilization', *Amer. Econ. Rev.*, vol. 51, p. 126.

WORLD HEALTH ORGANIZATION (1965), *European Symposium on the Estimation of Hospital Bed Requirements*, WHO.

# 8 H.E.Klarman, J.O'S.Francis and G.D.Rosenthal

Efficient Treatment of Patients with Kidney Failure

Herbert E. Klarman, John O'S. Francis and Gerald Rosenthal, 'Cost effectiveness analysis applied to the treatment of chronic renal disease', *Medical Care*, vol. 6, 1968, pp. 48–54.

This paper attempts to answer one question: Under existing conditions of knowledge regarding the cost and end-results of treating patients with chronic renal disease, what is the best mix of center dialysis, home dialysis, and kidney transplantation? The question is explored through the application of cost-effectiveness analysis.

## Dimensions of the problem

It is estimated that in the United States perhaps 6000 persons whose life spans could be appreciably prolonged through treatments already known die every year from chronic renal diesase. A large majority of these persons are 15–54 years old. Currently, it is estimated, approximately 1,000–1,100 receive available treatments – 850 are on dialysis and 150–200 receive kidney transplants annually.

Treatment is expensive. On the average, a kidney transplantation costs $13,000, and the annual cost of dialysis is $14,000 at a hospital centre and $5000 in the patient's home.

Costliness of treatment coupled with lack of adequate health insurance coverage is a major factor in the Federal government's support of a substantial proportion of total expenditures, through its accepted role as sponsor of medical research demonstrations of new methods of treatment and new ways of delivering health services. The Federal government also faces decisions regarding the size and scope of such programs in its own hospitals.

Other Western nations, including Great Britain and Sweden, have assumed a commitment to provide treatment for all persons with chronic renal disease who are eligible to receive it from a medical standpoint.

## Why cost-effectiveness analysis?

Cost-effectiveness analysis is a special, narrower form of the cost-benefit approach that economists have evolved in the past generation. Much of the original work was done in the field of water resources.

The cost-benefit approach represents an attempt to apply systematic measurement to projects or programs in the public sector, where market prices are lacking and external effects in production or consumption loom important (so that individual decisions do not reflect true economic values). The cost-benefit approach is characterized by (1) the objective of enumerating as completely as possible all costs and all benefits expected and (2) the recognition that costs and benefits tend to accrue over time.

In principle, cost-effectiveness analysis partakes of both of these characteristics: a complete listing of inputs and outputs and recognition of time. The time dimension is treated by means of the discount rate, which serves to convert a future dollar into its present value. Under cost-effectiveness analysis the benefits need not be so complete as under the cost-benefit approach. Rather, certain results are specified and all other results are regarded as held constant or perhaps of secondary importance.

Cost-effectiveness, rather than cost-benefit, is employed when various benefits are difficult to measure or when the several benefits that are measured cannot be rendered commensurate. Under cost-effectiveness analysis costs are calculated and compared for alternative ways of achieving a specific set of results.

In performing a cost-effectiveness analysis it is taken for granted that the results sought can be 'afforded'.

## Available treatments

Chronic renal disease, resulting in irreversible kidney failure, stems from a variety of disease processes. No measures known today can be applied to a population with the reasonable expectation that the number of persons who develop chronic renal disease will be reduced.

In some patients kidney function deteriorates to the point of cessation. The patient dies of poisoning within a short time, unless certain relatively new and radical treatments are applied. Two specific modalities are available: hemodialysis (the patient's blood is cleansed of impurities by an artificial kidney) and kidney transplantation. As previously implied, dialysis can take place at a hospital center or in the patient's home. The center may be a teaching hospital or a community hospital related to it. Dialysis at home usually is performed under close supervision of hospital center personnel. In transplantation the kidney may be taken from a live donor, usually a blood relative, or from a cadaver just deceased with kidneys intact.

An obvious difference between dialysis and transplantation is that dialysis continues over the patient's lifetime, whereas transplantation is a one-time procedure, with due allowance for the careful and prolonged follow-up that it requires. When a transplanted kidney fails, the patient may survive and can submit to another operation or shift to dialysis permanently.

### Measures of end results

What is uniquely significant in both dialysis and kidney transplantation is their capability for prolonging lives that otherwise would be cut short. It is no oversimplification to express their contributions in terms of the number of life-years gained by beneficiaries.

It is possible to make some allowance for certain differences in life-style between patients on dialysis and those with an effective transplanted kidney. The latter have greater vitality, escape restrictive regimens, can continue to live in the same community, yet are free to travel without encumbrance or special arrangements. They enjoy a differential in the quality of life, which may be quantified as a fraction of each life-year gained. In this paper the differential is set at one quarter of a life-year. Other values may be posited; the implications of the findings are not affected.

Consideration was given to drawing a similar distinction between life-years on dialysis at the center and at home. It appears that although treatment at home is preferable for some patients, treatment at the center is preferable for others. There is yet no clear-cut evidence in either direction; accordingly, it seems best at this time to give equal value to a life-year gained at either location.

### Measures of cost

Cost is measured in terms of the present value of life-time expenditures for two cohorts of equal size, say 1000 persons, each embarking on treatment with dialysis or kidney transplantation. Expenditures depend on unit cost, previously presented, and on the volume and timing of services used.

It should be noted that total expenditures are calculated, regardless of who pays for them. It is desirable – and has been found feasible – to separate the question of sources and mechanisms of financing from that of economic efficiency.

Since dialysis is a continuing treatment over the patient's lifetime, the number of life-years gained is a necessary element of its cost while the same gain also serves as the measure of end results. To estimate the present value of the cost of transplantation, it is necessary to develop rates of retransplantation and of life years spent on dialysis by members of this cohort whose transplanted kidneys fail, who survive, and do not receive second kidney transplants. The cost of maintenance drugs is also taken into account.

For both cohorts it is important to tag the time when expenditures are incurred, so that they may be discounted to the present. It is realized that the choice of an appropriate rate of social discount is problematical, for there do not yet exist objective criteria for choosing one that commands general assent. In this paper a rate of 6 per cent is employed, because for diverse reasons it appears frequently in this type of analysis. Selection of alternative rates would affect the dollar amounts calculated in this paper but not the rank order of costs.

In order to facilitate calculations, projected future percentage increases in relative unit cost are combined with the initial discount rate of 6 per cent to yield a net discount rate. For transplantation and for center dialysis an extra annual rate of increase of 2 per cent (above any rise in the general price level) is posited and for home dialysis, which has a much lower labor component, an extra annual rate of increase of 1 per cent. The net rates of discount are, therefore, approximately 4 and 5 per cent, respectively.

Since transplantation occurs in the present, its estimated cost for a cohort can be estimated with greater certainty than that of dialysis, which takes place over a long time period. Reductions in the future cost of dialysis, if any, may be offset by the tendency to accept for treatment more patients with complications from other diseases.

The indispensable requirement for calculating the present value of expenditures expected to be incurred by each cohort, as well as for calculating the end results of treatment, are survivorship tables, with separate specification of years spent on dialysis and years with a functioning, transplanted kidney.

It will be noted that the total number of patients cared for has no bearing on the results of the cost-effectiveness analysis. The total cost of treatment is, of course, in part a function of the number of patients, and total cost does influence the determination of what can be afforded.

**Table 1 Life years – cohort of 1000 individuals starting on a chronic hemodialysis program**

| End of year | Number of individuals | | Average dialysis life years |
|---|---|---|---|
| | Dead | On dialysis | |
| 1 | 150 | 850 | 925 |
| 2 | 85 | 765 | 808 |
| 3 | 77 | 688 | 727 |
| 4 | 69 | 619 | 654 |
| 5 | 62 | 557 | 588 |
| 6 | 56 | 501 | 529 |
| 7 | 50 | 451 | 476 |
| 8 | 45 | 406 | 428 |
| 9 | 41 | 365 | 385 |
| 10 | 37 | 328 | 346 |
| 11 | 33 | 295 | 311 |
| 12 | 30 | 265 | 280 |
| 13 | 27 | 238 | 251 |
| 14 | 24 | 214 | 226 |
| 15 | 21 | 193 | 203 |
| 16 | 19 | 174 | 183 |
| 17 | 17 | 157 | 168 |
| 18 | 16 | 141 | 149 |
| 19 | 14 | 127 | 134 |
| 20 | 13 | 114 | 120 |
| 21 | 11 | 103 | 108 |
| 22 | 10 | 93 | 98 |
| 23 | 9 | 84 | 89 |
| 24 | 8 | 76 | 80 |
| 25 | 8 | 68 | 72 |
| 26 | 7 | 60 | 64 |
| 27 | 6 | 54 | 57 |
| 28 | 6 | 49 | 52 |
| 29 | 5 | 44 | 47 |
| 30 | 4 | 40 | 42 |
| 31 | 4 | 36 | 38 |
| 32 | 4 | 32 | 34 |
| 33 | 3 | 29 | 30 |
| 34 | 3 | 26 | 28 |
| 35 | 3 | 23 | 25 |

Table 1 – continued

| | | | |
|---|---|---|---|
| 36 | 2 | 21 | 22 |
| 37 | 2 | 19 | 20 |
| 38 | 2 | 17 | 18 |
| 39 | 2 | 15 | 16 |
| 40 | 2 | 13 | 14 |
| 41+ | 13 | | 160 |
| Total | 1000 | | 9005 * |

* 9005 ÷ 1000 = 9·005 years of life expectancy for each individual.

## Basic data

Table 1 presents life years gained by a cohort of 1000 individuals embarking on a chronic hemodialysis program.[1] This table is based on two assumptions: (1) the death rate in the first year is 15 per cent; (2) the death rate in every subsequent year is 10 per cent. For the first six years the survival estimates are based on data accumulated from various operating dialysis centers in hospitals in the United States. Life expectancy in the longer run must be predicated on speculation, for actual experience with chronic dialysis has not yet reached 10 years, much less the 30–40 years shown in the table.

Table 4 shows the disposition of a cohort of 1000 persons who embark on transplantation. In evaluating the experience of individuals on transplantation, it became evident that several alternatives must be considered. Patients starting on transplantation may have a successful first transplantation, may require a second transplantation, may die, or may move on to a program of long-term hemodialysis.

Here, too, experience has been too short to enable one to generate an expected life table with great accuracy or confidence. The assumptions taken from the Committee are that at the end of two years approximately 50 per cent of the cohort will have a surviving first transplanted kidney, 10 per cent will have a surviving second kidney transplant, 20 per cent will have died, and 20 per cent will be on long-term dialysis.

1. The authors had access to the data developed for and by an expert Committee on Chronic Kidney Disease, convened by the Bureau of the Budget. Since this paper draws heavily on the Committee's data it is not necessary to present here as detailed a documentation of sources and bases for assumptions as would be required otherwise. See Committee on Chronic Kidney Disease (1967).

It must be emphasized that kidney failure following transplantation signifies loss of the donated kidney, not death of the patient. In case of such failure, some patients die whereas others move into a dialysis pool.

Owing to the additional alternative, given failure of a transplanted kidney, it was essential to develop criteria for dividing the failures occurring after year 2 into two categories – those dying and those moving into dialysis programs. An annual failure rate of 5 per cent was posited. The procedure adopted in this analysis follows from the evidence that the median age of people who have chronic uremia is approximately forty-five years. To facilitate calculations it was assumed that the mortality rate for each age class would be approximately twice the rate for that age class in the US population as a whole. Table 2 presents the expected mortality by five-year intervals from age forty-five to sixty-nine, translated into annual rates. Table 3, derived from Table 2, distributes the annual kidney failure rate of 5 per cent between death and dialysis for each age class.

Table 2 **Expected annual mortality rates for kidney failures by five-year intervals, ages 45–69**

| Age (years) | Range of annual mortality rates per 1000 population | Assumed annual mortality rates per 1000 pop. (normal ×2) | Adjusted rate per 100 pop. (per cent) |
| --- | --- | --- | --- |
| 45–49 | 4·75– 6·89 | 11·64 | 1·2 |
| 50–54 | 7·58–10·72 | 18·30 | 1·8 |
| 55–59 | 11·63–16·03 | 27·66 | 2·8 |
| 60–64 | 17·31–24·17 | 41·48 | 4·1 |
| 65–69 | 26·42–35·93 | 62·35 | 6·2 |

Source: *Statistical Abstract of the United States*, 1966.

From the life tables for the dialysis cohort in Table 1 and the transplantation cohort in Table 4 it was possible to calculate the average life expectancy of an individual in each cohort. This was done by summing the total number of life years gained (or, where possible, taking the limit of the sum of a geometric progression) and dividing by 1000, the number of individuals in the initial cohort. This exercise yields a life expectancy gain of 9·0 years for an individual in the dialysis cohort. The life expectancy gain for an individual entering the transplantation cohort is approximately 17·2 years – 13·3 additional years on a successfully transplanted kidney and almost four years on dialysis, after the failure of a transplanted kidney. The added life years for a cohort embarking on transplantation are almost twice those of a cohort on dialysis alone, given the above assumptions.

When the adjustment is introduced for the qualitative differences between life after transplantation and life on dialysis, the differences between the results of transplantation and dialysis increases. Table 5 summarizes the calculations of cost and life years gained for each cohort.

Table 3 **Assumed distribution of annual kidney failures of five per cent between dialysis and mortality in each five-year survivorship period**

| Five-year survivorship period* | Proportion dying | Proportion to dialysis |
| --- | --- | --- |
| 1 | 1/4 | 3/4 |
| 2 | 2/5 | 3/5 |
| 3 | 1/2 | 1/2 |
| 4 | 4/5 | 1/5 |
| 5 | All | — |

\* Period starts at the end of year two in Table 4.
Source: Last column, Table 3.

The average increase in life expectancy with chronic hemodialysis alone is estimated to be nine years and that for transplantation, combined with dialysis when appropriate, is seventeen years. The present value of the *per capita* cost of the several treatment modalities is approximately $44,500 for transplantation, $38,000 for home dialysis, and $104,000 for center dialysis. If the conservative assumption of a 50–50 mix between home and center dialysis is made, the present value of the *per capita* cost of caring for the dialysis cohort is $71,000.

By almost every measure the maximum transplantation route appears to be the more effective way to increase life expectancy at a given cost. Further, the cost incurred is not appreciably greater than that of the least expensive dialysis program, that is, a program of home dialysis exclusively – which is not practicable.

Notwithstanding, it is noteworthy that the present value of the cost of a transplantation program does not differ a great deal

Table 4 **Disposition and average life years of transplantation cohort of 1000 by treatment modality**

| End of year | On transplanted kidney | Lose kidney during interval Aggregates in interval Total | Total | Move to dialysis | Die | Average life years Transplantation | Dialysis* |
|---|---|---|---|---|---|---|---|
| 1 | — | — | — | — | — | 875 | 55 |
| 2 | 600** | 400 | 400 | 200 | 200 | 675 | 200 |
| 3 | 570 | 30 ⎫ | | | | | |
| 4 | 552 | 28 ⎪ | | | | | |
| 5 | 524 | 28 ⎬ † | 137 | 105 | 32 | 2617 | 105 |
| 6 | 498 | 26 ⎪ | | | | | |
| 7 | 473 | 25 ⎭ | | | | | |
| 8 | 449 | 24 ⎫ | | | | | |
| 9 | 427 | 22 ⎪ | | | | | |
| 10 | 406 | 21 ⎬ † | 106 | 65 | ·41 | 2035 | 65 |
| 11 | 386 | 20 ⎪ | | | | | |
| 12 | 367 | 19 ⎭ | | | | | |
| 13 | 349 | 18 ⎫ | | | | | |
| 14 | 332 | 17 ⎪ | | | | | |
| 15 | 315 | 17 ⎬ † | 83 | 42 | 41 | 1579 | 42 |
| 16 | 299 | 16 ⎪ | | | | | |
| 17 | 284 | 15 ⎭ | | | | | |
| 18 | 270 | 14 ⎫ | | | | | |
| 19 | 256 | 14 ⎪ | | | | | |
| 20 | 243 | 13 ⎬ † | 65 | 13 | 52 | 1219 | 13 |
| 21 | 231 | 12 ⎪ | | | | | |
| 22 | 219 | 12 ⎭ | | | | | |
| 23 | 208 | 11 ⎫ | | | | | |
| 24 | 198 | 10 ⎪ | | | | | |
| 25 | 188 | 10 ⎬ † | 19 | — | 49 | 943 | — |
| 26 | 179 | 9 ⎪ | | | | | |
| 27 | 176 | 9 ⎭ | | | | | |
| 28+ | Less 5% annually | | | | | | |
| Total | | | | | | 3407 13,350+(480×8)/ 1000 = 17·2 | |

* Represents persons moving to dialysis, surviving eight years.
** Assumes no information until end of year two.
† Five-year survivorship groups (see Tables 2 and 3).

from the present value of the cost of a home dialysis program. This emphasizes the degree to which it is possible to underestimate the true cost of transplantation by omitting additional hemodialysis as part of the expected experience of the transplantation cohort. It will be recalled that the additional seventeen life-years accruing to the transplantation cohort consist of approximately thirteen years as the result of a successful transplantation plus four years on a long-term dialysis, following kidney failure.

## Implications

On the basis of the above findings it is concluded that transplantation is economically the most effective way to increase the life expectancy of persons with chronic kidney disease.

Certain factors constrain the expansion of transplantation capability. Removal of these constraints has the priority for action in the foreseeable future. More kidneys will be needed; it will be necessary to change certain state laws concerning autopsy and donation of organs and to improve the storage and preservation of kidneys. The last will depend on the outcome of research.

Successful research in tissue typing will serve to increase further the difference in cost per life-year gained between transplantation and dialysis. Any improvement in the technology of dialysis might reduce the difference.

Table 5 **Present value of expenditures and life years gained per member of cohort embarking on transplantation and on center and home dialysis**

| Modality | Present value of expenditures | Life years gained | Cost per life year |
|---|---|---|---|
| Dialysis | | | |
| Center | $104,000 | 9 | $11,600 |
| Home | 38,000 | 9 | 4200 |
| Mean | 71,000 | 9 | 7900 |
| Transplantation | | | |
| Unadjusted | 44,500 | 17 | 2600 |
| Adjusted for quality | 44,500 | 20·5 | 2200 |

Note: The cost of transplantation incorporates $24,500 for dialysis, based on a 50-50 per cent distribution of patients between the center and home.

It should be noted that the amount to be spent on research in an area cannot be expressed simply as a percentage of expenditures for services. Rather, research expenditures are properly a function of the size of the problem (measured by the sum of costs due to expenditures plus cost due to loss of earnings plus cost due to pain and suffering), multiplied by the probability of accomplishing successful research and of applying it. The probability of successful outcome in research, in turn, depends on what is already known and on the availability of trained scientific manpower to exploit it.

The large difference in cost between dialysis at the center and at home suggests that it may be worthwhile to explore the factors conducive to an expansion of home dialysis. It is obvious that one limitation on the performance of dialysis at home is the condition of housing. Accordingly, it may be desirable to consider alternative ways to improve the housing of patients with chronic renal disease and their families.

*Reference*

COMMITTEE ON CHRONIC KIDNEY DISEASE (1967), *Report*, Bureau of the Budget.

# Part Three
## Hospitals

Part Three continues to integrate theory with application, this time with explicit emphasis on the most important part of the health care sector – the hospitals. In the British National Health Service, hospitals account for about 60 per cent of total public expenditure on health and they are also the biggest users of manpower.

Newhouse (Reading 9) develops an economic model of a hospital. The characteristic hospital, whether in Britain or the the USA, is a non-profit institution which raises immediate problems of analysis since this fact appears to render the established economic theory of the firm, based as it is on profit-maximizing assumptions, inapplicable. Newhouse develops a utility maximizing model which, while it is clearly only a first attempt in this difficult area, appears to hold out the promise of further developments. One assumption implicit in the Newhouse model, in particular, is that hospitals will minimize the costs of each activity they engage in which, if false, is an area ripe for further study. Most existing costing studies of hospitals, however, do assume them to be efficient in this cost minimizing sense. Reading 10 is one of the earliest attempts to interpret the hospital cost data collected in the National Health Service and in it Martin Feldstein shows how, if sensible comparisons are to be made between different hospitals in the NHS, adjustments must be made to allow for differences in the kinds of 'output' produced by them. He also presents a workable way in which this can be done. The reading by Judith Mann and Donald Yett (Reading 11) is a recent survey of most of the material that, up till 1968, had appeared on hospital costs. It surveys both the empirical results obtained and also discusses some of the conceptual problems, integrating modern cost theory with the real world problems facing applied econometricians.

# 9 J. P. Newhouse

## An Economic Model of a Hospital

Joseph P. Newhouse, 'Toward a theory of non-profit institutions:
an economic model of a hospital', *American Economic Review*, vol. 60,
1970, pp. 64–74.

The private non-profit firm has been ignored by economic theory
until very recently. It was easy for economists to overlook such
firms in the past because of their relative unimportance, at least
for the past century and a half.[1] But presently this sector has
grown to a position of importance. In 1966, nearly $15 billion was
spent on hospital care, not including expenditures on construction, research, or insurance administration charges (Somers and
Somers, 1967, p. 43). Hospitals employed nearly 1·3 million people
in 1963, over twice as many as 'Blast Furnace and Basic Steel
Products' and nearly twice as many as 'Motor Vehicles and
Equipment (US Bureau of Labor Statistics, 1963). Since decisions
made by non-profit institutions affect the allocation of resources,
it is important that their decision-making process be understood.

In this paper a very simple model of a hospital is developed, and
its implications are considered at some length. An attempt is
made to justify the realism of this model, though like any model
it cannot be entirely realistic. To develop the model, we will make
the particularly unrealistic assumption that hospital expenses are
financed by the consumer and not by a third party. We do this in
the hope that this simple model may prove applicable to other
non-profit institutions where third party payments are not as
important; such as colleges and universities, the performing arts,
and museums. Later, however, we remove the assumption that
the consumer pays his own bill.

We are concerned with the relationship between a hospital's
non-profit status and economic efficiency. To understand that
relationship, we must postulate a maximand for the hospital
decision-maker. The first element in the maximand is quantity of
services provided. Hospital services seem to be desirable in some

1. There is some evidence that the non-profit corporation was the
dominant form of business organization in the colonial period. See Davis
(1917).

ethical sense which justifies the claim that consumers have a 'right' to medical care. It is the basis for granting hospitals certain tax and other legal privileges, such as exemption from the Robinson–Patman and Taft–Hartley Acts, and it seems to be the *raison d'etre* for philanthropy. Apparently it is felt that the public is better off if it consumes more hospital services (as well as more of the services provided by other non-profit institutions).[2] No doubt the public would be better off (and think itself better off) if it consumed more of many different kinds of products. Yet that is irrelevant to a decision-maker at a hospital. If his institution exists for a social purpose and because of that can ask for gifts and tax privileges, he is likely to be concerned about the quantity of the service provided. Therefore, we take quantity as one element in the decision maker's maximand. Maximizing quantity implies (on the assumption of a downward-sloping demand curve) keeping price as low as possible. It may also involve price discrimination such as charity care (or scholarships based on need).

To understand why the second element, quality, belongs in the maximand, it is necessary to examine the locus of decision-making in a hospital. One characteristic of non-profit hospitals is that usually control formally resides in a board of trustees or similar group. The board in turn appoints an administrator who is in charge of day-to-day decisions. The medical staff also generally exerts influence over resource allocation decisions. It is important to know what incentives these various parties face in making decisions regarding resource allocation.

If the administrator is not to make a 'profit', his performance cannot be judged by the profit criterion. Therefore, his salary and promotional chances must be a function of some other variable or variables. It seems plausible to assume that the prestige of the institution is prominent among these other variables. The trustees, insofar as they participate in the decision-making process, may also be influenced by this variable. Prestige, in turn, is affected by the size of the institution, but probably even more by the quality of the product produced.

There may be other reasons why the trustees and the administrator would give weight to both quantity and quality.[3] There may be a pursuit of status quite independent of any managerial reward.

2. Apparently the public is better off if it consumes less of some other services.

3. The remainder of this paragraph is based on references found in Fritz Machlup's article (1967, pp. 1–33).

There may be a desire to serve society independent of the desire to preserve existing tax and legal privileges. There may be a desire to show professional excellence or technical virtuosity by stressing quality. In short, while we have derived a maximand based on quantity and quality by considering the self-interest of the administrator (and trustees) narrowly defined, such a maximand is consistent with other motivations.

The maximand is reinforced by whatever role the medical staff may play in the decision-making process. They have a strong interest in the quality of the facilities available since it is one determinant of the quality of care they can give and of their professional standing. Further, the existing staff will find it easier to attract additional staff (and so ease their own work load) by maintaining high quality facilities. The medical staff is also interested in quantity, since each physician wants a bed available should a patient of his require hospitalization (Stevens, 1968).

The administrator, the trustees, and the medical staff may, of course, weigh quality and quantity considerations differently, but that need not impair the theory. We assume that some final resolution is obtained among the tastes of the administrator, the trustees, and the medical staff, so that we can speak of the tastes of the hospital decision-maker.

Support for the notion that decision-makers perceive both quality and quantity to be in their maximand can be found in the hospital trade literature. One prominent hospital administrator wrote, 'No one can seriously believe that the public would knowingly permit any step to be taken that would lead to the slightest sort of deterioration of quality' (Brown, 1959, p. 35). And as Jerome Rothenberg said

... medical ethics and collective concern for quality significantly modify free enterprise. . . . In medicine we are not free to envisage saving resources by lowering the quality of care. Less than the highest quality care often represents a total waste[4] (1951, p. 676).

Another leading hospital administrator has written:

The hospital is the community trustee responsible for a large amount of the definitive medical care provided in a community. Its first responsibility is to program its service to meet community needs, and its second is to conduct such services with suitable efficiency and economy, always with great sensitivity toward its responsibility and authority to meet high standards of both quality and quantity of services. . . . The

4. It is not clear why a concern for quality should modify free enterprise.

patient expects that hospital services will be of high quality[5] (Dixon, 1961, p. 284).

A voluminous study of the medical market done for the State of Michigan said: 'From the community's viewpoint, the hospital is most effective ... when it admits the greatest number of patients who need admission ...' (Pauly, 1967).

Yet quality and quantity cannot be maximized without limit. The nonprofit institution faces a budget constraint; its deficit cannot be larger than a certain amount. We therefore postulate a model of constrained quantity-quality maximization. Millard Long has informally put forth a similar hypothesis, but he does not draw any conclusions from his model.[6] He saw the 'guiding principle' of the hospital as a

... desire to maximize the number of patients seen subject to several constraints. There is a financial constraint; operating deficits cannot go beyond a point specified by the sponsoring agency. Another constraint is that the quality of care should be the best possible with available equipment and personnel; hospitals seldom cut corners when doing so would reduce the quality of care (1964, p. 212).

Our model differs in an important respect from Long's by making quality a variable of choice rather than a constraint. The existence of accreditation bodies, however, may make some minimum standard of quality necessary. Insofar as it does, a constraint does exist[7] (Feldstein, 1967, ch. 7).

How are quality and quantity measured? One can think of

5. The first part of this quotation ignores the vital question of how one defines community needs and whether needs are different from community demands. Nevertheless, we are interested in the light it sheds on the maximand. The administrator of a different non-profit institution has said, 'As dean of a Graduate School of Public Health, reasonably alert to the attractiveness of having the largest possible number of tuition-paying students that his facilities can accommodate ...' (Crabtree 1963, p. 1179).

6. Baumol and Bowen (1965) also emphasize both quality and quantity in the non-profit area generally, but do not formalize their ideas.

7. Feldstein has postulated a maximand for a hospital decision maker in the British National Health Service which is somewhat similar to ours, but used for a different purpose. Feldstein discovered that the number of cases treated in a region was more responsive to bed availability than was length of stay. He found that such behavior was consistent with a three-variable maximand, which was maximised subject to a budget constraint. The maximand included length of stay, number of cases treated, and a quality variable. Our interest, however, is in a different question, namely, the trade-off between quality and quantity.

certain criteria which are indicative of quality: personnel/patient ratios or professional personnel/patient ratios or the availability of certain laboratory or other facilities. There are, however, several difficulties associated with the use of such criteria. First, do high personnel/patient ratios indicate high quality or merely substitution of labor for capital (or low-skilled labor for high-skilled labor) in the hospital production function?[8] Similarly, is the availability of certain facilities also merely a substitution in the production function? Second, how may these criteria be combined in any meaningful fashion? The weight each criterion would receive in a weighted average is ambiguous, as is the meaning of any such average. Finally, there are intangibles associated with the notion of quality.

To avert these difficulties, at least in part, we assume quality to be represented by a vector of characteristics, some of which may not be quantifiable except in the sense of being present or absent. Further, we assume that the demand for the services of each institution depends upon quality as well as price. The justification for this assumption is that physicians probably prefer higher quality hospitals and so are more inclined to seek staff privileges there. Also, if the physician has multiple privileges, he may prefer working in the higher quality hospital (and given the extent of hospital insurance, he probably will not find it too difficult to convince the patient). When two quality vectors have the same cost, we assume that the hospital decision-maker chooses that quality vector which maximizes quantity bought at a given price. The implication of these assumptions is that an increase in quantity demanded at each price which is brought about by an increase in quality can only be accomplished at an increased cost. Restricting ourselves to this subset of quality vectors which has the property of maximizing quantity demanded at a given price, we can associate each quality vector with a level of cost. We can then attach an arbitrary set of numbers to each quality vector, which serve as an ordinal measure of quality. The only restriction on the numbers is that they must increase as cost increases. For convenience we shall use the costs themselves as measures of quality.[9]

8. Feldstein (1967, ch. 4) finds that a modified Cobb–Douglas production function with nurses, physician beds, and other supplies as explanatory variables fits data generated by the British National Health Service rather well. In the modified form, nursing services are not substitutes for other inputs, but the other inputs are substitutes for each other.

9. This is another formulation of a problem which has caused some controversy in the literature, namely, how to measure quality. J. L. Nichol-

This approach averts the problem of measuring quality directly but unfortunately measurement difficulties are not restricted to that variable. Quantity supplied and demanded, while seemingly straightforward, also presents an analytical problem. We take it to mean the number of patient-days in the case of a hospital. (One could measure the number of students attending a medical school.) However, the 'product' of a hospital may vary so much depending on the diseases its patients have that a simple measure of patient-days cannot accurately reflect the output of the hospital. (Feldstein, 1967, ch. 2). This is an aggregation problem which is inherent in a multiple-product firm, since the treatment of each diagnosis can be seen as a distinct product.

If there are distinct demand and cost curves for various diagnoses, each must be analysed as a separate product with any interdependencies acknowledged. To take account of subproducts and interdependencies here would complicate the analysis, but would not alter the conclusions. Therefore, we shall continue to speak of the hospital as though it were a single product firm whose physical output were unambiguously measurable.

Suppose quality is given, say, at the minimum permissible level for accreditation. This determines an average cost curve – call it $AC_0$. At this quality, income and all other relevant variables except price held constant, there is a certain demand at each price which determines a demand curve, call it $d_0$. Assume for now that the decision-maker cannot run a deficit – all his costs must be met from revenues. Then, given that he wants to maximize the quantity of output (in physical terms) provided at that quality, and, assuming a downward sloping demand curve, he produces at the quantity $q_0$ for which $AR = AC$. If there is more than one point where $AR = AC$, he chooses the one associated with the largest quantity. Such an outcome is graphed in Figure 1.

Suppose that a higher quality product is available at a cost $AC_1$,

---

son (1967) has criticized Gilbert (1961) for using cost rather than price to measure the contribution to welfare of a change in quality. Since cost equals price in our model, this criticism presents no problem to it; one could merely say that the assumptions imply that an increase in quality, quantity held constant, implies an equal increase in both cost and price. Our analysis is really in the same spirit as Nicholson's by proposing a criterion which relates to the consumer's preferences as revealed in the market-place; that is, that the decision-maker is in equilibrium at the quality level which maximizes quantity bought at a given price when two quality levels have the same cost. Gilbert's measure, on the other hand, seems to be more a technological criterion.

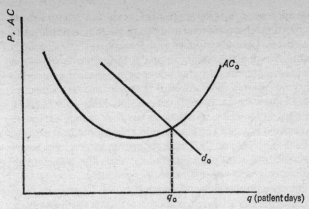

Figure 1

a cobalt radiation machine can be bought or more nurses can be hired. This higher quality product raises the demand curve to $d_1$, so that there is a new equilibrium output $q_1$ as shown in Figure 2.

Depending upon the relative movement of the demand curve and cost curve and their shapes, the new equilibrium point may lie to the right or left of the old one. As the quality variable runs over its potential range of values, the locus of equilibrium quantity-quality combinations is traced out. If, after a certain point, further increases in quality shift demand up less and less while raising costs more and more, the trade-off curve will eventually bend back as is illustrated in Figure 3 (see Theil, 1952; Hirshleifer, 1955).

The decision-maker will choose the point on this trade-off curve which yields him the highest utility. That will be where the curve is tangent to the highest attainable indifference curve, $I_o$. (We assume the decision-maker's indifference curves have the usual shape.) This outcome is shown at point $A$ in Figure 3.

Suppose that the decision-maker is told he may run a deficit of a certain size. Then, instead of producing the quantity in Figures 1 and 2 where $AR = AC$, the decision-maker produces a sufficiently larger quantity to exhaust the subsidy given him. This shifts the trade-off curve to the right at each quality level (or, alternatively, up at each quantity level), thereby enabling the decision-maker to attain a higher indifference curve. Suppose the deficit is not given to the decision-maker, but is affected by his actions. Such would be the case if the decision-maker conducted fund-raising drives whose success depended upon the effort he

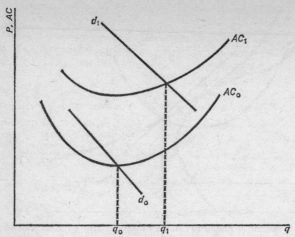

Figure 2

put forth. The fund-raising drive will be carried on until the marginal benefit to the decision-maker of shifting the trade-off curve out by the amount the marginal dollar would do so equals the marginal cost of raising that dollar.

We are interested in using this model to assess the effect of the hospital's non-profit status upon efficiency. First, note that this model implies least-cost production insofar as the decision maker pursues his maximization goals. Suppose that the marginal revenue product of a factor exceeded its marginal factor cost. A profit-maximizing firm would expand production to the point of equality, thereby achieving a socially optimal allocation of factors.[10] A constrained quantity-quality maximizer will also expand production to the point of equality. He can use the 'profit' the profit-maximizing firm would have gained to shift his quantity-quality trade-off curve out and thereby reach a higher indifference curve. When the equalities hold for all factors, the trade-off curve cannot be shifted out any more.

Even though the model implies least cost production, there are two reasons why it does not lead to an optimal outcome. (These reasons also apply to a model based on simple cost reimbursement by a third party.) The two reasons are a bias against producing lower quality products and barriers to entry resulting from non-profit status. Up until now we have treated the hospital as if

10. Assuming perfect product and factor markets and no externalities.

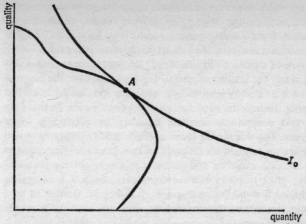

Figure 3

it had produced only one quality. In reality it produces several. From a normative standpoint one would desire that the hospital produce all qualities (all products) which were profitable when price equalled marginal cost, just as a profit-maximizing firm would. How likely is this outcome in the non-profit sector? To bring out the essence of the problem, we assume all quality vectors have demand and cost functions which are independent of those associated with other quality vectors. This assumption is made for ease of exposition.

Different quality levels generate demand which can be measured in the same units of quantity, for example, patient-days. This makes it possible to derive total or aggregate quantity; that is, quantity summed over all quality levels. Will the decision maker try to maximize this figure subject to the constraint that all qualities produced at least break even? If he does, the outcome is similar to that predicted by traditional theory in a profit-maximizing sector.[11] The answer is no, he will not necessarily do so. This is a major difference between the implications of this model and those of the profit-maximizing model, and so from a positive point of view constitutes one test of the model. The reason why the decision maker does not produce all profitable qualities lies in the quality variable which is in his maximand. An example

11. Obviously this will not be the outcome in the profit-maximizing sector if the demand and cost functions for various products are not independent. But that does not affect the conclusion.

should make this clear. A hospital can produce hospital care in wards, semi-private rooms, or private rooms, where quality increases from ward to private room. Why should the hospital produce care in a private room when the same patient-day would be counted a patient-day in a ward? Because if the patient is willing to pay the additional cost of private room care, the hospital can raise its quality level without changing its quantity level. But suppose the hospital produces only top quality care. In that case it could conceivably increase quantity by producing lower qualities, but this would lower average quality. Whether it will produce lower qualities depends on how much inferior qualities will increase quantity and on how much weight the decision-maker gives quantity relative to quality. Such a bias against producing low-quality products, even if they are demanded by a certain segment of the population, does not exist for a profit-maximizing firm.

Is such a bias observed? First, proprietary hospitals (or hospitals for profit) are thought to produce lower quality care than voluntary short-term general hospitals. There is a lower percentage of accreditation among the proprietaries than among the voluntaries. Of all the short-term hospitals listed by the American Hospital Association in 1965, 62 per cent (with 87 per cent of the beds) were accredited, but only 34 per cent of the proprietaries (with 60 per cent of the proprietary beds) were accredited. (Somers and Somers, 1967, p. 77).

Second, one thinks of the description of medical care as a 'Cadillac only' industry.[12] 'The potential for "Cadillac only" medicine is nowhere more real than in the American hospital' (Rosenthal, 1966, p. 109). Part of the reason for Cadillac only medicine may be that it tends to maximize the skilled labor input, and the physician's preferences may affect resource allocation. Nevertheless, a bias toward high quality hospitals is what the model would predict.[13]

12. Recall Long's observation, quoted earlier in this section, that '. . . hospitals seldom cut corners when doing so would reduce the quality of care.'

13. Although non-profit educational institutions are not all of high quality, this does not mean that the bias does not exist there also. Many of the observed quality differences in education may be due to differences in the position of the trade-off curve; high endowment institutions have curves which are farther from the origin. The bias toward high quality which we believe exists for non-profit institutions is for a given trade-off curve. Since the variance in trade-off curves for hospitals is probably less than the

Third, evidence from the nursing home industry agrees with the prediction of the model that non-profit institutions will emphasize quality. More non-profit nursing homes have a registered nurse as the top nursing skill level than proprietary homes. (Solon, 1963).[14] This is shown in Table 1.

Table 1 **Top nursing skill level among full-time staff in skilled nursing homes***

|  | Proprietary homes (per cent) | Non-profit homes (per cent) |
| --- | --- | --- |
| Registered nurse | 44 | 67 |
| Licensed practical nurse | 42 | 22 |
| No RN or LPN | 14 | 11 |

* Based on the 1961 National Inventory, conducted by the Public Health Service.

Last, the model predicts the often maligned duplication of sophisticated and expensive equipment in voluntary hospitals (Dunlop, 1965; Rosenthal, 1966). According to the de Bakey Commission on Heart Disease, Cancer, and Stroke, 30 per cent of the 777 hospitals equipped to do open-heart surgery had no cases in the year under study. Of the 548 hospitals that did have cases, 87 per cent did less than one operation per week (Rosenthal, 1966). The prestige accruing to the voluntary hospital possessing advanced equipment (and the value its decision-maker gives that prestige) may also be the reason for greater capital intensity in the voluntary hospitals than the proprietaries.[15] An alternative explanation is that capital is relatively cheaper for the voluntaries so that cost minimization would lead to greater capital intensity (Berry, Jr, 1965, p. 117 ff). Cost minimization, however, is neutral with respect to duplication of equipment, since output level is not specified. However, the interest of the decision-maker in the voluntary hospital in quality as well as quantity may well be causing the duplication of equipment which in turn is causing the greater capital intensity.

variance for educational institutions, the bias appears in the hospital sector as Cadillac only hospitals.

14. This index of quality is subject to the qualification noted above about indices of quality.

15. Presumably more prestige comes from advanced capital equipment than additional labor. For figures on the greater capital intensity of the voluntaries, see Somers and Somers (1967, p. 49).

In normative terms, the problem is that the decision-maker has picked a point on the quantity-quality trade-off curve which is optimal for him but not necessarily socially optimal.[16] Are there any factors which might induce a socially optimal choice by the decision maker? First, the possibility of entry exists. We show below that this is unlikely to correct the problem. Second, philanthropy, insofar as its gifts are for a specific purpose, places a constraint on the point on the trade-off curve which the decision maker selects.[17] Unfortunately, the projects for which funds are given are usually those which will increase the quality of the output, whereas, as we have seen, the danger is that the decision-maker will on his own choose too high a quality level. Thus, philanthropy does not help very much either in remedying this defect of the organization of the industry.[18]

The second reason why non-profit status hinders economic efficiency is the barriers to entry which result from it. Consider the possibility of entry by other hospitals. If highly unusual entry conditions existed, the hospital sector might still be considered efficient. Suppose that a hospital would enter if it thought it would undersell hospitals already in the industry, even though it would not make a profit from so doing, since it would set price at average cost. In other words, there would be a number of potential quantity-maximizing hospitals, all of whom would now be outside the industry and so producing a zero quantity. Since they are quantity maximizers, they can better their condition by entering the industry and beginning production. In so doing, they force the price of hospitals already producing down to minimum average cost and force them to produce lower quality products. *Mirabile dictu*, the non-profit hospital sector would be efficient.

While this type of entry may sound strange, before dismissing it out of hand, one should consider what attracts resources into the hospital sector (and other non-profit sectors) now. Evidently it is not the opportunity for profit. Perhaps it is not too wide of the

16. The socially optimal point would be the outcome observed in a market dominated by knowledgeable consumers which functioned so as to satisfy their tastes (assuming the income distribution is optimal).

17. After receiving a tied philanthropic gift, the decision-maker is in exactly the same position as a consumer who is given more of one particular good.

18. However, if the philanthropist derives benefit from gifts which raise the quality level, optimality requires a higher quality level than if he did not. The argument here is that such gifts do not correct an already existing bias towards too high quality.

mark to suggest that the chance to provide a service will lead some altruistic citizens to try to establish a hospital.[19] This does not appear to be such a far fetched explanation for the founding of either hospitals or private colleges. They are often started by civic-minded individuals who organize a fund drive.

The problem is whether it is realistic to rely on this type of entry to assure satisfaction of demand and least cost production. For the possibility of entry by other non-profit firms seems to be weak support indeed for the proposition that the hospital sector, left to its own devices, will reach a social optimum. It is one thing to say concern for the common weal is responsible for the establishment of hospitals, but quite another to say that it does so in a manner that we might term optimal.

We have spoken throughout in terms of a decision-maker. Yet the theory of the firm assumes that an entrepreneur, not a decision-maker or an administrator, will seize a profitable opportunity for entry. There is no position in the hospital (or non-profit) sector for an entrepreneur. The entrepreneurs in this case are the civic-minded organizers, but they may not be present when an opportunity for entry exists. This has two consequences. Since there is no mechanism analogous to the possibility of profit which makes the threat of entry credible to existing institutions, there is less of a spur to least cost production. Inefficient but already established firms may continue to exist. Also, demand must generally be met by existing firms, which means some consumer demands for hospital care may not be met. If the non-profit form of organization is to be retained, there is a need for government policies to promote entry, for example, by continuing tax write-offs to philanthropists or by providing funds for hospital construction.[20]

However, there may be mechanisms other than entry by non-profit hospitals for driving average revenue to minimum average cost and for satisfying consumer demands.[21] Suppose hospitals are being operated at an average cost above minimum average

19. 'Back in the nineteen-twenties, a group of eight or ten collectors in New York decided [to establish the Museum of Modern Art]. . . . The Metropolitan would not show any so-called modern art. They would not collect it and they would not show it, and one of the reasons the Museum of Modern Art was established was that this otherwise great institution was not ready to move into this field' Nelson A. Rockefeller.

20. Even if non-profit status is not retained, the role physicians play in resource allocation may lead to a quality bias.

21. Or at least to a point on the average cost curve if indivisibilities are important.

cost. An opportunity would exist for the entry of a profit-making firm. Why do we not observe this? That is, why does this sector of the economy continue to be organized primarily on a not-for-profit basis? One possibility is, of course, that hospitals are operating at minimum average cost and consumer demands are satisfied, so there is no opportunity for entry for a profit-making firm. If so, the existence of a profit-making sector keeps the non-profit sector efficient in the same way that non-union firms may place a constraint on wage changes in unionized firms. But this is at best an explanation of why non-profit and profit-making firms might co-exist. It does not explain why so very few profit-making hospitals exist.

One possible explanation has been advanced by Kenneth Arrow. He views the notion of profit in medicine as incompatible with the delegation of choice the consumer makes to the physician; that is, as incompatible with the trust the consumer must have that the physician is deciding solely in the interests of the consumer. Hence, hospitals are non-profit. This view, while not without some intuitive appeal, does not withstand close scrutiny. The argument about trust, if it is true at all, is only true for medicine. Yet schools and universities, museums, symphony orchestras, and theater groups are also often organized on a non-profit basis. Hence, some explanation of the phenomenon more general than trust must be found. Also, the patient places his trust in the physician. It does not logically follow that the hospital or the medical school must be non-profit. The existence of profit-making firms in medicine – most notably pharmaceutical manufacturers and distributors, but also private laboratories and private nursing homes – tends to indicate that there must be other reasons for hospitals' being non-profit. Thus, we cannot rely on this hypothesis to explain why we do not observe the entry of profit-making firms.

There are other, simpler explanations. One is merely that there may be legal barriers to entry for profit-making firms. Another has to do with the subsidies the hospital receives from private philanthropy and its favourable tax status (See Arrow, Reading 1). This permits the hospital some deviation from the minimum average cost of a private firm and hence some scope for inefficiency. The non-profit hospital might be run more inefficiently than a hypothetical profit-making one and yet be able to charge a price equal to or below that of a private firm. The difference in costs would simply be made up by the subsidy. Nor should it be thought that philanthropy is negligible; for all non-federal short-term hospitals in 1964 there was a capital input of $1·68 billion, 38 per cent of which or over $630 million came from philanthropy. The 38 per cent is up from 25 per cent in 1958 (Somers and Somers, 1967, p. 211). The argument here is not that philanthropy directly causes inefficiency, but that it hinders selection of the fittest.[22] Good management is not always rewarded, which may explain the persistent calls for strengthening hospital management. (Somers and Somers, 1967, pp. 39–55, 121–6, 247–50, 286–88).

Philanthropy thus has its drawbacks. Perhaps philanthropy's favored tax status should be discontinued. Its existence, which provides some shelter for the non-profit hospital, raises the barriers to entry by profit-making firms.

The analysis up to this point has assumed that the consumer pays his own bill. The importance of third party schemes such as Medicare makes it important to modify the model to take account of their existence. It should be clear that so long as resources are constrained, the quality-quantity trade-off is an inherent one; these are simply two commodities to which the decision-maker can allocate his resources. The effect of changing the basis of payment may be merely to alter the location and shape of the trade-off curve and doing that alters none of the conclusions reached above.

However, simple charge or cost reimbursement by a third party introduces a further potential inefficiency. Under this system the decision-maker could conceivably push both quality and quantity to the point where the additional utility to him was zero. What would keep him from doing so? To do so would naturally lead to relatively high insurance rates, and this might lower the quantity demanded.[23] Would the decision-maker take account of this effect? If there were many hospitals in one area, any one hospital's contribution to the high insurance rates would be negligible so that no single decision-maker would take account of his contribution to them (Olson, 1965). Thus, quality may be even higher and quantity lower than all would desire. If rates were based on the experience of a small number of hospitals,

22. There is some reason to think, however, that operation of the market may not lead to selection of the fittest even under competitive conditions in any simple way. See Winter Jr (1960).

23. It might also have the opposite effect. By making insurance more attractive to previously uninsured risk-averters, effective price could be lowered and demand raised.

the effect each hospital has on insurance rates is more noticeable and so more likely to be taken into account. The growth of hospital planning councils may be viewed as a step to make the large-group case similar to the small-group case.

One implication of the large-group case is that there is no incentive to the decision-maker to minimize cost. In effect, resources are no longer constrained to the individual decision-maker; the trade-off curve can be shifted out at will. This, of course, is the extreme case: nevertheless, the real world may be quite close to it. Even in a world in which resources are treated as free, however, lower qualities may have a negative marginal benefit to the decision-maker and so not be produced. Thus, the cost-reimbursement model can generate the same quality bias that the demand-curve model shows.

To summarize the conclusions of this discussion: We have examined ways in which the non-profit status of voluntary hospitals may cause misallocation of resources. First, there is a bias against producing lower quality products (a bias in the sense that a profit-maximizing firm would produce such qualities). Second, there is little reason to think that a non-profit hospital will enter in response to a profitable opportunity (which may exist either because consumer demands are not being satisfied or because inefficient hospitals are providing the product). Philanthropy gives the non-profit hospital some latitude for inefficiency, and this, among other things, tends to forestall entry by profit-making firms. An additional problem exists if the hospital is simply reimbursed by a third party for its costs. By removing the budget constraint, incentives for least cost production are weakened.

References

ARROW, V. J. (1963), 'Uncertainty and the welfare economics of medical care', *Amer. Econ. Rev.*, vol. 53, pp. 941–73.

BAUMOL, W. J., and BOWEN, W. G. (1965), 'On the performing arts', *Amer. Econ. Rev. Proc.*, vol. 55, pp. 495–502.

BERRY, R. E. Jr (1965), 'Competition and efficiency in the market for hospital services', unpublished doctoral dissertation, Harvard University.

BROWN, R. E. (1959), 'Let the public control utilization through planning', *Hospitals*, vol. 33, pp. 34–9.

CRABTREE, J. A. (1963), 'Plans for tomorrow's needs in local public health administration,' *Amer. J. Pub. Health*, vol. 53, pp. 1175–81.

DAVIS, J. S. (1917), *Essays on the Earlier History of American Corporations*, Harvard University Press.

DIXON, J. P. (1961), 'Hospitals and the community', in E. A. Confrey (ed.), *Administration of Community Health Services*, International City Managers' Association.

DUNLOP, J. T. (1965), 'The capacity of the United States to provide and finance expanding health services', *Bull. N.Y. Acad. Medicine*, vol. 41, pp. 1325–37.

FELDSTEIN, M. S. (1967), *Economic Analysis for Health Service Efficiency*, Amsterdam.

GILBERT, M. (1961), 'The problem of quality changes and index numbers', *Econ. Devel. and Cult. Change*, vol. 9, pp. 287–94.

HIRSHLEIFER, J. (1955), 'The exchange between quantity and quality', The *RAND* Corporation (P-406).

LONG, M. F. (1964), 'Efficient use of hospitals', in S. J. Axelrod (ed.), *The Economics of Health and Medical Care*, University of Michigan Press.

MACHLUP, F. (1967), 'Theories of the firm: marginalist, behavioral, managerial', *Amer. Econ. Rev.*, vol. 57, pp. 1–33.

NICHOLSON, J. L. (1967), 'The measurement of quality changes', *Econ. J.*, vol. 77, pp. 512–30.

OLSON, M. Jr (1965), *The Logic of Collective Action*, Harvard University Press.

PAULY, M. V. (1967), 'Efficiency in public provision of medical care', unpublished doctoral dissertation, University of Virginia Press.

ROCKEFELLER, N. A. (1967), 'The governor lectures on art', *New York Times Magazine*, April 9th.

ROSENTHAL, G. D. (1966), 'The public pays the bill', *Atlantic Monthly*, vol. 218, pp. 107–10.

ROTHENBERG, J. (1951), 'Welfare implications of alternative methods of financing medical care', *Amer. Econ. Rev. Proc.*, vol. 41, pp. 676–87.

SOLON, J. A. (1963), 'Nursing homes and medical care', *New England J. Medicine*, vol. 269, pp. 1067–74.

SOMERS, H. M., and SOMERS, A. R. (1967), *Medicare and the Hospitals*, The Brookings Institution.

STEVENS, C. (1968), 'Hospital market efficiency: the anatomy of the supply response', paper presented at the second Conference on the Economics of Health, Baltimore, Dec. 5–7th.

THEIL, H. (1952), 'Qualities, prices and budget inquiries', *Rev. Econ. Stud.*, vol. 19, pp. 129–47.

WINTER, S. G. Jr (1960), 'Economic natural selection and the theory of the firm', The RAND Corporation (P-2167).

US Bureau of Labor Statistics (1963), *Employment and Earnings for the United States*, 1909–1962, Government Printing Office.

# 10 M. S. Feldstein

## The Effects of Case-Mix on Hospital Costs

Excerpt from Martin S. Feldstein, 'Hospital cost variation and case-mix differences', *Medical Care*, vol. 3, 1965, pp. 95–103.

[. . .] Hospital costs have long been a subject of concern to the Ministry of Health and the Treasury. Rapidly increasing expenditure led in 1953 to an official study of the cost of the National Health Service by the Guillebaud Committee (1956), assisted by Richard Titmuss and Brian Abel-Smith (1956). In 1956–57, a Select Committee on Estimates held lengthy hearings on hospital running costs[1] (see also Feldstein, 1963).

One of the important results of these enquiries has been the introduction of 'departmental costing'. In place of the older 'subjective' accounting procedures, in which input costs are grouped together regardless of their use, 'departmental costing' assigns an appropriate proportion of hospital expenditures for nursing salaries, medical salaries, maintenance, heating, etc. to the departments in which they are used: ward, out-patient, X-ray services, etc. It was intended that such information would permit useful comparison of the cost performance of different hospitals. Costs that diverged substantially from national or regional averages could stimulate local departments to seek improved efficiency and provide regional authorities with a basis for following-up high cost hospitals. In this way, the Government hoped that inter-hospital variation in costs would be reduced.

This paper examines the extent of variation in different types of ward costs, measured on both a per patient week and a per case basis. The first section shows the existence of substantial variation and indicates that there was little reduction in variation during the first five years of the departmental costing scheme. Although the study is restricted to large, acute, non-teaching hospitals, there are substantial differences among the hospitals in the composition of the cases treated; this is shown in the second section. If cost variation reflects differences in case-mix, it is important

1. Reports are tabulated and published annually in 3 volumes as *Hospital Costing Returns*, by H M S O. Also, see Montacute (1962).

that this be taken into account explicitly whenever hospital costs are compared. The third section presents estimates of the extent to which different categories of costs are influenced by case-mix; certain types of costs are shown to be substantially affected, while others are not. A final section discusses some of the ways in which the statistical relationship between costs and case-mix can be used; several research studies currently in progress are described.

## Variation in costs

To assess the extent of cost variation in hospitals of a similar type, attention was focused on large (i.e. with expenditure exceeding £50,000 per year), acute, non-teaching hospitals. Information about 177 such institutions was published in the hospital costing returns for the fiscal year ended 31st March 1961 (Ministry of Health, 1961). Table 1 presents the mean and coefficient of variation for each of several types of ward costs in these 177 hospitals; separate figures are given for costs per patient week and per case.

Most cost types show substantial variation. The coefficient of variation of Total Ward Cost per case, 25·2 per cent, indicates that approximately one third of the hospitals have costs that are 25 per cent above or below the average. Figure 1 shows that the frequency distribution of hospitals by total ward cost per case is somewhat skewed; fifteen hospitals have costs of less than £40 per case and eighteen have costs of more than £70. The range extends from less than £35 to more than £110. The individual cost types in Table 1 reveal greater variability than the total.

Although costs per patient week are less varied than costs per case, there are still substantial inter-hospital differences. Figure 2 shows that total ward cost per patient week has a range from £19 to £41. Again, the individual cost types are relatively more varied than the total.

Variation decreased little during the first five years of the costing scheme. The annual coefficients of variation for the 125 large, acute, non-teaching hospitals that were included in the departmental costing scheme from 1957–8 to 1961–2 are presented in Table 2. In evaluating this information it should be borne in mind that the individual hospitals' figures for the first year were subject to substantial error; the reduction in variation between 1957–8 and 1958–9 may largely reflect this. After that year, the relative variation in ward cost per case remained completely stable. Even for such household activities as laundry (per patient

Table 1 **Variation in ward cost per case and ward cost per patient week**\*

| Cost type | Cost per patient week | | Cost per case | |
| | Average† (£) | Coefficient of variation‡ (%) | Average† (£) | Coefficient of variation‡ (%) |
|---|---|---|---|---|
| Total | 28·42 | 12·2 | 54·62 | 25·2 |
| Medical | 3·02 | 21·5 | 5·71 | 25·0 |
| Nursing | 7·02 | 16·2 | 13·50 | 26·3 |
| Domestic (172) | 1·74 | 53·1 | 3·49 | 67·4 |
| Nursing and Domestic (172) | 8·73 | 17·7 | 17·01 | 31·2 |
| Professional and Technical | 0·13 | 84·4 | 0·26 | 107·3 |
| All staff (172) | 11·75 | 15·4 | 22·75 | 27·5 |
| Clothing, bedding and linen | 0·23 | 35·1 | 0·45 | 43·0 |
| Drugs | 0·93 | 25·0 | 1·77 | 27·5 |
| Dressings | 0·32 | 32·5 | 0·60 | 33·3 |
| Medical and surgical appliances and equipment | 0·90 | 33·6 | 1·68 | 32·5 |
| Furniture etc. | 0·30 | 52·3 | 0·58 | 59·9 |
| Water, rates and other direct | 0·80 | 32·0 | 1·52 | 38·5 |
| Total direct | 15·86 | 13·6 | 30·44 | 25·6 |
| Dispensary (175) | 0·25 | 33·1 | 0·47 | 38·1 |
| Cleaning, portering and transport (176) | 1·38 | 57·8 | 2·64 | 64·6 |
| Medical records service (176) | 0·25 | 47·5 | 0·49 | 58·5 |
| Works and maintenance | 1·39 | 36·0 | 2·71 | 49·3 |
| Power, light, heat, etc. | 1·41 | 23·8 | 2·72 | 36·8 |
| Laundry (176) | 0·92 | 23·5 | 1·77 | 33·8 |
| Catering | 4·79 | 16·2 | 9·24 | 29·1 |
| Total indirect | 12·54 | 16·4 | 24·14 | 28·8 |

\* In 177 large, acute, non-teaching hospitals, 1960–61. Numbers in parenthesis indicate that one or more hospitals reported no costs in category and were omitted from calculation.

† An unweighted mean of the hospitals' average costs.

‡ Coefficient of variation = $\dfrac{\text{standard deviation}}{\text{mean}} \times 100$

week), boiler (per 1000 lb of steam raised). and catering (per person fed per week), relative variation showed little change.

It would be incorrect to regard the observed variation in costs as indications of differences in the efficiency with which hospitals are run. Hospitals differ in the facilities with which they are endowed, the composition of the caseload that they treat, and the quality of the service that they give. Each of these may affect the hospital's costs. To assess the *costliness* of a hospital, costs must be purged of the effects of case-mix differences; if medical cases are more costly than surgical cases, a hospital's proportion of medical and surgical cases should be explicitly taken into account in any consideration of its cost performance. Other factors outside the control of the hospital's administrators and staff may also influence costs, e.g. hospital size, age and location. These must be recognized and their importance evaluated if we are to go beyond measuring the costliness of a *hospital* and consider the costliness of its *management*. Variation in 'management costliness' would then reflect differences in the quality of service and the efficiency of operation.

The extent to which acute hospitals differ in their case-mix composition is commonly underestimated. The current system of hospital costing and the usual process of comparing hospital costs with national averages indicate a tacit assumption that case-mix differences are either not substantial or have little influence on costs. The next section shows that neither assumption is justified.

### Differences in case-mix

Hospitals are required to present annual reports (Annual Hospital Return, Form SH3) of the number of cases treated in each specialty. To illustrate the substantial variation among large, acute, non-teaching hospitals in the proportional composition of the case-mix, we have grouped the various specialties into eight mutually exclusive categories: general medicine, pediatrics, general surgery, ENT (including tonsils and adenoids), traumatic and orthopaedic surgery, other surgery, gynaecology and obstetrics. A small number of cases (less than 10 per cent) are considered as a residual.

The proportion of cases in each category during the year 1960

Table 2 **Coefficients of variation in hospital costs***

| Cost type | Fiscal year | | | | |
| | 1957–8 | 1958–9 | 1959–60 | 1960–61 | 1961–2 |
| --- | --- | --- | --- | --- | --- |
| Ward cost per case | 24·84 | 22·01 | 22·58 | 22·58 | 22·79 |
| Ward cost per week | 13·87 | 11·85 | 9·96 | 12·47 | 10·01 |
| Laundry per week | 24·75 | 23·89 | 22·79 | 22·56 | 24·11 |
| Boiler cost per 1000 lb steam | 37·15 | 29·82 | 30·04 | 26·18 | 28·41 |
| Catering per person fed per week | 11·23 | 10·58 | 14·22 | 9·42 | 9·61 |

* 125 large, acute, non-teaching hospitals which participated in the hospital costing scheme during the first five years.

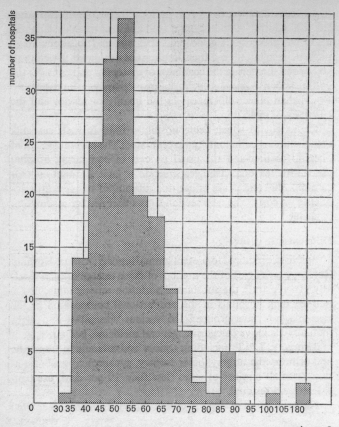

Figure 1 Total ward cost per case

was calculated for the 177 hospitals discussed above.[2] Table 3 presents the mean and coefficient of variation of each of these proportions. The very high values of the coefficients of variation (for all categories except general medicine and general surgery) must be interpreted cautiously; the actual distributions are bimodal (many hospitals do no work in a particular category) and highly skewed (a few hospitals concentrate a much higher than average proportion of their work in these areas). Tables 4 and 5 indicate more clearly the extent of variation by presenting for

2. I am grateful to the Ministry of Health for providing this data.

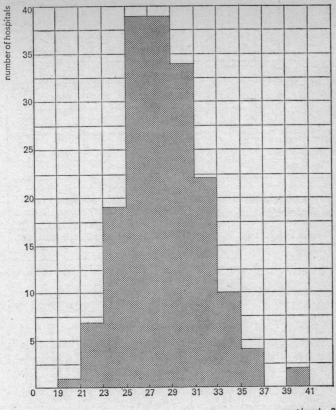

cost/week, £

Figure 2  Total ward cost per patient week, 1960–61

each of the case categories the distribution of hospitals by the proportion of their case-mixes in that category. Thus, the general medicine column of Table 4 indicates that in 10·16 per cent of hospitals medical cases constituted less than a proportion of 0·1 of total caseload, while in an additional 7·91 per cent of hospitals medical care accounted for between 10 and 12·5 per cent of total caseload; in contrast, in 2·25 per cent of hospitals, more than 30 per cent of the caseload was general medical cases. Figures 3, 4 and 5 illustrate the distribution for general medicine, general surgery, and traumatic and orthopedic surgery.

The variation in each of the eight proportions is not attenuated by any substantial tendency for the proportions of different types

Table 3 **Case-mix proportions**

| Speciality | Mean proportion | Coefficient of variation (%) |
|---|---|---|
| General medicine | 0·174 | 40·5 |
| Pediatrics | 0·034 | 113·3 |
| General surgery | 0·324 | 35·1 |
| ENT | 0·088 | 98·5 |
| Traumatic and orthopedic surgery | 0·095 | 86·7 |
| Other surgery | 0·066 | 106·6 |
| Gynaecology | 0·082 | 78·2 |
| Obstetrics | 0·077 | 130·8 |

Table 4 **Variation in hospital case-mix: general medicine, general surgery and obstetrics**

| Proportion of total caseload | Percentage of hospitals with indicated case-mix proportion | | |
|---|---|---|---|
| | General medicine | General surgery | Obstetrics |
| <0·025 | 6·21 | 1·69 | 58·19 |
| 0·025— | — | — | 1·69 |
| 0·050— | — | — | 0·56 |
| 0·075— | 3·95 | 1·13 | 2·82 |
| 0·100— | 7·91 | 0·56 | 2·26 |
| 0·125— | 12·99 | 0·56 | 5·08 |
| 0·150— | 20·33 | 1·69 | 7·91 |
| 0·175— | 15·82 | 4·52 | 5·08 |
| 0·200— | 12·99 | 6·78 | 7·91 |
| 0·225— | 10·17 | 7·34 | 2·26 |
| 0·250— | 4·52 | 9·04 | 1·69 |
| 0·275— | 2·82 | 4·52 | 1·69 |
| 0·300— | 0·56 | 13·56 | 1·69 |
| 0·325— | — | 10·73 | — |
| 0·350— | 1·13 | 15·82 | 0·56 |
| 0·400— | — | 11·30 | 0·56 |
| 0·450— | 0·56 | 7·34 | — |
| 0·500— | — | 1·13 | — |
| 0·550+ | — | 2·26 | — |

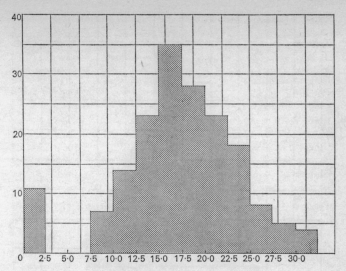

Figure 3 Distribution of hospitals by percentage of caseload
in general medicine

to vary together. The correlations between the proportions, presented in Table 6, indicate that although they are not statistically independent of each other (15 of the 28 correlations exceed the 5 per cent significance level of $r = \pm 0.145$), neither is there a high degree of correlation among them. While hospitals with a higher proportion of obstetrical cases tend to do relatively more gynaecology ($r = 0.315$), and relatively less general surgery ($r = -0.398$), other categories such as general medicine and general surgery show no correlation ($r = 0.005$).

A general assessment of the extent of intercorrelation among all eight proportions may be made by a statistical method known as 'principal component analysis' (Kendall, 1957, ch. 2; Lawley and Maxwell, 1963, ch. 4). By this method we associate with the eight proportions a set of eight 'principal component variables'; this is similar to the way in which factor analysis associates a set of factor values with the original observed variables. Each principal component variable is a weighted average of the eight case proportions.[3] Instead of describing the case-mix of each hospital by the eight proportions, we may use the eight principal com-

3. The specific nature of these weights need not be described here; they are derived from a calculation involving the latent vectors of the correlation matrix of the eight case proportions.

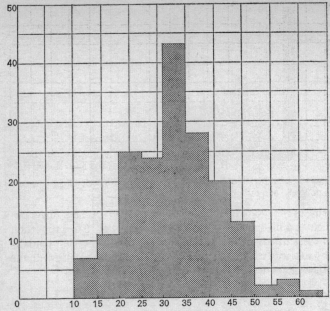

Figure 4 Distribution of hospitals by percentage of caseload in general surgery

ponent variables. If the eight proportions were highly associated with each other, it would be possible to define one or two principal component variables that represented a very high percentage of the total variation in all eight proportions. This would be analagous to finding one or two 'factors' that characterized the case-mix composition of the hospitals. In contrast, if all eight proportions were completely uncorrelated with each other, each of the principal component variables would represent one eighth of the total variation. Table 7 shows the percentage of total variation represented by each principal component variable. The two largest together account for only 46·1 per cent, which must be compared with the 25 per cent that would be achieved if the eight case proportions were completely uncorrelated.[4]

We may therefore conclude that when the case-mixes of large,

4. I hope that readers already familiar with principal component analysis will forgive the lack of precision in the above description. Although several of the statements might have been expressed more accurately, I believe the general idea is best conveyed as presented.

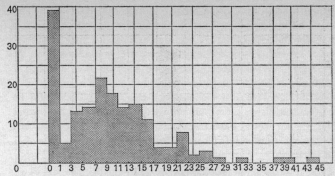

Figure 5 Distribution of hospitals by percentage of caseload
in traumatic and orthopedic surgery

acute hospitals are represented by eight broad specialty categories
there is a high degree of interhospital variation. The proportion
of cases in each of the individual categories varies substantially
and in a way which is, in general, not strongly correlated with the
other categories.

### Effects of case-mix differences on cost variation

The evidence of the previous section suggests that substantial
differences in case-mix proportions may be responsible for part
of the observed differences in case costs and costs per patient
week. In this section we present estimates of the extent to which
case-mix differences can explain the observed cost variations.

#### Method

The method used has been to estimate the 'least squares' linear
regression equation relating each cost type to the eight case-mix
proportions. The multiple correlation coefficient ($R$) of the equation is a measure of the extent to which the cost variation is
associated with the case-mix differences. More specifically, the
square of the multiple correlation coefficient ($R^2$) is the proportion
of the total variation in the particular cost that has been explained by the equation relating cost to the eight case types (For
the best understanding of calculation of $R^2$ etc., see Hoel, 1962,
ch. 7; Yule and Kendall, 1950, ch. 12).

Before turning to the results presented in Tables 8 and 9, it is
worthwhile to note some additional properties of this measure.
First, the value of $R^2$ reflects not only the association between the
dependent variable (cost) and the explanatory variables (case

proportions), but also the relative numbers of observations and explanatory variables. Even if there were no real association between the costs of the 177 hospitals and the proportions of their cases in each of the eight categories, we would expect an $R^2$ greater than zero. Indeed, if we divide cases into not nine but 177 mutually exclusive types, we would obtain an $R^2$ of exactly one, even if there were no association between costs and case-mix! To correct for this we present an adjusted value ($\bar{R}^2$) which indicates the $R^2$ that would have been obtained if the sample had been extremely (infinitely) large instead of containing only 177 hospitals.

**Table 5 Variation in hospital case-mix: traumatic and orthopedic surgery, other surgery, gynaecology, ENT (including tonsils and adenoids) and pediatrics**

| | *Percentage of hospitals with indicated case-mix proportion* | | | | |
|---|---|---|---|---|---|
| *Proportion of total caseload* | *Traumatic and ortho-pedic surgery* | *Other surgery* | *Gynae-cology* | *ENT (inc. tonsils and adenoids)* | *Pedi-atrics* |
| <0·01 | 22·03 | 22·60 | 23·73 | 23·73 | 42·94 |
| 0·01— | 2·82 | 9·04 | 3·39 | 3·95 | 2·82 |
| 0·03— | 7·34 | 13·56 | 4·52 | 9·04 | 6·78 |
| 0·05— | 7·91 | 17·51 | 7·34 | 9·04 | 8·47 |
| 0·07— | 12·43 | 13·56 | 10·73 | 10·17 | 9·60 |
| 0·09— | 10·17 | 10·73 | 16·38 | 11·30 | 9·04 |
| 0·11— | 7·91 | 1·69 | 14·69 | 4·52 | 6·78 |
| 0·13— | 8·47 | 3·39 | 9·60 | 9·04 | 4·52 |
| 0·15— | 6·21 | 0·56 | 5·08 | 6·78 | 0·56 |
| 0·17— | 2·26 | 1·69 | 1·13 | 4·52 | 1·13 |
| 0·19— | 2·26 | 1·69 | 1·13 | 2·26 | 1·69 |
| 0·21— | 4·52 | 0·56 | 0·56 | 1·13 | 1·13 |
| 0·23— | 1·13 | 1·13 | 0·56 | 1·69 | 1·13 |
| 0·25— | 1·69 | 0·56 | 1·13 | 0·56 | 1·13 |
| 0·27— | 0·56 | 1·69 | | 0·56 | 1·13 |
| 0·29— | 2·26 | | | 1·13 | 1·13 |
| 0·31+ | | | | 0·56 | |

Second, the calculated multiple correlation coefficients are only sample estimates based upon the particular costs and case-mix quantities observed in the 177 hospitals in 1960–61 and are therefore subject to sampling errors. To indicate whether the sample $R^2$ differs significantly from zero, we present the $F$–value and indicate the probability that such a value would have been obtained if the true $R^2$ were really zero.

Third, the calculated values of $\bar{R}^2$ may systematically overestimate the true associations between costs and the specified case-mix. This will occur if there are other variables (e.g. hospital size) that also influence costs, and these variables are correlated with any of the case proportion variables. To the extent that such a correlation exists the explanatory effects of the omitted variables will be attributed to the case-mix variables. The importance of omitted variables and their relation to case proportions is currently being investigated.

Against this possibility of overestimation must be balanced two reasons why the calculated $\bar{R}^2$ values are actually underestimates of the association between costs and case-mix. The relationships which we assumed in calculating the regression equations were arbitrarily kept linear; a non-linear equation (including, for example, the squares of some of the proportions) would probably increase the ability to explain cost variation by eight case proportions. We might also be able to increase the equation's explanatory power by selecting a different set of eight categories or by dividing cases into a larger number of types. Our selection of eight case types, although perhaps not the best for explaining cost variations, does however provide a medically meaningful way of dividing a hospital's case-mix. Experiments with larger numbers of case proportions do not show very much greater explantory power. While the relationship between ward cost per case and the eight case proportions shows an $\bar{R}^2$ of 0·275, a relationship with twenty-seven case proportions shows only 0·320. Although this increase is 'statistically significant' ($p > 0·10$), the difference is not very substantial when weighed against the computational difficulties of using the larger number of case types.

Problems such as these are inherent in any statistical study. If they are borne in mind, the method of multiple correlation analysis is a powerful and useful tool for describing the association between cost variations and case-mix differences.

*Results*

Table 8 presents the results for various categories of cost per case. Case-mix differences have explained 27·5 per cent of the variation in overall ward costs per case. Even more sensitive to case-mix differences is medical cost per case; here 37·6 per cent of inter-hospital variation is explained. At the other extreme only 7·6 per cent of variation in expenditure for medical and surgical appliances is accounted for. In such things as medical salaries and drug expenditures, case-mix differences have a direct effect on patients in different specialties requiring different kinds and amounts of these services. In contrast, variations in cost per case of such things as domestic services and patients' clothing are more likely to reflect case-mix differences indirectly through their effect on patients' average durations of stay.

This is confirmed by Table 9 which presents the results for various costs on a per patient week basis. Here only 2·1 per cent of the variation in overall ward costs is accounted for by cost differences. Certain cost categories – those in which the effect of case-mix was indicated as more direct – are more substantially influenced: 24·7 per cent of the variation in medical costs and 14·0 per cent of the variation in expenditure for dressings are explained by case-mix differences. The small effect on nursing costs ($\bar{R}^2 = 0·045$) is rather surprising. Although several interpretations are possible, the result may indicate that nursing staffs are not varied between hospitals in response to differences in the types of patients being treated.

The general conclusions to be drawn from these results is quite clear. Ward costs per case and, to a lesser extent, per patient week, are substantially and significantly influenced by the case-mix composition of the hospital's workload. Any attempts to compare hospitals' cost for administrative or research purposes, or to establish relationships between costs and other characteristics (e.g. number of beds), should therefore generally take case-mix into account. But although there are important associations between costs and case-mix, the porportion of total variation that remains unexplained is, in all cases, quite large. Thus, inter-hospital cost variations are not merely a reflection of case-mix but indicate differences in hospital efficiency, management efficiency, and standards of service

**Table 6 Correlations among case proportions***

| | Pediatrics | General surgery | ENT | T and O surgery | Other surgery | Gynaecology | Obstetrics |
|---|---|---|---|---|---|---|---|
| General medicine | −0·076 | 0·005 | −0·381 | −0·142 | −0·207 | 0·013 | −0·059 |
| Pediatrics | | −0·211 | −0·131 | −0·105 | −0·204 | 0·113 | 0·154 |
| General surgery | | | 0·023 | −0·100 | −0·246 | −0·335 | −0·398 |
| ENT | | | | 0·050 | 0·119 | −0·316 | −0·352 |
| T and O surgery | | | | | 0·035 | −0·330 | −0·335 |
| Other surgery | | | | | | −0·201 | −0·234 |
| Gynaecology | | | | | | | 0·315 |

* In 177 large acute hospitals, 1960.

Table 7 **Proportion of total case-mix variation associated with each principal component**

| Principal component number | Proportion of total variation |
|---|---|
| 1 | 0·268 |
| 2 | 0·194 |
| 3 | 0·142 |
| 4 | 0·136 |
| 5 | 0·087 |
| 6 | 0·083 |
| 7 | 0·071 |
| 8 | 0·020 |

Table 8 **Effects of case-mix differences on ward costs per case***

| Cost type | Average (£) | Coefficient of variation (%) | Effect of case-mix ($\bar{R}^2$) | F-value | Probability (<) |
|---|---|---|---|---|---|
| Total | 54·62 | 25·2 | 0·275 | 9·33 | 0·001 |
| Medical | 5·71 | 25·0 | 0·376 | 14·27 | 0·001 |
| Nursing | 13·50 | 26·3 | 0·223 | 7·32 | 0·001 |
| Domestic (172) | 3·49 | 67·4 | 0·131 | 4·32 | 0·001 |
| Nursing and domestic (172) | 17·01 | 31·2 | 0·237 | 7·82 | 0·001 |
| All staff (172) | 22·75 | 27·5 | 0·264 | 8·91 | 0·001 |
| Clothing, bedding and linen | 0·45 | 43·0 | 0·129 | 4·25 | 0·001 |
| Drugs | 1·77 | 27·5 | 0·303 | 5·83 | 0·001 |
| Dressings | 0·60 | 33·3 | 0·169 | 5·49 | 0·001 |
| Medical and surgical appliances and equipment | 1·68 | 32·5 | 0·076 | 2·80 | 0·01 |
| Total direct | 30·44 | 25·6 | 0·285 | 9·79 | 0·001 |
| Catering | 9·24 | 29·1 | 0·235 | 7·75 | 0·001 |
| Laundry (176) | 1·77 | 33·8 | | | |
| Total indirect | 24·14 | 28·8 | 0·223 | 7·31 | 0·001 |

* In 177 large, acute, non-teaching hospitals, 1960–61. Numbers in parenthesis indicate that one or more hospitals reported no costs in category and were omitted from calculation.

## Table 9 Effects of case-mix differences on ward costs per patient week*

| Cost type | Average (£) | Coefficient of variation (%) | Effect of case-mix ($\bar{R}^2$) | F-value | Probability (<) |
|---|---|---|---|---|---|
| Total | 28·42 | 12·2 | 0·021 | 1·47 | 0·20 |
| Medical | 3·02 | 21·5 | 0·247 | 8·20 | 0·001 |
| Nursing | 7·02 | 16·2 | 0·045 | 2·04 | 0·05 |
| Domestic (172) | 1·74 | 53·1 | 0·046 | 2·05 | 0·05 |
| Nursing and domestic (172) | 8·73 | 17·7 | 0·049 | 2·13 | 0·05 |
| All staff (172) | 11·75 | 15·4 | 0·049 | 2·14 | 0·05 |
| Clothing, bedding and linen | 0·23 | 35·1 | 0·005 | 1·10 | † |
| Drugs | 0·93 | 25·0 | 0·002 | 1·05 | † |
| Dressings | 0·32 | 32·5 | 0·140 | 4·57 | 0·001 |
| Medical and surgical appliances and equipment | 0·90 | 33·6 | 0·053 | 2·22 | 0·05 |
| Total direct | 15·86 | 13·6 | 0·061 | 2·43 | 0·05 |
| Catering | 4·79 | 16·2 | 0·007 | 1·15 | † |
| Laundry (176) | 0·92 | 23·5 | 0·117 | 3·92 | 0·001 |
| Total indirect | 12·54 | 16·4 | 0·036 | 1·83 | 0·10 |

* In 177 large, acute, non-teaching hospitals, 1960–61. Numbers in parentheses indicate that one or more hospitals reported no costs in category and were omitted from calculation.

† $p > 0.20$.

### References

ABEL-SMITH, B., and TITMUSS, R. (1956), *The Cost of the National Health Service in England and Wales*, Cambridge University Press.

FELDSTEIN, M. S. (1963), 'Developments in health service administration and financial control', *Medical Care*, vol. 1, no. 3.

GUILLEBAUD COMMITTEE (1956), *Report of the Committee of Enquiry into the Cost of the National Health Service*, Cmd 9663, HMSO.

HOEL, P. G. (1962), *Introduction to Mathematical Statistics*, Wiley & Sons.

KENDALL, M. G. (1957), *A Course in Multivariate Analysis*, Charles Griffin & Co.

LAWLEY, D. N., and MAXWELL, A. E. (1963), *Factor Analysis as a Statistical Method*, Butterworth.

MINISTRY OF HEALTH (1961), *Hospital Costing Returns for the Year Ended March 31st*, part 1. HMSO.

MONTACUTE, C. (1962), *Costing and Efficiency in Hospitals*, Oxford University Press.

SELECT COMMITTEE on ESTIMATES (1956–7), *Sixth Report: Running Costs of Hospitals*, HMSO.

YULE, G. U., and KENDALL, M. G. (1950), *An Introduction to the Theory of Statistics*, Griffin & Co.

# 11  J. K. Mann and D. E. Yett

Hospital Costs

Judith K. Mann and Donald E. Yett, 'The analysis of hospital costs:
a review article', *Journal of Business*, vol. 41, 1968, pp. 191–202.

Perhaps no aspect of inflation in recent years has received more
attention and concern than the rapid rise in the price of hospital
services. During the fifteen years between 1950 and 1965, the
Hospital Daily Service Charge component of the Consumer Price
Index (CPI) rose by 165 per cent. By comparison, the All Medical
Care component and the overall CPI increased during the same
period approximately 65 and 30 per cent, respectively (US Public
Health Service, 1967, p. 27). During 1966 alone, the index of
hospital charges rose by 16·5 per cent (as compared to a 3·3 per
cent increase in overall consumer prices) (US Department of
Health, Education and Welfare, 1967, p. 31).

The pronounced upward trend of hospital charges has per-
sisted despite a concerted effort to increase the available 'supply'
of hospital care. With the assistance of federal financing (largely
through the Hospital Survey and Construction Act), a total of
nearly $17 billion was expended on hospital construction, expan-
sion, and replacement between 1950 and 1965 (US Department
of Health, Education and Welfare, 1966, pp. 5–32). Large as it
was, it is apparent that this effort did not increase supply sufficiently to satisfy rapidly expanding demand without a profound
rise in prices. Moreover, from all indications, public policy should
be expected to stimulate an even greater increase in the demand
for hospital services during the next decade.[1] And, since all seg-
ments of the population are unanimous in the desire to stem the
upward spiral of hospital rates, attention is being focused more

1. Consider, for example, the following report: 'The fact that hospital
charges rose especially rapidly in the second half of 1966 suggests that
Medicare, which came into effect July 1st, contributed to the increase.
Medicare raised hospital occupancy rates in many places. The total occu-
pancy rate was 4 per cent higher in August 1966 than in August 1965'
(US Department of Health, Education and Welfare, 1967, *A Report to the
President* . . ., p. 31). Even greater increases in occupancy rates have been
predicted for the future (see Somers and Somers, 1967 pp. 239–43).

and more on ways in which anticipated demand increases can be matched by an equal expansion of supply.

The most obvious methods of increasing supply are to enlarge the total bed capacity of the hospital industry and to make more effective use of existing facilities. Since the number of hospital beds can be increased either by adding to existing facilities or by building new ones, two issues are of considerable importance: (1) is there an optimum size for hospitals? and (2) how large is the maximum potential gain from increased utilization? The economist's approach to both questions has been to explore the nature of the relevant long-run and short-run cost curves. In recent months, three excellent empirical studies of this sort have been reported. Unfortunately, they all lead to different conclusions regarding the impact of scale and utilization on hospital expenses.

The purposes of this paper are:

1. To review these studies with an eye toward clarifying the sources of their apparently conflicting results and

2. To present an alternative theoretical formulation of cost behavior for use in future research.

Accordingly, Section I summarizes the works of W. John Carr and Paul J. Feldstein, Martin S. Feldstein, and Mary Lee Ingbar and Lester D. Taylor. Section II evaluates these studies in terms of their differing institutional settings, methodologies, and policy implications. Section III presents our conclusions and recommendations for future hospital cost analyses.

## I The empirical evidence
### W. John Carr and Paul J. Feldstein

In their study Carr and Feldstein (1967, pp. 45–65) analysed nationwide data on 3147 US voluntary short-term general hospitals. Their goal was to determine the optimal hospital size for purposes of area-wide planning. In the process, they also derived estimates of the approximate effects of a number of other factors upon costs. In general, their conclusions support the traditional economic postulate that unit costs tend to decline, and then rise, as 'size' is increased.

Using the technique of multiple regression, Carr and Feldstein isolated the partial relationship between total operating expenses and hospital size by holding constant such variable characteristics as the number of out-patient visits, the range and scope of service facilities available, and the presence or absence of training and research activities. Their measure of cost, taken from reports of expenses for 1963 submitted to the American Hospital Association, was adjusted for differences in factor prices by replacing the average wage rate for employees of each specific hospital with the average wage for all hospital employees. Their measure of 'size', the average daily patient census, was based upon a desire to specify scale in terms of the hospital's ability to provide care, rather than its physical capacity.

Carr and Feldstein's estimated 'cost function' expressed a quadratic relationship between total adjusted operating expenses and average daily patient census (holding constant the other specified cost-determining characteristics). The partial regression coefficients of both the first- and second-degree terms in size were found to be highly significant with positive signs, and since the constant term was negative, a U-shaped *average* cost curve was implied. Setting the number of services offered equal to their mean value (14·15), and ignoring all other factors, they concluded that the long-run average cost function reached its minimum at an average daily census of approximately 190 patients. Apparently, hospitals designed to operate at a higher census level incur diseconomies and, therefore, should be avoided.

### Martin S. Feldstein

Martin Feldstein's *Economic Analysis for Health Service Efficiency* is one of the most comprehensive works in the field of empirical hospital research (Feldstein, 1967). Combining technical prowess with a broad understanding of the institutional structure of the British National Health Service, Feldstein analysed the hospital as a production unit in almost all possible aspects and delineated its role in a general model for planning the supply and use of health services within that system. However, we must limit our attention to that phase of his work which presents his estimation of the hospital cost function.

Like the previous investigators, Feldstein employed multiple regression analysis in fitting a quadratic relationship between operating expenses and hospital size. However, his model differed from Carr and P. J. Feldstein's in several essential respects. First, M. Feldstein estimated per-unit costs directly, rather than deriving them from a total cost function; accordingly, his dependent variable was operating expenses per medical case. Second, he specifically distinguished between size and utilization – taking the number of beds as his measure of the former, and the flow of cases per bed per year as his measure of the latter. Third, he standardized for variation in service capability indirectly by including in his regression the proportion of patients in selected diagnostic categories, rather than absolute numbers of services available. Finally, in view of the National Health System's uniform salary scale, no attempt was made to adjust 'costs' for factor price differences.

Feldstein fitted progressively more elaborate equations to his data from 177 short-term, non-teaching, general hospitals. His final estimate expressed cost per case as a quadratic function of both the number of beds and the flow of cases per bed per year (with case-type proportions included linearly). Although the partial coefficients of the first- and second-degree terms in beds indicated a U-shaped average cost curve, the minimum point was reached at slightly over 1000 beds, near the upper limit of observed hospital size. Thus, the U-shape is strictly an artefact of the quadratic function fitted. Recognizing this fact, Feldstein estimated semilogarithmic and logarithmic cost functions which decreased monotonically and predicted with equal confidence. Given the lack of evidence for diseconomies of large scale within the relevant range, the general conclusion of his investigation is that, if the rate of treating patients was identical for hospitals of all sizes, larger hospitals would achieve substantial economies of scale. The tendency of large institutions to lengthen the average patient stay and, thus, treat cases at considerably slower rates is responsible for higher-than-predicted unit costs. If such hospitals raised their case flows to the average, Feldstein's estimates show that they could reduce their cost per case by as much as 12 per cent.

*Mary Lee Ingbar and Lester D. Taylor*

In their investigation of *Hospital Costs in Massachusetts*, Ingbar and Taylor (1968) analysed a more extensive array of variables than were included in any previous hospital cost study. Data on over one hundred operating characteristics of seventy-two short-term general hospitals for the years 1958 and 1959 were pooled and subjected to principal component analysis. In this manner, the potential number of independent variables was reduced to fourteen major factors which accounted for 85 per cent of the variation in the original list. From these, the following eleven were 'identified' on the basis of their simple correlation with the initial 100 or so variables: (1) Size-Volume, (2) Utilization,

(3) Length of Stay, (4) Laboratory Activity, (5) Radiology Activity, (6) Surgical Activity, (7) Maternity Activity, (8) Pediatric Activity, (9) Ambulatory Activity, (10) Private Service, and (11) Ward Services.

From each of the identified factor sets, the most significant measure was selected for use in a multiple regression analysis of per-unit costs. Three separate cost models were delineated. For the first, in which operating expense per *available bed day* was specified as the dependent variable, the only measure associated with the factor 'size-volume' found to be significant was medical and surgical physician expense per patient day. No more obvious measure of size or utilization (e.g., beds or occupancy rates) appeared as an important determinant of cost. 70 per cent of the total variation in this particular definition of average cost was explained by the indicated 'size-volume' factor and measures for Radiology, Surgical and Ambulatory Activities.

The second model estimated by Ingbar and Taylor employed expense per *patient day* as the dependent variable. It is interesting that, in addition to the above four factors, both beds and beds-squared appeared as significant variables in this regression. Contrary to expectation, the signs of the coefficients were such that an inverted U-shaped function, with a maximum at 150 beds, was indicated. However, the magnitude of the potential cost reduction for hospitals of more than 200, or less than 100, beds is extremely small – so small, in fact, that the authors concluded average cost in this sense was virtually constant with respect to size.

In their final model, Ingbar and Taylor related cost per patient day to utilization (measured by occupancy rates). As anticipated, the coefficient of utilization was negative and highly significant. Consequently, although they did not find size to be a major factor in explaining average cost behavior (in terms of either actual or available patient days), they did provide additional evidence that higher utilization is associated with lower unit costs for hospitals of all sizes.[2] These conclusions were tested and confirmed on the basis of similar data for 1962–3.

2. The same three models were also used to estimate average costs for separate service categories and individual departments within the hospitals studied. In addition, average revenue was substituted for average expenses (on the grounds that revenue is determined by costs for non-profit organizations), and parallel analysis was performed. Neither extension substantially modified their conclusions regarding the effects of scale and utilization on unit costs.

## II An evaluation of the evidence

The contrasting implications of the foregoing hospital studies might, of course, be due to differences in terms of empirical settings, the selection of measures to represent cost and output, and/or statistical methodologies. Certainly, there is no obvious reason to suppose that British and American hospitals function alike – or even that Massachusetts hospitals are typical of American hospitals in general. If, in fact, there are differences either in their production functions or in their incentives to minimize costs, these would be expected to have significant effects on the estimated cost functions.[3]

Specifically, the declining average cost curve depicted by M. Feldstein could be explained if British hospitals characteristically exhibit greater production indivisibilities, along with higher incentives to minimize costs, than do their American counterparts. However, the essential difference between the two institutional settings is that the former is financed by the British Treasury while the latter has no such single source of support. It is difficult to see how this fact alone might introduce indivisibilities, and it is more likely to create lower than higher British incentives to minimize costs.[4] Consequently, it is implausible to attribute Feldstein's findings to the institutional characteristics of the British system. Similarly, no evidence exists which suggests that Massachusetts hospitals have atypical production functions, or cost-minimizing incentives different from those of other American hospitals. Yet, one or both of these conditions would be necessary to explain the divergence between the Ingbar–Taylor and the Carr–Feldstein findings in terms of institutional setting alone.

A second explanation of the multiplicitity of outcomes could lie in the authors' different measures of 'cost'. Although each

3. Several writers have discussed the implications of the absence of cost-minimizing incentives in the hospital industry. Carr and Feldstein, in restricting their sample to voluntary short-term hospitals, argued that variations in efficiency (if not dependent on size) could be considered random, and thus dismissed them. Another point of view was adopted by K. K. Ro (1966). He asserted that 'there is no great incentive to minimize cost' (p. 12). For this reason, and because hospital output is difficult to define and measure, he relegates the estimation of a cost function to secondary position in his study (p. 42).

4. Even if the institutional setting of British hospitals were responsible for indivisibilities, it is unlikely that M. Feldstein would have captured this effect. The cost of most of the factors typically characterized as indivisible were directly excluded from his analysis.

employed, essentially, direct operating expenses, M. Feldstein excluded outpatient expenses and depreciation (in addition to construction and expansion costs excluded from the other studies); and Carr and Feldstein altered actual labor costs by using the national average of hospital earnings. Unfortunately, without access to their original data, it is impossible to estimate the relative importance of these alterations in expense figures. Furthermore, while the adjustments that were made solved some problems, they increased the necessity to examine carefully the sorts of 'cost functions' which were actually estimated.

For example, M. Feldstein's exclusion of depreciation expense was intended to avoid the well-known inadequacy of accounting data as a measure of capital usage[5] and to focus attention on the independent effects of utilization and scale on day-to-day operating expenses. In pursuing the latter goal, he makes a useful distinction between the very short-run and a quasi-long-run. However, by omitting any measure of capital cost, he ignores an essential character of the traditional concept of long-run: the change in *all* 'fixed costs' associated with increasing scale.

Similarly, while Carr and Feldstein's substitution of national average for actual salary figures represents a commendable attempt to overcome the serious problem of differences in relative factor prices, it is unlikely that they were completely successful. This technique does adjust for a subset of absolute factor prices, but does not standardize their relative values.[6] Therefore, they not only failed to capture the long-run expansion path (and thereby 'the' long-run cost function), but they may have created a distorted representation of the least-cost combination of inputs.

The third, and most significant, reason for the variety of 'cost function' results is the fact that each author applied an entirely different model of cost behavior. Under these circumstances, even if adjustments could be made to remove the influence of the various institutional settings and accounting measures of cost, their differing interpretations of a long-run cost function would still preclude them from reaching the same conclusion. This is not to detract from the many valuable insights into the nature of hospital operating expenses provided by each of the studies reviewed. Rather, our intent is to emphasize the importance of

5. The bias inherent in accounting data is widely recognized. See, for example, Walters (1963, pp. 39–41).

6. For a similar treatment of wage differentials, see Cohen (1967, pp. 355–8). The same criticism is applicable to this aspect of both studies.

uniform theory if the results of cost analyses are to be sufficiently consistent to serve as effective decision-making tools. It should not be supposed, however, that the authors are solely responsible for the lack of uniformity in their respective interpretations of cost theory; at least part of the blame is attributable to the ambiguous state of cost theory itself.

It is widely recognized that theorists disagree on such issues as whether cost should be defined as a stock or a flow and whether, in measuring opportunity cost, one should consider a factor's current use as a 'foregone alternative'.[7] However, such sources of theoretical disagreement could not have been responsible for the divergent hospital cost descriptions since none of the authors explored the implications of opportunity cost applications.

For these studies, a more fundamental methodological issue is the appropriate specification of 'output' relative to cost. In this context, there are two levels of difficulty: one conceptual and one statistical. The basic conceptual issue is the specification of the time dimensionality of output. Is it a stock or is it a flow? Is there a clear-cut demarcation between the short-run and the long-run? Of what relevance is calendar time to cost-output behavior? These questions can best be discussed within the context of the output measures which are generally selected for analysis. For hospital cost studies, such a measure is particularly elusive. Accordingly, we turn our attention first to the statistical problems of measurement.

Ideally, hospital output should be measured in terms of homogeneous units of service rendered.[8] Numerous approaches to developing such a measure have been proposed, but none has been unanimously accepted – primarily because none is without its limitations. In addition to those discussed here, others include S. R. Gottlieb, *et al.* (1964); R. E. Berry Jr (1967); D. Saarthof and R. Kurtz (1962). All of the studies reviewed above made major contributions toward the eventual solution to this prob-

7. For differing views of the definition of cost, cf. Alchian and Allen (1967, pp. 222–43, and 285); Joe S. Bain (1953, pp. 83–5); Friedman (1955, pp. 230–38); Leftwich (1964, pp. 136–41), Stigler (1966, pp. 104–14).

8. There are those who argue that the output of a health facility should be specified in terms of its effect on the patient (see, for example, Scitovsky, 1964, p. 136); Martin (1963, pp. 101–6); Donabedian (1966, pp. 167–70); Auster, Leveson, and Sarachek (1966, pp. 4–8) and Ro (1966, p. 43).

We reject this definition of hospital output for the same reason that we do not regard the output of a beauty salon as beauty.

lem. Nevertheless, it is instructive to examine certain pitfalls that were not completely avoided.

Ingbar and Taylor attempted to standardize their primary output measure (bed days) through the explicit recognition of differences in the services rendered by hospitals. However, the inclusion in their regression analysis of such variables as the number of X-rays taken, operations performed, and babies delivered probably goes beyond merely standardizing the unit of output. In view of the fact that each of these services was the most significant variable in its set, and that the combined factor sets completely characterize the range of hospital operations, their procedure amounts to measuring the product directly in terms of its component parts. They not only 'standardized' for the *type* of output but for the *amount* as well.

Having characterized the cost-output relationships through the use of factors, it is not surprising that Ingbar and Taylor found no relationship between average cost and beds. Beds was meant to measure scale; but the theory of long-run costs presumes an explicit relationship between output and scale. If measures for *both* variables are included in a regression analysis of firms which are operating efficiently at various sizes, the strong correlation between them will make one of the measures redundant, and it will always be insignificant. If their choice of factors can be regarded as a composite measure of output, a surprising implication of the Ingbar–Taylor study is that hospitals apparently operate efficiently.[9] Unfortunately, since they did not include a quadratic term in a weighted average of the factors, they did not, in effect, test the same hypothesis as the other authors, namely, that economies of scale exist and decrease with hospital size.

While Carr and Feldstein also recognized that variations in services is a source of heterogeneity, their approach to standardization was substantially different from Ingbar and Taylor's. Using average daily patient census as a measure of scale (i.e. efficient output), they held the effect of services constant by including as an explanatory variable a simple count of the number of services and facilities available.[10] As they pointed out, this

9. Strictly speaking, the fact that beds, on the one hand, and the combined weighted factors, on the other hand, are highly correlated implies that hospitals are either operating efficiently or that their inefficiency is significantly non-random.

10. Carr and Feldstein extended their investigation of service effects by disaggregating their sample into five service capability groups and running separate regressions in each. Their results confirmed their initial findings.

measure is limited in the sense that it assumes that all facilities and services have an equal impact on cost. On the other hand, it clearly captures some aspects of the heterogeneity of care without being a redundant measure of output. In this respect, Carr and Feldstein came closer to identifying the independent effect of scale on average hospital costs.

While accounting for the number of services available is certainly a step in the right direction toward establishing a homogeneous unit of output, including a measure of their utilization would probably yield even better results. The problem is to find a technique which accomplishes this goal without at the same time obscuring the independent cost-output relationship. In this regard, M. Feldstein provides a promising approach. Recognizing that the services rendered to a patient are dependent upon the patient's diagnosis, he incorporated the proportion of cases in various medical categories. By using relative as opposed to absolute magnitudes, he avoided the collinearity problem encountered by Ingbar and Taylor. On the other hand, by implicitly including varieties of treatment, he was able to standardize for service variability. Future investigators may find it profitable to combine the Carr–Feldstein and M. Feldstein approaches in order to obtain a measure of output which is more homogeneous both in terms of case mix and service provided (see Yett and Mann, 1967, pp. 41–52).

In addition to his contribution in standardizing hospital output, M. Feldstein made a valuable distinction between the cost effects of hospital size and those of care intensity, given size. In the process, however, he probably overestimated the extent of potential scale economies. It will be recalled that Feldstein omitted from his measure of cost certain major capital expenditures. Consequently, perhaps his cost curve should not be directly evaluated as a long-run function. Suppose, for instance, that the inclusion of beds was regarded as standardizing for any capital-cost variations which had not been eliminated from expense figures. His estimated relationship between cost per case and cases per year, holding bed capacity constant, would then be interpreted as a short-run cost curve. Using his derived regression coefficients, it can be shown that each member of the family of such curves generated by changing bed capacity reaches it minimum point at a level of 32·75 cases per year times the total number of hospital beds.[11]

11. Feldstein's estimated cost function yields the following equation:

Given this constant proportionality between beds and the number of cases at alternative short-run minimum costs, it follows that the partial relationship between unit cost and beds which Feldstein presented as a long-run function actually depicts a curve connecting these minimum points. However, the appropriate theoretical construct is the envelope of short-run total cost curves.[12] If there is such a thing as optimal output for a given size, Feldstein's 'long-run function' is misleading in two respects. First, in omitting some major capital items, his short-run functions can only be regarded as average variable cost. Since these curves fall further and further below average total cost as scale increases, they could suggest constantly declining long-run average cost even if the 'true' long-run function were U-shaped. Second, since the minimum points of successively lower short-run functions lie to the right and below the appropriate points of tangency, a curve connecting these low points will be steeper over this range than the long-run envelope. For both these reasons, policy makers should be wary of concluding that the economies for larger-sized hospitals are as great, or exist over as wide a range, as Feldstein's estimates appear to indicate.

From the preceding discussion, it seems clear that the incompatible implications of the studies reviewed above are fundamentally due to the authors' individual and differing methodologies. Their alternative techniques for reducing the heterogeneity in the measure of output go a long way toward explaining the lack of uniformity in their conclusions. But there is another issue concerning the measurement of output which may provide even more

$$\frac{C}{K} = -3\cdot54(10)^{-2}B + 1\cdot96(10)^{-5}B^2 - 7\cdot14\frac{K}{B} + 0\cdot109\left(\frac{K}{B}\right)^2,$$

where $C$ is cost, $K$ is cases per year, and $B$ is beds. Differentiating with respect to $K$ gives:

$$\frac{\delta(C/K)}{\delta K} = -7\cdot14\frac{1}{B} + 0\cdot218\frac{K}{B^2}.$$

Setting this expression equal to zero and solving for $K$ gives the minimum point in terms of $B$. Thus,

$$K = \frac{7\cdot14}{0\cdot218}B = 32\cdot75B.$$

This is obviously a minimum, as the second partial with respect to $K$ is

$$\frac{\delta^2(C/K)}{\delta K^2} = 0\cdot218\frac{1}{B^2} > 0.$$

12. This interpretation of Feldstein's model is, of course, only valid under the assumption of cost minimization on the part of hospital administrators. If such incentive is lacking, there is no way to apply the traditional theory.

insight: To what extent does time dimensionality affect the theory and estimation of cost behavior?

Carr and Feldstein obtained their estimates by using a stock measure of output (average daily patient census). Ingbar and Taylor experimented with a stock and flow separately (available bed days in one model; patients per year times days per year in another). M. Feldstein used both a stock measure for 'scale' (beds) and a flow measure for 'output' (cases per bed per year). If the shape of the cost function for any firm depends upon the time dimensionality of output, it is clear that a stock measure might not yield the same estimate as would a flow. It is precisely this issue which is pursued in a recent contribution to cost theory developed by Armen A. Alchian (1959) and expanded by Jack Hirshleifer (1962). The model which they exposited reinterprets the 'classical' cost function as dependent on both the stock, or volume, of output and the rate at which it is produced.

In brief, the rate-volume theory states that a larger anticipated volume of production has a per-unit cost-reducing effect if the rate at which it is produced is fixed. Conversely, the rate of production has a per-unit cost-increasing effect if volume is held constant. The proportionate variation of both rate and volume (i.e., holding time constant) can then be expected to produce a U-shaped per-unit cost curve, with the volume effect predominant over low ranges, and rate effect predominant over high.

The application of the rate-volume model to continuously producing firms is perhaps not so obvious as its application to industries which tend to produce in batches (such as the contract-based aerospace industry). In the latter case, volume can be readily identified as rate times time, whereas in the former the absence of a specified period of production presents a conceptual difficulty.[13] However, the model does suggest an interpretation of cost behavior which resolves many of the intractibilities associated with the traditional 'long-run' function. First, it defines in

13. Consider the following example of an intuitively appealing application of the rate-volume model to a continuously producing firm: 'It is clear . . . that a publisher will incur higher costs if he prints and binds short novelettes than if he produces only lengthy books, even when the rate at which he prints the pages is the same in both cases. Because of the set-up costs involved in the binding, packaging and distribution of his product, the length of the book is an important determinant of his costs. Moreover, it is our contention that the length of the book in this example is analogous to the volume or size of a batch of output in terms of the way in which it affects costs' (Yett, 1967, p. 8).

specific terms the meaning of output. Second, it explicitly incorporates time and information costs, which, after all, are decision parameters to a firm, but which traditional theory, with its rigid dichotomy between short and long run, has difficulty explaining. Finally, it clarifies the causal relation between 'scale of production' and cost by emphasizing the cost effects of the planned volume of output.

For the hospital industry, it may be illuminating to regard the number of beds as a proxy for the anticipated volume of output, and the number of cases per unit time as the rate at which hospital services are produced. Indeed, M. Feldstein's recognition of the importance of the rate of production is what led him to include a flow variable of cases per bed per year in his analysis of the cost-bed relationship. Since traditional theory suggests that only one of these variables is the output to which cost is related, Feldstein regarded the partial function between cost and beds as 'the long-run cost curve'. However, if the rate-volume model is a better explanation of cost behavior, such a partial relationship (between cost and volume, *holding rate constant*) would yield constantly decreasing unit cost – exactly as Feldstein found.

As encouraging as is this outcome in establishing the usefulness of a rate-volume approach, Feldstein's estimated cost curve when rate and volume are varied proportionately is even more convincing. Expressing his flow variable as a constant proportion of beds (that proportion calculated from his reported mean figures), we find the average cost function reaches a minimum at 438 beds.[14] This figure is well within his range of observations, the mean of which was 310 beds. Our result tends to support Feldstein's contention that many hospitals have not taken full advantage of available 'economies' but modifies his conclusion that the average cost curve declines continually over the entire size range.[15]

14. The calculations are as follows:

$$\left(\frac{\bar{K}}{B}\right) \Big/ \bar{B} = \frac{23 \cdot 18}{300} = 7 \cdot 727 (10)^{-2}$$

$$C/K = [-3 \cdot 54 - 7 \cdot 14 (7 \cdot 73)](10)^{-2} B + [1 \cdot 96 + 1 \cdot 09 (7 \cdot 73)^2](10)^{-5} B^2$$
$$= -58 \cdot 73 (10)^{-2} B + 67 \cdot 09 (10)^{-5} B^2$$

$$d\left(\frac{C}{K}\right) \Big/ dB = -58 \cdot 73 (10)^{-2} + 134 \cdot 18 (10)^{-5} B = 0$$

$$B = \frac{58 \cdot 73 (10)^3}{134 \cdot 18} = 438.$$

15. It should be emphasized that Feldstein's finding of an L-shaped cost

## III Conclusions and recommendations

It is evident from the innovative nature and technical sophistication of the works reviewed that the analysis of hospitals costs has made remarkable progress in recent years. Each of these studies has contributed new insights into the problems of measuring and estimating the potential effects of varying scale in this industry despite the fact that, at least superficially, they reached entirely different conclusions.

It is our contention that the differences in their findings cannot be attributed to any institutional peculiarities of the hospitals studied by the various authors. Nor is it likely that the relatively minor variations in their cost measures are the explanation. What does seem to be responsible is their differing interpretations of the relation between 'output' and 'scale'. With this fact in mind, it is less surprising that they did not reach similar conclusions, since, implicitly, each tested a different hypothesis.

Carr and Feldstein focused exclusively on the long run and made the assumption that, on the average, hospitals operated with economic efficiency (i.e., at a point on their long-run cost curve). Consequently, they defined scale in terms of a hospital's output – the ability to provide care for a given number of patients. M. Feldstein, on the other hand, noted that observed differences in intensity of care could be regarded as short-run fluctuations in output. He felt that such fluctuations are of interest in their own right and, moreover, must be removed if a long-run function in scale is to be independently estimated. Ingbar and Taylor also intended to treat separately the primarily short-run effects of

---

curve is not unusual. On the contrary, the vast majority of cost summaries in almost every industry have led to the same conclusion. (For a description of forty-four such studies, see P. J. D. Wiles, 1956.) Moreover, this is precisely what classical theory would lead us to expect. As Walters put it, 'The statistical L-shaped or constant cost conditions would not be inconsistent with a U-shaped long-run cost curve. Using the "naive" argument, why should any competitive entrepreneur expand and stay on the rising part of the cost curve?'

Considering the improbability of testing the validity of the classical U-shape from direct empirical observations, the major value of the rate-volume approach is readily apparent. By estimating the independent cost effects of variations in both measures of output and then imposing mathematical proportionality between them, the existence of any 'diseconomies' can be verified despite the fact that firms do not behave irrationally. For further discussions of this point, see Alchian, *op cit.*, p. 30; and Hirshleifer, *op cit.*, pp. 254–5.

utilization and the long-run influence of size. Had their technique for standardizing output not interfered with this intent, it is likely that their results would have been similar to those of M. Feldstein.

A strict application of the conventional dichotomy between short run and long run in the estimation of cost functions leaves little choice but to follow either the approach of Carr and Feldstein (and assume observed output represents efficiency) or that of M. Feldstein (and partial out the effect of 'short-run' fluctuations).[16] We have argued, however, that the necessity of this choice may be avoided by explicitly including time as a variable in the analysis through the use of separate measures for both stock and flow.

Looking at M. Feldstein's stock measure alone, his results suggest an L-shaped function. However, using both his stock and flow, we demonstrated that the implications of a rate-volume model were supported, and a U-shaped cost curve was indicated. The compatibility of this result with that of Carr and Feldstein suggests that non-proportional variations in the rate and volume of production were not significant in their sample. Indeed, Carr and Feldstein present a persuasive argument that utilization and scale do move together in the hospital industry: small hospitals operate most efficiently at lower-than-average relative occupancy in order to adjust to demand fluctuations more economically. Under such conditions, it is immaterial, of course, which measure is used. Either the stock or flow would reflect the same cost-output relation.

Although it is clear that recent hospital cost investigations are not so inconsistent as at first they might appear, this does not mean that the issue to which they were addressed has been settled. No attempt has been made in this paper to explore such problems as how to obtain measures of economic cost, avoid the 'regression fallacy' bias, choose between simultaneous and reduced form systems, etc.[17] As important as these issues are, they will remain

16. It should be recognized, however, that observed differences in utilization need not represent movements along a 'short-run' cost curve. If costs do not immediately respond to temporary deviations from least-cost output, observed values of unit costs will be biased. This type of 'errors-in-variables' problem is often called the 'regression fallacy bias'. For a detailed explanation, see Friedman, op cit., pp. 232–4; and J. Johnston 1960, pp. 189–92).

17. These and other widely recognized problems are discussed at length in such works as: Walters, op cit., pp. 39–49; Johnston, op cit., pp. 26–43; Friedman, op. cit., pp. 230–38; Caleb A. Smith (1955), pp. 212–30.

unsolved until a consistent and definitive hospital cost model has been developed. It is our opinion that the Alchian–Hirshleifer model offers considerable promise in this direction, and we are currently engaged in an effort to specify its characteristics within the hospital setting and to employ it in the analysis of the costs of providing long-term in-patient care (see Yett and Mann, 1967).

## References

ALCHIAN, A. A. (1959), 'Costs and outputs', in *The Allocation of Economic Resources*, Stanford University Press.

ALCHIAN, A. A. and ALLEN, W. R. (1967), *University Economics*, 2nd edn, Wadsworth Publishing Co.

AUSTER, R., LEVESON, I., and SARACHEK, D. (1966), 'The production of health, an explanatory study', NBER.

BAIN, J. S. (1953), *Pricing, Distribution and Employment*, revised edn, Holt, Rinehart & Winston.

BERRY, R. E. Jr (1967), 'Returns to scale in the production of hospital services', *Health Research Service*, Summer.

CARR, W. J., and FELDSTEIN, P. J. (1967), 'The relationship of cost to hospital size', *Inquiry*, vol. 4, pp. 45–65.

COHEN, H. A. (1967), 'Variations in cost among hospitals of different sizes', *Southern Econ. J.*, vol. 33, pp. 355–8.

DONABEDIAN, A. (1966), 'Evaluating the quality of medical care', *Milbank Memorial Fund Q.*, vol. 44, pp. 167–70.

FELDSTEIN, M. S. (1967), *Economic Analysis for Health Service Efficiency*, North Holland Publishing Co.

FRIEDMAN, M. (1955), 'Comment', in *Business Concentration and Price Policy*, NBER, Princeton University Press.

GOTTLIEB, S. R., *et al.* (1964), *The Nature of Hospital Cost*, Bureau of Hospital Administration, University of Michigan.

HIRSCHLEIFER, J. (1962), 'A successful reconstruction?', *Journal of Business*, no. 35.

INGBAR, M. L., and TAYLOR, L. D. (1968), *Hospital Costs in Massachusetts*, Harvard University Press.

JOHNSTON, J. (1966), *Statistical Cost Analysis*, McGraw-Hill.

LEFTWICH, R. H. (1964), *The Price System and Resource Allocation*, revised edn, Holt, Rinehart & Winston.

MARTIN, L. M. (1963), 'Expenditures, prices and units of medical care', in R. M. Bailey, 'An economic analysis of private medical practice organization', unpublished D.B.A. dissertation, Indiana University.

RO, K. K. (1966), 'A statistical study of factors affecting the unit cost of short-term hospital care', unpublished Ph.D. dissertation, Yale University.

SAARTHOF, D., and KURTZ, R. (1962), 'Cost comparisons don't do the job', *Modern Hospital*, no. 94.

SCITOVSKY, A. A. (1964), 'An index to the cost of medical care – a proposed new approach', *The Economics of Health and Medical Care*, University of Michigan.

SOMERS, H. M., and A. R. (1967), *Medicare and the Hospitals: Issues and Prospects*, Brookings Institution.

SMITH, C. A. (1955), 'Survey of the empirical evidence on economies of scale', *Business Concentration and Price Policy*, Princeton University Press.

STIGLER, G. J. (1966), *The Theory of Price*, third edn, Macmillan.

US PUBLIC HEALTH SERVICE (1967), *Medical Care Financing an Utilization*, no. 947–1A.

US DEPARTMENT of HEALTH, EDUCATION and WELFARE (1967), *A Report to the President on Medical Care Prices*.

US DEPARTMENT of HEALTH, EDUCATION and WELFARE (1966), *Health, Education and Welfare Trends*, 1965 edn.

WALTERS, A. A. (1963). 'Production and cost functions; an economic survey', *Econometrica*, vol. 31.

WILES, P. J. D. (1956), *Price, Cost and Output*, Basil Blackwell & Mott.

YETT, D. E. (1967), 'An evaluation of alternative methods of estimating physicians' expenses relative to output', *Inquiry*, no. 4.

YETT, D. E., and MANN, J. K. (1967), *The Costs of Providing Long-Term Care: An Econometric Study*, Human Resources Research Centre, University of South California Research Institute for Business and Economics.

# Part Four
# The Value of Human Lives

The final section in this volume takes up the important question of the valuation of human life and, by implication, of improvements in health which was discussed in a preliminary way in the 1962 article by Mushkin (Reading 4). Lives saved clearly constitute an aspect of the 'output' of health services and the social value placed upon them can be used both to assess the productivity of the health 'industry' and can also be used to help establish priorities in health care investment plans. The current state of the measurement of the value of life is, as yet, imperfect and there is a great deal of work still to be done both in inventing procedures for improving current estimates of the pecuniary values of lives and in developing means for supplementing these (minimal) estimates with other social and humanitarian dimensions of 'output' such as reduction in suffering, pain and misery. We expect to see substantial progress in this area over the next decade.

The first paper in this section, by Schelling (Reading 12), is a wide ranging discussion of how and why one might wish to measure the value of preventing a death and of the enormous difficulties, both technical and emotional that must be overcome. The next two papers, by Michael Jones-Lee and R. F. F. Dawson (Readings 13 and 14) relate explicitly to the valuation of life as used in road investment decisions. Currently, the value used in actual investment calculations is £17,000 per life. Enke (Reading 15) looks at the analogous problem, not of saving life, but of preventing birth. A major difference between the two is that the cost-benefit of birth prevention does not need to include the costs and benefits of life to the unborn whereas the cost-benefit of death prevention clearly needs to include the costs and benefits of life to the person who may die.

This area is, of course, a controversial one and economists have yet to reach a consensus as to the appropriate means of measurement. The selection here gives the reader some idea of the possible angles from which the problem can be, and has been, attacked.

# 12 T. C. Schelling

The Value of Preventing Death

Excerpt from T. C. Schelling, 'The life you save may be your own',
in S. B. Chase (ed.), *Problems in Public Expenditure Analysis*,
The Brookings Institution, Washington DC, 1968, pp. 127–62.

This is a treacherous topic, and I must choose a nondescriptive title to avoid initial misunderstanding. It is not the worth of human life that I shall discuss, but of 'life-saving', of preventing death. And it is not a particular death, but a statistical death. What is it worth to reduce the probability of death – the statistical frequency of death – within some identifiable group of people none of whom expects to die except eventually?

Worth to whom? Eventually I shall propose that it is to the people who may die, or who may lose somebody who matters to them. But the subject is surrounded by so much mystery, sentiment, moral consideration, husbandry, and paternalism, that some of the fringe issues need to be discussed first, if only to identify what the subject is not. Some of these issues are exciting, more exciting than the economics of life expectancy. They involve the special qualities that make an individual's life unique and his death an awesome event, that make hangmen's wages a special market phenomenon and murder the only crime worth solving in a detective story.

The first part of the paper examines society's interest in life and death; the second part surveys the economic impact of untimely death, viewing it more as a loss of livelihood than as a loss of life, seeing how the losses and any possible gains are distributed among taxpayers, insured policyholders, and others who have no personal connection with the deceased. The third part deals with the consumer's interest in reduced mortality and how that interest can be identified, expressed, or allowed for in government programs that, at some cost, can raise life expectancy. It is here that we recognize that life as well as livelihood is at stake; so is anxiety, and the life at risk concerns the consumer personally.

## Social interest in life and death

'Pain, fear, and suffering,' we are told, '. . . are considered of great importance in a society that values human life and human welfare' (D. J. Reynolds, 1956). They are important, too, to ordinary people who do not like pain and suffering. We have been told that the value of a human life ought to be considered, at least partially, without regard to whether the person who might die is a producer or not, that this value should result from a collective decision concerning the 'expense that the nation is willing – as a moral judgment – to undertake, to save one of its members' (Selma Mushkin, 1962). Why a moral judgment? Why not a practical judgment – a consumer choice – by the members of society about what it is worth to reduce the risk of death? Is death so awesome, so frightening, and so remote, that in discussing its economics we must always suppose it is someone *else* who dies?

[. . .] 'For a variety of reasons it is beyond the competence of the economist to assign objective values to the losses suffered under [pain, fear, and suffering].'[1] The same is true of cola and Novocain, one of which puts holes in children's teeth and the other takes the pain out of repairing them. If they were not for sale it would be beyond our competence, as economists, to put an objective value on them, at least until we took the trouble to ask people. Death is indeed different from most consumer events, and its avoidance different from most commodities. There is no sense in being insensitive about something that entails grief, anxiety, frustration, and mystery, as well as economic privation. But people have been dying for as long as they have been living; and where life and death are concerned we are all consumers. We nearly all want our lives extended and are probably willing to pay for it. It is worth while to remind ourselves that the people whose lives may be saved should have something to say about the value of the enterprise and that we analysts, however detached, are not immortal ourselves.

### Individual death and statistical death

[. . .] I am not going to talk about the worth of saving an identified individual's life. Amelia Earhart lost in the Pacific, a score of Illinois coal miners in a collapsed shaft, an astronaut on the tip of a rocket or the little boy with pneumonia awaiting serum sent by dogsled – even the heretofore anonymous victims of a Yugoslavian earthquake – are part of ourselves, not a priceless part but a private part that we value in a different way, not just quantitatively but qualitatively, from the way we measure the incidence of death among a mass of unknown human beings, whether that

1. Reynolds, *op. cit.*

population includes ourselves or not. If we know the people, we care. Half the entertainment industry and most great literature is built on this principle. But our concern in this paper will be statistical lives.

We must recognize, too, that the success of organized society depends on traditions, attitudes, beliefs and rules that may appear extravagant or sentimental to a confirmed materialist (if there is one). The sinking of the Titanic illustrates the point. There were enough lifeboats for first class; steerage was expected to go down with the ship. We do not tolerate that any more. Those who want to risk their lives at sea and cannot afford a safe ship should perhaps not be denied the opportunity to entrust themselves to a cheaper ship without lifeboats; but if some people cannot afford the price of passage with lifeboats, and some people can, they should not travel on the same ship.

[. . .] Most of us have very special feelings about suicide and euthanasia, birth control and abortion, bloodsports and capital punishment, and there is no way to deny these feelings in the interest of 'rationality' without denying most of what makes us human. We go to great lengths to recover dead bodies. We give a firing squad one blank cartridge so that every member can pretend he did not take a life.

Responsibility for death introduces special problems. A man can be sent on a mission or on repeated missions with small probability of survival, but sending a man to certain death is different. The 'chance' makes the difference, apparently because people can hope – the people who go and the people who send them. Guilt is involved; one of the reasons for having a book of rules about when to run the risk and when not to – when to land the disabled aircraft and when to abandon it and take to para-chute – is to relieve the man who gives the orders, the man in the control tower, of personal guilt for the instruction he gives.[2] Safety regulations must be partly oriented toward guilt and responsibility. A window washer may smoke on the job until he gets lung cancer, and it is no concern of his employer; but his safety belt must be in good condition.

To evaluate an individual death requires attention to special feelings. Most of these feelings, though, involve some connection between the person who dies and the person who has the feelings; a marginal change in mortality statistics is unlikely to evoke these

2. This important point was brought to my attention by Jack Carlson, whose Ph.D. thesis (1963) dealt with the subject.

sentiments. Programs that affect death statistically – whether they are safety regulations, programs for health and safety, or systems that ration risk among classes of people – need not evoke these personal, mysterious, superstitious, emotional, or religious qualities of life and death. These programs can probably be evaluated somewhat as we evaluate the commodities we spend our money on.

What is the alternative to death? It depends. For the paralytic it is a life of paralysis; for someone who escapes a highway accident it is the same life as before, unless the near miss changes his behavior. The type of risk that might be reduced is likely to be correlated with age, sex, income level, number of dependents, and life expectancy. Any program that reduces the risk of death will be discriminatory. Infant mortality affects infants and those who have them; motor accidents affect people who use the roads; starvation kills the poor, and a regulation that surrounds swimming pools with fences will affect different age groups according to the height of the fence. Even lightning is not random in its choice of victims; and any analysis that initially ignores the specific group affected has to be adaptable to the specific deaths that would be averted by a given program.

Where does the problem arise? It arises in disease, road accidents, industrial safety, flood control, the armed services, safety regulations, personal protection, and all the things that people do that affect their life expectancy. In the marketplace it arises in the choice of hazardous occupations; in home safety; in residential location and in risky everyday enterprises like diving and swimming. It is often hard to discern, though, or to separate, the things that people do to save their own lives or that governments do to save the lives of citizens, because mortality is so closely correlated with other things that concern people. We eat for satisfaction and avoid starvation, heat our homes to feel warm and avoid pneumonia; we buy fire and police protection to save economic loss, pain, embarrassment and disorder, and in the process reduce the risks of death. When we ride an airplane, death is about the only serious risk that we consider; but if we compare an advanced country with a backward one the difference in safety to life is correlated with so many comforts, amenities, and technological advances that it is hard to sort out life-saving and life-risking components. The impact on life expectancy of, say, the electric light, is so cumulative and indirect that it would hardly be worth sorting out if we could sort it out.

[. . .] Who loses if a death occurs (or has to be anticipated)? First, the person who dies. Exactly what he loses we do not know. But, before it happens, people do not want to die and will go to some expense to avoid death. Beyond the privation that death causes the person who dies there is the fear of death. The anxieties are visible and are real. [. . .] If we ask, who is willing to make an economic sacrifice to prevent a death, in most societies there is at least one unequivocal answer: the person who is to die. By all the standards that economists take seriously, the prospective victim loses.

Second, death is an event – and the prevention of death a consumer good – that in our society inextricably involves the welfare of people close to the person who dies. Death is bereavement and disturbance of integral small societies – families – where people play roles that are often unique and always difficult for others to fill.

Finally, there is 'society' – other people. They can lose money or save as a result of a death with which they have no personal connection. In a few dramatic cases – the inventor of a wonder drug, a poet, statesman, or a particularly predatory criminal – the impact of a death may be out of all proportion to the victim's personal economics – to his earnings, expenditures, taxes, contributions and his exploitation of public programs and facilities. The rest of us, though, are known to the economy mainly by the money we earn and spend and the money that is spent upon us; and an accounting approach will uncover most of the impact.

Death is a comparatively private event. Society may be concerned but is not much affected. There is a social interest in schools and delinquency, discrimination and unrest, infection and pollution, noise and beauty, obscenity and corruption, justice and fair practices, and in the examples men set; but death is usually a very local event. The victim and his family have an intense interest; society may want to take that interest seriously, but it is hard to see that society has a further interest of its own unless, as in military service or public orphanages, there is an acknowledged public responsibility. Society's interest, moreover, may be more in whether reasonable efforts are made to conserve life than in whether those efforts succeed. A missing man has to be searched for, but whether or not he is found is usually of interest – intense interest, to be sure – to a very few.

But the taxes we pay and the school lunches we eat have their impersonal ramifications and can motivate someone else to take an economic interest in our longevity. The accounting for those ramifications is the subject of the next section.

### Economic interest in lost livelihoods

When we consider the cost of a death to society – the costs that might be decreased by a program that reduces deaths – it is as important to discover where the costs fall as to aggregate them. There is a convention that nations are the bases of aggregation, but costs can be local, regional, or national; they can fall on particular sectors of the economy, particular levels of income, particular groups of taxpayers or welfare recipients.

Especially if there is an opportunity to prevent the death – to reduce the incidence of death within some part of the population – there is as much interest in who would have borne the cost of the death as in what the total cost would be. First, interested parties may have to be identified, to persuade them that they should bear the cost of reducing some mortality rate. [. . .] Second, if the losses are to be compensated, their location and size must be known. Third, if a sense of justice or social contract requires that the beneficiaries pay for the benefits, we want to know who benefits.

Someone may care about the effect of a death on the gross national product, though I doubt that anyone cares much. Still, the GNP is so often taken as the thing we care about that at least passing attention should be devoted to the aggregate effect of death and its postponement on the economy.

### *Population economics*

At the GNP level, death is mainly a matter of population economics. There may be scale effects in efficiency or in the provision of public services, but it is hard to tell whether the United States is richer as it becomes more dense and more congested. Military considerations aside, it is not obvious that in a country like this the number of people makes much difference.

If it did, we would probably have a conscious policy of migration. We might also have a conscious policy of family incentives, subsidizing children or taxing their parents. It is hard to escape the conclusion that if people are what we want, programs to reduce mortality are a sluggish way to get them.

A question that has received some attention is how to calculate the worth of a child. There has been some investment in the child and this investment is lost if the child dies. Alternatively, the child will produce income in the future; and his discounted net contribution, positive or negative, goes with him. This is complicated: if he lives he will produce and he will procreate; if he dies he may leave dependents of his own.

I doubt whether this kind of population economics is worth the arithmetic. At best, it is the way a family deals with the loss of a cow, not the loss of a collie. Though children are not pets, in the United States they are more like pets than livestock, and it is doubtful whether the interests of any consumers are represented in a calculation that treats a child like an unfinished building or some expensive goods in process.

## Assessing the costs of a death

If a lonely, self-sufficient hermit dies – a man who pays no taxes, supports no church, is too old for military service and leaves no dependents, owning nothing but a burial plot and a prepaid funeral – there are no costs or benefits. Whatever he would have paid, to make his life safer and to increase his life expectancy, he is dead now and no one knows the difference.

If a Harvard professor dies – a taxpaying man with a family, who contributes to the United Fund and owns twice his salary in life insurance, is eligible for social security and has children who may go to college – the accounting of gains and losses is complicated.

The largest losses will fall on his family, and we should distinguish at once between his life and his livelihood. His family will miss him, and it will miss his earnings. Let us for the moment leave aside the grief, the loneliness, the loss of direction or authority in the family, the emotional privation, and all the things the man represented except his income. The reason for leaving them out at this point is not that they are unmeasurable, or none of our business, but that they are non-transferable and non-marketable, and there is no 'accounting' way to estimate them. For the moment look at the material losses, and get the pure accounting out of the way.

How much of the loss of livelihood falls on the family depends on institutional and market arrangements. In an extremely communal society or an extremely individualist one, there may be a rule or tradition for sharing the loss: orphans may be supported by contributions, rotated among the neighbors, taken in by next of kin, absorbed in a communal orphanage, or otherwise supported at the expense of society at large or of a select responsible group. Alternatively, life insurance may accomplish somewhat the same thing. Whether a 'protective benevolent society' is a genuinely fraternal institution or a modern insurance company with a quaint name, the effect is to share the costs.

It is somewhat arbitrary to say that the cost 'really' falls on the family and the rest is redistribution, or the cost 'really' falls on the committed members of the community, or on the policyholders whose premium payments will reflect the death. The family, the community, and the insurance market are all social institutions characterized by a system of enforceable or honored obligations. The important question is who pays the costs or suffers the losses, not which losses are original and which are transferred.

Life insurance offers a straightforward way of identifying a group of people who have a financial interest in each other's longevity, and to whom the cash value of improved mortality has an unmistakable meaning. (Insurance-company campaigns to keep us from getting fat reflect this interest.) Thus, the extent to which people share the burden of lost livelihoods in society is not altogether determined by social philosophy and legislation but can be determined by individual choices in an organized market where people can hedge against death somewhat the way they can hedge against crop failure, inflation, or fluctuating exchange rates.

### Insurance and national policy

[. . .] If there were a national policy on life insurance, it could be interpreted as a national policy on sharing the financial losses that result from a man's death. (In fact, if there were mandatory life insurance in an amount determined by a man's income, life insurance could almost be dispensed with by merely revising the tax schedules. This is what, to a large extent, is done with retirement insurance.) If that were done, the cost of a man's death to the nation at large would be substantially reflected in the survivor's benefits paid out under the program, plus the lost taxes. [. . .] One who believes instead that insurance is a private matter, not one for national policy or government intrusion, should concern himself with whether the market for life insurance is well organized and consumers are properly knowledgeable, and with how policyholders – the people who pay the premiums that are geared to mortality rates – get their interests represented, or could get their interests represented, in government or private programs that reduce the risk of death.

## Noncontractual claims

[. . .] Less contractual are a variety of claims on relatives, friends and welfare agencies. The family may cease to be a net contributor to a church, possibly become a beneficiary. The children's eventual claims for college scholarships will be enhanced, unless they are obliged to give up college altogether. The United Fund, the Girl Scout Cookie Drive, time volunteered to civic programs, and all the other informal taxes and transfer payments that people participate in, will be affected. These are not trivial: there are crude data to suggest that the impact of voluntary 'social security' and voluntary 'taxes' are at least of the order of magnitude of, say, a fairly progressive state income tax.

It is interesting that some of the claims a man's dependents may make on others are themselves insurable, although brothers apparently do not insure each other's lives to protect themselves against having to care for each other's children at their own expense. Corporations insure the lives of employees, naming the survivors as beneficiaries, partly as a way – I have been told by a corporation executive who dealt with these matters – to minimize their vulnerability to the importunities of a man's dependents – to the claim of a widow, for example, that the corporation ought to give her a job.

## Taxes

Turn now to the real taxes that a man would have paid. These taxes are a man's share in the overhead cost of government, in the provision of public goods and services that are not used up by the taxpayer himself. When a man dies he stops paying his share in the space program, and the rest have to make it up.

The man's taxes are positive or negative according to whether he is a net contributor or a net recipient, and according to how much cost his very presence in society imposes on government. Dead, he won't drive, steal, go to school, or leave unextinguished campfires. (His death can be a gain to federal taxpayers and a loss to his city, or the other way around.)

These costs or losses, positive or negative, due to a man's death, could be approximately offset by replacing the man. In principle, selective immigration might compensate society for the man's death. The main reason why immigration could not in principle handle the problem is that there is one obligation of citizenship that the immigrant is unlikely to assume. That is the family obligation of the man who dies. There have been frontier societies that imported wives, even husbands. But to achieve a genuine economic replacement for the taxpaying father who dies, one would have to find bachelors and widowers seeking ready-made families to marry into; this is undoubtedly asking more than either the free market or individually negotiated immigration could manage. Most income-tax payers probably spend more to support families than to support their government, and that contribution is a hard one to replace.

What are the taxes to be accounted for, and how are they to be accounted for? The man's property taxes can be excluded; the taxes will go on being paid by whoever owns his property – his family or the person who buys his house or automobile. (There will be a slight change of interest to local governments, a tendency for property assessments to change with the turnover of real estate, or for values to be depressed by an increment in the supply of houses – a matter of elasticity estimates, not of accounting.) The issues mainly concern federal and state income taxes, employment taxes, excise and sales taxes, net of the costs of collecting them and net of transfer receipts; and the subject of inquiry is the difference between the taxes (net of transfers) that he and his family would have paid had he not died and the taxes they go on paying, and the man's (or the child's) utilization of government benefits, valued at marginal cost.

The difficult problems relate to the income tax. One set of problems relates to how taxable incomes are; this depends on source of income, the jurisdiction a man lives in, and what constitutes taxable income. Another set relates to the distribution of taxable income in an economy like ours. What happens to taxable income when the Harvard professor dies? Is there merely a subtraction from the tax rolls of one income in a fairly high bracket? Or are there economic laws that impose a shape on the distribution of income independently of who dies? The professor will be replaced by a man who in turn may be replaced by the institution he left to go to Harvard. Even if marginal productivity theory states that the GNP goes down by approximately what the man was being paid, it will not say that taxable income goes down accordingly. If there is a loss to the economy because the man is replaced by a marginally less competent man at the same salary, this would show up as quality depreciation of Harvard's product, and would be of interest to the Internal Revenue Service only as it influences future tax rates.

If one takes the extreme position that the distribution of taxable income is unaffected by the particular incidence of death by tax brackets, the reduction in income tax would be proportionate to the man's income, not to the taxes he paid. Thus, if the Harvard professor has twice the income of a high school teacher and pays four times the income tax, the impact on income tax revenues of his disappearance from the tax base is only twice that of the high school teacher, not four times. The alternative bench mark is the hypothesis that the remaining distribution of income is unchanged – there is just a little nick in the frequency distribution at the income of the man who died, and a little cusp at the new level of income for his family – and everybody else's tax return goes on being just what it would have been. I doubt whether the state of economic analysis permits us to identify which of these two hypotheses is the more plausible or what compromise is most valid.

## Taxes and fiscal policy

To Massachusetts the man's taxes were spendable revenue, just as his contribution to the United Fund was spendable revenue to that organization. State governments cannot engage in functional finance, accommodating fiscal and monetary policies to the tempo of economic activity. National governments can.

It is saving that causes the problem here. If the man and his family always consumed exactly the amount of their income after taxes, the government could marginally adapt to the man's death by reducing expenditure (or raising other people's taxes) in an amount equal to the man's income tax. But if the man saved part of his income, and with the loss of his income there is a reduction in saving, the difference between the decline in (full-employment) GNP and the decline in consumption is greater than the income taxes the man paid.

A reduction of saving due to death need not have an impact different from the reduction in saving due to some economic casualty – loss of a car or loss of a business – or due to any other change in tastes, institutions, or the distribution of income. But that is a topic to be treated by someone else at another time.

### Consumer interest in reduced risk

The avoidance of a particular death – the death of a named individual – cannot be treated straightforwardly as a consumer choice. It involves anxiety and sentiment, guilt and awe, responsibility and religion. If the individuals are identified, there are many of us who cannot even answer whether one should die that two may live. And when half of the children in a hospital ward are to get the serum that may save their lives, half a placebo to help test the serum, the doctor who divides them at random and keeps their identities secret is not exclusively interested in experimental design. He does not want personally to select them or to know who has been selected. But most of this awesomeness disappears when we deal with small increments in a mortality rate in a large population.

Suppose a program to save lives has been identified and we want to know its worth. The dimensions of the risk to be reduced are fairly well known, as is the reduction to be achieved. Suppose also that this risk is small to begin with, not a source of anxiety or guilt.

Surely it is sensible to ask the question: What is it worth to the people who stand to benefit from it? If a scheme can be devised for collecting the cost from them, perhaps in a manner reflecting their relative gains if their benefits are dissimilar, it surely should be their privilege to have the program if they are collectively willing to bear the cost. If they are not willing, perhaps it would be a mistake to ask anybody else to bear the cost for them; they, the beneficiaries, prefer to have the money or some alternative benefits that the money could buy. There are reasons why this argument has to be qualified, but there is no obvious reason why a program that reduces mortality cannot be handled by letting the beneficiaries decide whether it is worth the cost, if the cost falls on them.

There are two main ways of finding out whether some economic benefits are worth the costs. One is to use the price system as a test. It is possible to see what people are willing to pay for the privilege of sitting at tables rather than counters in a restaurant, what they are willing to pay to use library books or to save an elm tree in the front yard. Sometimes the market is poor; sometimes analysis is confused by joint products; sometimes consumer behavior is subject to inertia and the information is needed before the market adjusts. But at least we can try to observe what people will pay for something.

Another way of discovering what the benefits are worth is to ask people. This can be done by election, interview, or questionnaire; the more common way is to let people volunteer the information, through lobby organizations and letters to congressmen or to newspapers.

It is sometimes argued that asking people is a poor way to find out, because they have no incentive to tell the truth. That is an important point, but hardly decisive. It is also argued, and validly, that people are poor at answering hypothetical questions, especially about important events – that the mood and motive of actual choice are hard to simulate. While this argument casts suspicion on what one finds out by asking questions, it casts suspicion too on those market decisions that involve remote and improbable events. Unexpected death has a hypothetical quality whether it is merely being talked about or money is being spent to prevent it. Asked whether he would decline to fly an aircraft that had a statistically higher accident rate than another if it would save an overnight stop, a man may not give the same answer that his actions in the airport would reveal; he still might not feel that his actual decision was authoritative evidence of his values or that, had mood and circumstance been different – even had the amount of time for consultation and decision been different – his action might not have been different too.

Voting behavior is probably to be classed somewhere between a purchase and a questionnaire: an individual's vote is indecisive, while the election as a whole is conclusive.

*Small probability of large events*

[. . .] A difficulty about death, especially a minor risk of death, is that people have to deal with a minute probability of an awesome event, and may be poor at finding a way – by intellect, imagination, or analogy – to explore what the saving is worth to them. This is true whether they are confronted by a questionnaire or a market decision, a survey researcher or a salesman. It may even matter whether the figures are presented to them in percentage terms or as odds and whether charts are drawn on arithmetic or logarithmic scales.

[. . .] What it would be like to grow old without a companion, to rear a family without a mother or father in the house, to endure bereavement, is something that most of us have no direct knowledge of; and those who have some knowledge may not yet know the full effects over time. Many of us think about it only when we make a will or buy life insurance, or witness the bereavement of a friend or neighbor.

As consumers we can investigate the subject but most of us have not investigated; the cost of doing so is high, and there is not much fun in it. Furthermore, this is, more than most decisions, a family one, not an individual one.[3] Nearly every death involves at least two major participants, typically the immediate family. It is not even clear who it is that has the greater stake in a person's not dying – himself, his spouse if he has one, his children if he is a parent, or his parents if he is a child – and the subject is undoubtedly a delicate one for the members of the consuming unit to discuss with each other. Whatever the motives of a respondent when being interviewed alone about a safety program or a hazardous occupation, his motives are surely complex when he talks to his wife about how much he would miss her or she would miss him, the likelihood of a happy remarriage, or which of them would suffer more if one of the children died.

## Death versus anxiety

The problem is even harder if the risk to be attenuated is large enough, or vivid enough, to cause anxiety. In fact, the pain associated with the awareness of risk – with the prospect of death – is probably often commensurate with the costs of death itself. A person who sooner or later must undergo an operation that carries a moderate risk of being fatal will apparently sometimes choose to have the operation now, raising the stakes against himself in the gamble, in order to avoid the suspense. Wives of men in hazardous duty suffer; and most of us have sat beside someone on an airplane who suffered more with anxiety than if he had been drilled by a dentist without Novocain, and who would have paid a fairly handsome price for the Novocain. Let me conjecture that if one among forty men had been mistakenly injected with a substance that would kill him at the end of five years, and the forty were known to the doctor who did not know which among them had the fatal injection, and if the men did not know it yet, the doctor would do more harm by telling them what he had done than he had already done with the injection.

This anxiety is separate from the impact of death itself. It applies equally to those who do not die and to those who do, to people who exaggerate the risk of death as much as if their estimates were true. It counts, and is part of the consumer interest in reducing the risk of death. It is not, or usually not, any kind of double counting to bring it into the calculation. But it is – except

3. The family gets little attention in economics. It is an income-sharing unit, a consumption-sharing unit, and a welfare-sharing unit. That is, they live off the same income, share the same bathroom, and care about each other.

where knowledge of risk permits people to make better economic decisions, or exaggerations of risk lead them to hedge excessively and uneconomically – almost entirely psychic or social. Relief from anxiety is a strange kind of consumer good. What the consumer buys is a state of mind, a picture in his imagination, a sensation. And he must decide to do so by using the same brain that is itself the source of his discomfort or pleasure. However much 'rationality' we impute to our consumer, we must never forget that the one thing he cannot control is his own imagination. (He can try, though; this accounts for the business in tranquilizers, and for the readiness of airlines to serve their passengers alcoholic beverages.)

## Consumer choices and policy decisions

These, then, are some of the reasons why it is hard for our consumer to tell us intelligently what it is worth to him to reduce the risk of death, why it may even be hard to get him to make a proper try. These are also reasons why the consumer may be poor at making ordinary choices about death in the marketplace. He may not do much better in buying life insurance or seat belts, using or avoiding airplanes, flying separately or together with his wife when they leave the children behind, selecting cigarettes with or without filters, driving under the influence of liquor when he could have taken a taxi, or installing a fire alarm over the basement furnace.[4] Some of his marketplace decisions may be more casual (perhaps out of evading his responsibilities, not meeting them) but they may be no better evidence than the answers he would give to questions.

Consumers apparently do often evade these questions when they have a chance. In matters of life and death doctors are not merely operations analysts who formulate the choice for the executive; they are professional decision makers who not only diagnose but decide for the consumer, because they decide with

4. Many parents try not to fly on the same plane (although they usually drive home together on New Year's Eve). I took for granted that this was sensible, though extravagant – until Richard Zeckhauser suggested I think it over. Should one double the risk of losing one parent to eliminate the risk of losing two? I decided then that the answer was hard to be sure of, and probably sensitive to the number of children and their ages, even if only the welfare of the children is taken into account, and more so of course when the parents' welfare is too. (Evidently happily married childless couples should travel on the same plane.) I still do not intend to discuss it with my wife, especially in the presence of the children.

less pain, less regret, cooler nerves, and a mind less flooded with alternating hopes and fears.

Still, in dealing with death-reducing programs, these are the kinds of decisions that somebody has to make. We can do it democratically, by letting the consumers decide for themselves through any of the marketplace or direct-inquiry techniques that we can think of. Or we can do it vicariously, by making some of these highly introspective and imaginative decisions for them, briefing ourselves on the facts as best we can.

If then it turns out that the safety device or health program is a public good and not everybody wants it at the price, or that the tax system will not distribute the costs where the benefits fall, so that we are collectively deciding on a program in which some of us have a strong interest, some a weak interest, and some a negative interest, that makes it rather like any other budgetary decision that the government takes. Divergent interests are almost bound to arise when the decision involves restricting the activities of some people for the safety of others. We need not get all wound up about the 'pricelessness' of human life nor think it strange that the rich will pay more for longevity than the poor, or that the rich prefer programs that help the rich and the poor those that help the poor. There may be good reasons why the poor should not be allowed to fly second-class aircraft that are more dangerous, or people in a hurry should not be allowed to pay a bonus to the pilot who will waive the safety regulations; but these reasons ought to be explicitly adduced as qualifications to a principle that makes economic sense, rather than as 'first principles' that transcend economics.

## Some quantitative determinants

What results should we anticipate? Is there any *a priori* line of reasoning that will help us to establish an order of magnitude, an upper or lower limit, a bench mark, or some ideal accounting magnitude that ought to represent the worth, to a reflective and arithmetically sophisticated consumer, of a reduction in some mortality rate? Is there some good indicator – life insurance, lightning rods, hazardous duty pay – that will give us some basis for estimate? Is there some scale factor, like a person's income, to which the ideal figure should be proportionate or of which it should be some function?

At the outset, we can conjecture that any estimate based on market evidence will at best let us know to within a factor of two or three (perhaps only five or ten) what the reflective individual would decide after thoughtful, intensive inquiry and good professional advice. This conjecture is based on the observation that most of the market decisions people make relate to contingencies for which the probabilities themselves are ill-known to the consumer, sometimes barely available to the person who seeks statistics, invariably applicable in only rough degree, and mixed with joint products that make the evidence ambiguous. What will somebody pay for a babysitter who, in case of fire, will probably save the children or some of them? With a little research one can find out the likelihood of fire or other catastrophe during the time that one is away from home, the likelihood that they would be saved if a babysitter were on guard, and the likelihood that they would save themselves or otherwise be saved if no one were home. It would take a good deal more research to relate this to the age and type of furnace, the shape and composition of the house and the location of roofs and windows, the performance of babysitters of different ages and sexes, the ages and personalities of the children, the season of the year, the quality of the fire department, the alertness of neighbors, and the hour of day or night that one is going to be away. The evidential value of this 'market test' will barely give us an estimate to within a factor of two or three.

*Worth as a function of income*

Is there some expectable or rational relation between what a man earns and what he would spend, or willingly be taxed, to increase the likelihood of his own survival or the survival of one of his family? Specifically, is there any close accounting connection between what he might spend and what he can hope to earn in the future, or what he owns?

So many examinations of the worth of saving life are concerned with the fraction of a man's income that he in some way contributes, that there may be a presumption that the outside limit of the worth of saving his life is the entirety of his expected future earnings. It does seem that if we ask ourselves the worth of saving somebody else's life, and he is somebody who personally makes no difference to us, his net contribution to total production may be the outside limit to what we can interest ourselves in. But when we ask the question, what is it worth to him to increase the likelihood of his own survival (or to us, our own survival), it is hard to see that his (our) future lifetime earnings provide either an upper or lower limit.

I am not saying that a man's expected lifetime income is irrelevant to an estimate of what he would pay to reduce fatalities in his age group. But discounted lifetime earnings are relevant only in the way that they are relevant to ordinary decisions about consumption, saving, quitting a job or buying a house. They are part of the income and wealth data that go into the decisions. Their connection is a functional one, not an accounting one. What a man would pay to avoid death, to avoid pain, or to modernize his kitchen, is a function of present and future income but need bear no particular adding-up relation.[5]

Let me guess. If we ask what it is worth to them to reduce by a certain number of percentage points, over some period, the likelihood that they will die, they will find it worth more than that percentage of the discounted value of their expected lifetime income. Arithmetically, if we tell a man that the likelihood of his accidental death over the next three years is 9 per cent and we can reduce this to 6 per cent by some measure we propose, and ask him what it is worth to reduce the probability of his death by 3 per cent over this period (with no change in his mortality table after that period), my conjecture is it is worth to him a permanent reduction of perhaps 5 per cent, possibly 10 per cent, in his income.

This is conjecture. The reader can determine what his own answer would be.

### Death itself versus anxiety

It is important to make the distinction mentioned earlier between death itself and anxiety about death. If one asks what it is worth to eliminate the fatality of certain childhood diseases he may discover that he is as preoccupied with the anxiety that goes with the risk as with the low-probability event itself.

A special difficulty of evaluating the anxiety and the event together is that they probably do not occur in fixed proportions. To

5. People get hung up, sometimes, on the apparent anomaly that if a man would yield 2 per cent of his income to eliminate a 1 per cent risk of death, he'd have to give up twice his entire income to save his own life – which he cannot do if his creditors are on their toes. But he doesn't have to. I'd pay my dentist an hour's income to avoid a minute's intense pain – even to prevent somebody else's pain – without having to know what I'd do if confronted with a lifetime of intense pain. This is why the worth of saving a life is but a mathematical construct when applied to an individual's decision on the reduction of small risks; it has literal meaning only if we mean that a hundred men would give up the equivalent of two incomes to save one (unidentified) life among them.

be specific, there are good reasons for considering the worth of risk-reduction to be proportionate to the absolute reduction of risk, for considering a reduction from 10 per cent to 9 per cent about equivalent to a reduction from 5 per cent to 4 per cent. There is no reason for the anxiety to follow any such rational rule. Even a cool-headed consumer who rationally examines his own or his family's anxiety will probably have to recognize that anxiety and obsession are psychological phenomena that cannot be brought under any such rational control. If they could be, through an act of judgment, an act of self-hypnosis, a ban on disquieting conversations, or the avoidance of factual and fictional stimuli, through surgery or through drugs, the anxiety could perhaps be wholly disposed of. A family that lives with a 'high' low probability of death in the family, high enough to cause anxiety but low enough to make it unlikely, may benefit as much from relief as from longevity if the risk can be eliminated.

The anxiety may depend on the absolute level of risk and the frequency and vividness of stimuli. There may be thresholds below which the risk is ignored and above which it is a pre-occupation. It may depend on whether the risk is routine and continuous or concentrated in episodes. It undoubtedly depends on what people believe about risks, and has no direct connection with what the risks truly are. The existence of one source of risk may affect the psychological reaction to another source of risk. Furthermore, the anxiety will be related to the duration of suspense and can even be inversely correlated with the risk of death itself.

In other words, a rational calculus of risks and values will be pertinent – not compelling, but pertinent – to the avoidance of the event of death, but may have little relevance to choices involving fear, anxiety, and relief. People may, however, by engaging in enough sophisticated analysis of risk, change their sensitivity to the perception of risk, possibly but not surely bringing the discomfort into a more nearly proportionate relation to the risk itself.

*Scaling of risks*

[. . .] There is a good case, though not necessarily persuasive, for scaling risks. It is illustrated as follows.[6] A person is asked what risk of death is equivalent to certain blindness – at what risk of

6. The 'scaling' principle sketched here follows from modern decision (utility) theory as presented in R. D. Luce and H. Raiffa (1957, pp. 23–31), and especially reflects the authors' assumptions $\neq$ 4 (substitutability) and

death he would prefer certain blindness, at what risk of death he would rather run the risk than be surely blind – and his point of indifference between the two is found. Since this is a decision that can arise, it is presumed that a man can answer the question – not offhand, but after some study and advice. Suppose he says that certain blindness balances out at about 1/10 chance of death; he would run the risk of death to avoid blindness if it were less than 1/10, not if it were more than 1/10. He is then informed that a 1/10 chance of blindness must be equivalent to 1 chance in 100 of death. If he denies this, insisting that what holds for large probabilities does not hold for small ones, or that certainty is different from risk, the first question is rephrased as follows: If he had to choose between pure blindness and some risk of death, what risk of death would be equivalent to certain blindness. He may say he does not know and cannot find out because a hypothetical question will not motivate a meaningful answer. To make it meaningful, he is told that it may be necessary to incur some fatal risk to avoid blindness; there is, for instance, a surgical operation that cures certain kinds of blindness but involves a certain risk of death; there is some likelihood that this person will prove upon further diagnosis to be faced with that choice and he must make his decision now in case the contingency arises. If he can answer this contingent question – if he can say for the event that he must choose between certain blindness and some risk of death, an event with a yet unspecified probability, what risk of death he is just willing to incur to avoid otherwise certain blindness – then he has in effect chosen between some (unspecified) probability of blindness and a probability of death equal to that same probability multiplied by the contingent risk he said he was just willing to incur. He is now told that there is a 50:50 chance, or

---

≠ 2 (reduction of compound lotteries). It is consistent with the conclusions reached by A. A. Alchian (1953, pp. 26–50, especially p. 43). It can be simply construed from the 'sure-thing' principle of L. Savage (1954, pp. 21 ff). It is being used here, though, to cover an irreversibility in the 'continuity' assumption (≠ 3) of Luce and Raiffa. That continuity assumption implies that the certainty of any finite loss of income is equivalent to some probability of death; it does not say that the consumer can identify some finite loss of income, the certainty of which is equivalent to some specified probability of death. If, though, he can identify a loss of income the certainty of which is equivalent to some specified probability of some specified larger loss of income, it may be possible to fill in these gaps in the consumers' utility map. Thus we have a technique for making roundabout comparisons when the individual is unable to make a direct comparison. It may or may not be helpful.

that there is 1 chance in 20, that the diagnosis will make his contingent answer relevant; if he lets his answer stand, he has, in effect, stated his indifference between a 0·5 chance of blindness and a 0·05 chance of death, and also between a 0·05 chance of blindness and a 0·005 chance of death.

The argument may not be compelling, but it helps in establishing at least a presumption in favor of a scaling principle that, at first glance, might have appeared implausible.

What has been said about anxiety, though, could interfere. It will probably not interfere much if the outcome is to be known soon; the discomfort of suspense probably depends on the duration, and ought to be negligible if the man will know the outcome the next day. It could be considerable if he will not know for a year or two and if he cannot keep his family from knowing the kind of risk he has accepted.

*An illustrative application*

Imperfect as it is, this argument can be a tool for helping some people think about unfamiliar probabilities. A man who cannot come to grips with 1 chance in 1000 of death may be able to come to grips with 1 chance in 10, or vice versa. He is asked, for example, what reduction in income after taxes he would incur in perpetuity to avoid a 10 per cent chance of death (his own or somebody's he cares about). Suppose he says that he will give up one third of his income to avoid an immediate 10 per cent chance of dying. How can it be calculated from this what he might give up to avoid 1 chance in 1000 of dying? Rather, how can he tell from the answer he has given what his answer ought to be to the question containing the 0·001 risk? Dividing both figures by 100, he would give 1/300 of his income. But if successive increments of income lost are of progressively larger concern to a man, a loss of 0·33 per cent of income will not look one hundredth as bad to him as the loss of 33 per cent of his income. He might, however, be asked what fraction of his income he would give up to avoid a one tenth chance of losing one third of his income. This is an ordinary insurance decision, which he can presumably make (and he may be expected to give an answer that exceeds one thirtieth of his income). The process could be repeated for a one hundredth chance of losing a third of his income, but possibly it is not necessary when it is a question of dealing with increments on the order of a few per cent. Suppose he says that he would give up 5 per cent of his income to avoid a 1/10 chance of losing 33 per cent. Is he willing to give up about 0·5 per cent to avoid a 10 per cent chance of losing 5 per cent? Not exactly; he may say approximately, perhaps somewhat more – say 0·6 per cent. There is now a series of statements about bets he would place, suggesting that he considers the loss of 0·6 per cent of his income (after taxes) in perpetuity about equivalent to 1 chance in 1000 of immediate death.[7]

Let it be assumed that the man is in his early forties, with expected lifetime earnings to accrue on a rising scale over twenty-five more years. Discounting this income at something like the mortgage rate of interest – lower than the rate on consumer credit, higher than the earnings on conservative retirement plans, say 7 per cent – its capitalized value would be about ten times a year's income; 0·6 per cent of that is about 6 per cent of a year's income.

If similar answers were obtained from 1000 men of similar incomes and ages, it could be concluded that they would together rather give up the equivalent of six discounted lifetime incomes than suffer one immediate accidental death. In the age group of our man, that turns out to be about sixty annual incomes. Does this look high? Does it look low? It is up to the reader what figure he finds plausible. (It is up to the reader both as an analytical reader and as a consumer of life-saving programs.) It is also up to the reader whether it is of any help to break the decision into a series of comparisons like this.

Turn the choice around and ask the man what compensation he demands for running some additional risk. Should there be, for small increments, the same figure of worth? Would he run an additional chance in a thousand for a bonus equal to 6 per cent of a year's income? Should the answer be symmetrical? Probably not for the anxiety, not for the superstitious element in gambling, not for any special sense of regret that might ensue if the death could actually be identified – in case it occurred – with his choice to incur it. Otherwise, although symmetry cannot be demanded, it should probably be treated as one more test.

As a check the sample of a thousand men could be asked whether they would in the end rather take the cash as compensation. Rather than pay six lifetime incomes in total to avert one death among the thousand, might they prefer to run the risk and put the proceeds into life insurance? That would compensate the bereaved family with a sixfold rise in its income.

7. This technique, whatever its strengths and weaknesses, does *not* treat the marginal utility of income as constant. It never 'scales' income, or any other quantitative variable except pure probabilities.

Or they might want to split the difference: to pay half the price they originally decided on, leave the risk intact, and triple the income of the family of the man who dies. If so, their best buy is life insurance; they gave a wrong answer in haste, and the exercise should be repeated. (If they retort that they are already insured up to that level, the inference is that their original answer was a financial calculation of what it was worth to save the cost of insurance.)

Is there some level of adequate compensation for the family? It is distasteful to ask how much monetary compensation a family needs in order to suffer no long-term loss in welfare when a member of the family dies; and an answer that makes a person priceless cannot be rejected.

[. . .] But a person can run a risk for cash. And he may prefer, if he runs the risk, to trade the cash for some still larger amount invested in life insurance, that is, for a greater 'expected value' correlated with death itself. If so, compensation tends to be commensurable with life-saving at the margin of small risks, and provides a helpful check on the consistency of a series of choices. Both introspectively and in conversation I have been surprised, in writing this paper, at how far life insurance can go toward meeting the demand of middle-aged fathers, after some sustained reflection, for their own mortality reduction.

## Discriminating for wealth

A special matter of policy is bound to arise here. If a government is to initiate programs that may save the lives of the poor or the rich, is it worth more to save the rich than to save the poor? The answer is evidently yes if the question means, is it worth more to the rich to reduce the risk to their own lives than it is to the poor to reduce the risk to their own lives. Just as the rich will pay more to avoid wasting an hour in traffic or five hours on a train, it is worth more to them to reduce the risk of their own death or the death of somebody they care about. It is worth more because they are richer than the poor. A hospital that can save either of two lives, but not both, has no reason to save the richer of the two on these grounds; but an expensive athletic club can afford better safety equipment than a cheap gymnasium; the rich can afford safer stoves in their homes than the poor; and a rich country can spend more to save lives than a poor one.

## Other members of the family

Most of this discussion has been focused on the man who earns a living for his family. To deal comprehensively with the subject, the problem should be recalculated from his point of view, but putting wife or child at risk, and from his wife's point of view putting her own life or one of the children's at risk. (To get a proper feel for the subject, the children might be given a chance to express their views; their immaturity should not offhand make what they say irrelevant.)

There is a qualification about families and children: the values placed on lives by members of the family, as well as the costs to society involved in somebody's death, are not additive, within the family. If death takes a mother, a father, and two children, each from a different family, the consequences are different from the death of a family of four in a single accident. This is true both of the costs to society, because of the differential impact of dependents' care, and of the personal valuations within the family. If a family of four *must* fly, and has a choice among four aircraft of which it is known that one is somewhat defective but not known which one it is, it should be possible to persuade them to fly together. 'Society's' interest, in support of the family's interest, should be to see that they are permitted to. Society's economic interest in this case will usually coincide.

## Conclusion

We have looked now at several ways to approach the worth of saving a statistical life. We have had to distinguish between the life and the livelihood that goes with it. We have had to distinguish between the loss of that livelihood to the consuming unit – the family – and the loss of the share that went to other members of the economy – the taxpayers, insurance policyholders, and kin. We have considered some of the ways that reduction of the risk of death differs from other commodities and services that consumers buy.

To recapitulate:

1. Death is an awesome and indivisible event that goes but once to a customer in a single large size.

2. For many people it is a low-probability event except on special occasions when the momentary likelihood becomes serious.

3. Its effect on a family is something that many consumers have little direct acquaintance with.

4. In an already advanced economy many of the ways of reducing the risk of death are necessarily public programs, budgetary or regulatory.

5. Reduction of risk is often a by-product of other programs that lead to health, comfort, or the security of property, though there are some identifiable programs of which the saving of lives is the main result.

6. Death is an insurable event.

7. Death is more of a family event than most other casualties that one might like to avert; its analysis requires more than perfunctory recognition that the family is the consuming unit, the income-sharing unit, and the welfare-sharing unit.

Still, though these characteristics are important, they do not necessarily make the avoidance of death a wholly different kind of objective from others to promote the general welfare. While it is important to be aware of how the avoidance of death differs from other programs, it is equally important to keep in mind in what respects it is similar. Society may indeed sometimes express its profoundest moral values in the way it deals with life and death, but in a good many programs to reduce fatalities society merely expresses the amount of trouble people will go to, or the money people will spend, to reduce the risks they run. There is enough mystery already about death, not to exaggerate the mystery.

[. . .] The difficult part of the problem is not evaluating the worth of a man's livelihood to the different people who have an interest in it, but the worth of his life to himself or to whoever will pay to prolong it. This is what is not insurable in terms that permit replacement. This is the consumer interest in a unique and irreplaceable good. His livelihood he can usually insure, not exactly but approximately, sharing the loss and making it a matter of diffuse economic interest; it is valuing his life that poses the problem.

And the difficulty is not just that, as with so many government budgetary and regulatory programs, the government has to weigh the divergent interests of various beneficiaries and taxpayers. Nor is it that, as with so many government programs, the government has to investigate how much the program is worth to people. The main problem is that people have difficulty knowing what it is worth to themselves, cannot easily answer questions about it, and may object to being asked. Market evidence is unlikely to reveal much.

Dealing with small changes in small risks makes the evaluation more casual and takes the pricelessness and the pretentiousness out of a potentially awesome choice. The question is whether the consumer, at this more casual level of straightforward risk reduction, has any sovereign tastes (or thinks he has) and can be induced to place his bets as calmly as he would fasten a seat belt or buy a lock for his door.

[. . .] In the end there may be a philosophical question whether government should try to adapt itself to what consumer tastes would be if the consumers could be induced to have those tastes and to articulate them. There may be a strong temptation to do the consumer's thinking for him and to come out with a different answer. Should one try to be guided by what the consumer would choose, when in fact the consumer may refuse to make the choice at all? If a doctor is asked to make a grave medical decision that a patient, or a patient's spouse, declines to make for himself, is the doctor supposed to guess what the patient, or the patient's spouse, would have decided if he'd had to decide for himself? Or is the doctor to decide as he thinks he would himself decide if he were in the patient's position. Or is he to make a welfare decision for the whole family or some other small society? Should the doctor ask the patient which among these criteria he wants the doctor to use, or does that merely upset the patient and lead to the doctor's having to decide how to decide on the criterion?

The gravity of decisions about life-saving can be dispelled by letting the consumer (taxpayer, lobbyist, questionnaire respondent) express himself on the comparatively unexciting subject of small increments in small risks, acting as though he has preferences even if in fact he does not. People do it for life insurance; they could do it for life-saving. The fact that they may not do it well, or may not quite know what they are doing as they make the decision, may not bother them and need not disfranchise them in the exercise of consumer-taxpayer sovereignty.

As an economist I have to keep reminding myself that consumer sovereignty is not just a metaphor and is not justified solely by reference to the unseen hand. It derives with even greater authority from another principle of about the same vintage, 'no taxation without representation'. Welfare economics establishes the convenience of consumer sovereignty and its compatibility with economic efficiency; the sovereignty itself is typically established by arms, martyrdom, boycott, or some principles held to be self-evident. And it includes the inalienable right of the consumer to make his own mistakes.

## References

ALCHIAN, A. A. (1953), 'The meaning of utility measurement', *Amer. Econ. Rev.*, March.

CARLSON, J. (1963), 'Valuation of life saving', Ph.D. thesis, Harvard University.

LUCE, R. D., and RAIFFA, H. (1957), *Games and Decisions: Introduction and Critical Survey*, John Wiley.

MUSHKIN, S. J. (1962), 'Health as an investment', *J. of Pol. Econ.*, Supplement, October, p. 156.

REYNOLDS, D. J. (1956), 'The cost of road accidents', *Journal of The Royal Statistical Society*, pp. 393–408.

SAVAGE, L. J. (1954), *The Foundations of Statistics*, John Wiley.

# 13  Michael Jones-Lee

Revealed Preferences and the Value of a Life

Michael Jones-Lee, 'Valuation of reduction in probability of death by road accident', *Journal of Transport Economics and Policy*, vol. 3, 1969, pp. 37–47.

In a recent paper Schelling suggests that 'There is no reason to suppose that a man's future earnings discounted in any pertinent fashion bear any particular relation to what he would pay to reduce some likelihood of his own death' (1968, and Reading 12).

The purpose of this paper is to show that, given certain assumptions about human preferences, one can measure the money value which an individual places upon a given reduction of the probability of his own death by road accident (or by any other cause). Since avoidance of certain death by road accident is simply the case in which the probability is reduced from one to zero, the value placed by an individual upon the avoidance of his own certain death by road accident may also be computed as a special case.

Information on private valuations can be useful in determining the public valuation of avoidance of death by road accident. Clearly the public valuation may be influenced by the public decision-maker's ethical predispositions; nevertheless, some notion of the values placed by individuals on specified reductions in the probability of their own death by road accident would be a valuable guide for public policy.

This paper is based upon the simple notion that all individuals prefer a lower to a higher probability of death by road accident and would be prepared to forfeit various combinations of income and leisure to reduce this probability by some given amount.

It might be objected that attempts to induce the individual to reveal his preferences would encounter the traditional 'public goods problem' (Musgrave, 1959), since safe roads once constructed do, by and large, afford 'safety' to all who use them. It may be possible, however, to induce individuals to reveal their preferences in the comparatively abstracted context of a Von Neumann–Morgenstern experiment. (Von Neumann–Morgenstern techniques are particularly suited to an analysis of this kind. If one is prepared to assume that the individuals involved obey the $N.M$ behaviour axioms concerning choice under conditions of risk, then a correct ranking of preferences amongst alternatives, each of which is described by a probability distribution of outcomes, is given by the mathematical expectation of $N.M$ utility for each alternative. Before the expectations operation can be performed, however, it is necessary to determine the $N.M$ utility index of each outcome in the probability distribution, and for this purpose we require an experimental procedure of the type described in the third section below.)

Private valuations are influenced by the prevailing distribution of income. Since the exercise is intended only as a guide to public decision-making and as an attempt to reduce the need for subjective value judgements, the distribution of income is taken as given.

### Assumptions and definitions

The following assumptions and definitions are used:

1. The term 'income' refers to a constant annual income having a present value, taken over expected life-span, equal to the present value of the individual's anticipated lifetime stream of income.[1]

2. The value which any individual places upon the permanent reduction in the probability of his own death by road accident from $p_1$ to $p_2$ $(p_1 > p_2)$ is the present value, taken over expected life span, of the difference between the maximum amount of income he would forego to reduce the probability from $p_1$ to zero and the maximum amount of income he would forego to reduce the probability from $p_2$ to zero.

The value which the individual places upon avoidance of his own certain death by road accident (defined as the maximum sum he would pay to avoid such a death) is simply the special case of the 'probability reduction value' in which $p_1 = 1$ and $p_2 = 0$.

3. All individuals are 'price takers' with respect to the rate[2] at

1. That is, $Y\left(\dfrac{1-(1+r)^{-n}}{r}\right) = \sum_{t=1}^{n} \dfrac{E_t}{(1+r)^t}$

where $Y$ = income
$\quad n$ = expected life-span
$\quad r$ = private time preference rate
$\quad E_t$ = expected income in year $t$

2. In the following pages this is referred to loosely as 'wage-rate'.

which they may transform leisure into income, and are completely free to decide upon the proportion of total time to be devoted to earning at this rate.[3]

4. All individuals satisfy the Von Neumann–Morgenstern behaviour axioms. Thus if we write the utility index of a situation in which the individual enjoys an income–leisure level $(Y, L)$ with death by road accident $(DR)$ a possible outcome with probability $p$ of occurrence, as:

$U[p : (DR), (Y, L]$,

then we have:

$U[p : (DR), (Y, L)] = p\ U(DR) + (1-p)\ U\ (Y, L)$

where      $U(DR) = N.M$ utility index of death by road accident

           $U(Y, L) = N.M$ utility index of income – leisure level $(Y, L)$ with no possibility of death by road accident

           $Y = $ income

           $L = $ leisure

Consider $U(Y, L)$ for various levels of $Y$ and $L$. The income-leisure utility function $U(Y, L) = f(Y, L)$ describes the individual's preferences in income and leisure when he faces a given set of prices and methods of use of leisure time. If the worst outcome which the individual contemplates is a slow death (which we assume will result from either income below some subsistence level and/or leisure time below some subsistence level), and more income and leisure are preferred to less, then we can place the following restriction upon the form of the utility function

$U(DS) = f(Y, l) = f(y, L)$

$$\frac{\partial f}{\partial Y} > 0\ , \frac{\partial f}{\partial L} > 0 \text{ for } L > l \text{ and } Y > y$$

$$\frac{\partial f}{\partial Y} = 0\ , \frac{\partial f}{\partial L} = 0 \text{ for } L < l \text{ or } Y < y$$

$U(DS) = N.M$ utility index of death by starvation or exhaustion

       $y = $ subsistence income

       $l = $ subsistence leisure.

If the utility function displays diminishing marginal utility of income and leisure, the utility of income schedules will have the general form shown in Figure 1.

3. We assume that all income is derived from wages and salaries: modification to include interest income would be relatively straightforward.

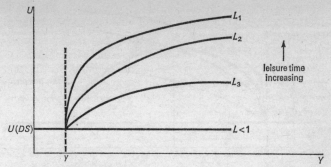

Figure 1  Utility of income schedules for zero probability of death by road accident, i.e. $U = f(Y,L)$

Now consider the wage rate constraint: denote the income level attainable for lesiure time $L_n$ as $Y_n$. We then have:

$$Y_n = (T - L_n)r$$

where $T$ is total time available to the individual for work or leisure and $r$ is the wage rate.

$$\text{Hence } L_n = \left(T - \frac{Y_n}{r}\right)$$

$$\text{and} \quad U(Y_n, L_n) = f\left(Y_n, \left(T - \frac{Y_n}{r}\right)\right)$$

$$\text{or} \quad U(Y_n, L_n) = \varnothing\,(Y_n)$$

describe the utility indices attainable within the total time and wage rate constraints. They may be regarded as the boundary of attainable utility indices, and may be superimposed on the curves of Figure 1 as shown in Figure 2.

$Y^*$ and $L^*$ represent the optimal income–leisure choice for the individual and $U(Y^*L^*)$ the optimal income–leisure choice utility index if death by road accident has zero probability of occurrence.

$Y_{T-L}$ is the maximum income which could be earned consistent with avoidance of death by fatigue.

$Y_T$ is the total income which could be earned if all available time were devoted to work.

### Value of reduction in probability of death by road accident

If the individual is subject to a probability $p$ of death by road accident for all income–leisure levels, his optimal income–leisure choice yields a utility level $U[p:(DR),(Y^*L^*)]$ given by

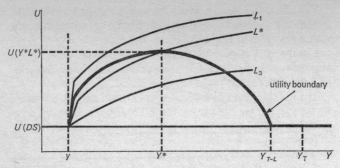

Figure 2 Utility boundary given by wage rate and total time constraints

$$U[p : (DR), (Y^*L^*)] = p\ U(DR) + (1-p)\ U(Y^*L^*)$$

Hence if $U(Y^*L^*) > U(DR)$, then

$$U[p : (DR), (Y^*L^*)] < U(Y^*L^*) \text{ for } p > 0$$

Now let us define $\bar{Y}_n$ as that level of income which, in conjunction with leisure $L_n$ and zero probability of death by road accident, is such that the individual is indifferent between it and his optimal income–leisure choice with death by road accident a possibility with probability $p$ of occurrence. For any given value of $p$ there is clearly a unique relationship between $\bar{Y}_n$ and $L_n$ given by

$$U[p : (DR), (Y^*, L^*)] = f(\bar{Y}_n, Ln).$$

Values of $\bar{Y}_n$ corresponding to various value of $L_n$ are shown in Figure 3 as the intersection of the $U[p : (DR), (Y^*L^*)]$ co-ordinate with utility of income curves within the utility boundary.[4]

Hence for leisure time $L^*$ the individual would be prepared to give up income $(Y^* - \bar{Y}^*)$ to reduce the probability of death by road accident from $p$ to zero. At leisure time $L_4$ he would be prepared to give up $(Y_4 - \bar{Y}_4)$. In general for leisure time $L_n$ he will be prepared to give up $(Y_n - \bar{Y}_n)$. Thus if the individual reduces leisure time from $L^*$ to $L_n$, increasing income from $Y^*$ to $Y_n$, and then forfeits income $(Y_n - \bar{Y}_n)$, he will be indifferent between his final position with zero probability of death by road accident and the situation in which his income–leisure level is $(Y^*L^*)$ but with probability $p$ of death by road accident.

4. Notice that a different value of $U[p : (DR); (Y^*L^*)]$ and hence a different set of $(\bar{Y}_n, L_n)$ combinations of income and leisure correspond to each value of $p$.

The maximum income which he would forego to reduce the probability of death by road accident from $p$ to zero is, then, the maximum value of $(Y_n - \bar{Y}_n)$.

Clearly, if it is possible to estimate maximum $(Y_n - \bar{Y}_n)$ for various values of $p$, then it is also possible to estimate the value of a reduction in the probability $p$.

The utility of income schedules and $U(DR)$ may be estimated by the appropriate $N.M$ experiment. Thus, given $p$, we can compute $U[p : (DR), (Y^*L^*)]$ and hence various values of $(Y_n - \bar{Y}_n)$. A tedious search for the maximum $(Y_n - \bar{Y}_n)$ may be avoided if we consider the first order conditions for a maximum

$$\frac{d(Y_n - \bar{Y}_n)}{dY_n} = 0$$

i.e. $\quad 1 - \dfrac{d\bar{Y}_n}{dY_n} = 0$

or $\quad 1 - \dfrac{d\bar{Y}_n}{dL_n} \cdot \dfrac{dL_n}{dY_n} = 0$

or $\quad \dfrac{d\bar{Y}_n}{dL_n} = -r$ .

Since, given $p$, values of $\bar{Y}_n$ are determined by the intersection of income utility schedules with the $U[p : (DR), (Y^*L^*)]$ coordinate (see Figure 3), the first order condition is (approximately) satisfied where a unit increment in $L_n$ yields a decrease in $\bar{Y}_n$ equal to the wage rate.

The second order condition for a maximum is:

$$\frac{d^2(Y_n - \bar{Y}_n)}{dY_n^2} < 0$$

or $\quad \dfrac{1}{r^2} \dfrac{d^2\bar{Y}_n}{dL_n^2} < 0$

or $\quad \dfrac{d^2\bar{Y}_n}{dL_n^2} < 0$ .

This condition is satisfied if, as is assumed, the utility function displays a diminishing marginal rate of substitution of income for leisure. (The analysis could be made purely positive at this stage by assumptions concerning the form of the utility of income and leisure schedules. It is shown in the Appendix that no more than diminishing marginal utility of income and leisure are required for an upward sloping 'maximum $(Y_n - \bar{Y}_n)$ vs $p$' relationship. Presumably stronger assumptions concerning second partial

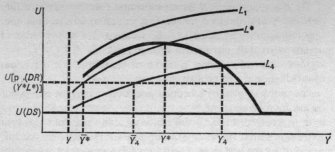

Figure 3

derivatives of the utility function would yield further results of a less obvious nature.) Hence,

if $\quad p = p_1$ yields maximum $(Y_n - \bar{Y}_n) = V_1$

and $\quad p = p_2$ yields maximum $(Y_n - \bar{Y}_n) = V_2$,

then the value of reduction from $p_1$ to $p_2$ is, by previous definition, the present value of $(V_1 - V_2)$ arising annually over the individual's expected life span.

If $p = 1$ then the maximum value of $(Y_n - \bar{Y}_n)$, for this value of $p$, is the sum which the individual would pay to avoid certain death by road accident. That is,

$$p = 1 \text{ yields maximum } (Y_n - \bar{Y}_n) = V_1$$

and $\quad p = 0$ yields maximum $(Y_n - \bar{Y}_n) = 0$

then $\quad (V_1 - V_2) = V_1$.

## The estimation procedure

(All income levels are net of tax.)

As an example of the computational procedure the suggested analysis was carried out for a university lecturer aged thirty.[5] Assuming a life span of seventy-five years, a typical lifetime stream of earnings, a private time preference rate of 5 per cent and an average working week of 40 hours, the deduced value of $r$ was £5500 p.a.[6]

5. Not the author!

6. This is the notional income this individual could earn if he devoted 24 hrs/day to earning. The notion of a constant opportunity cost of leisure for this type of profession is certainly dubious. We make the assumption largely for illustrative purposes.

By the appropriate $N$–$M$ experiments a set of income utility schedules was obtained for various values of leisure time with zero probability of death by road accident. The utility index of death by road accident was also estimated.

With this information a curve of maximum $(Y_n - \bar{Y}_n)$ was plotted against probability of death by road accident. Hence values were obtained for various reductions in the probability of death by road accident.

Essentially, estimation of the income utility schedules involved offering the individual a series of choices between, on the one hand, the certainty of relatively frugal income-leisure levels with zero probability of death by road accident and, on the other hand, a gamble involving two extreme outcomes (death by starvation and an income–leisure level of (£20,000 p.a., 24 hrs/day) with zero probability of death by road accident). By assigning arbitrary utility indices to the extreme outcomes in the gamble and by determining the odds[7] in the gamble which would just induce the individual to choose the gamble in preference to the certainty alternatives (see Table 1), it was possible to compute utility indices for the latter.

For example: Let $U(DS) = \theta$

$U(£20,000 \text{ p.a., } 24 \text{ hrs/day}) = \varphi$

Then for income–leisure level $(Y, L)$ determine $p$ such that the individual is indifferent between gamble $[p : (DS), (£20,000 \text{ p.a.,} 24 \text{ hrs/day})]$ and $(Y, L)$ with certainty.

Then $U(Y, L)$ is given by

$U(Y, L) = p\theta + (1-p)\varphi$

A utility index for death by road accident (presumably not generally equal to $U(DS)$, since a quick death is generally preferred to a slow death) was then estimated by inserting death by road accident in the gamble instead of death by starvation and determining the odds at which the individual was indifferent between the new gamble and some income-leisure level for which the utility index had already been estimated.

For example, for income–leisure level $(Y, L)$ of (known) utility

7. Probabilities were determined by asking the individual to decide upon the number of white counters to be included in a bag containing 10 black counters which would just induce him to take the gamble if drawing a black counter from the bag implied the death outcome while drawing a white counter implied the (£20,000 p.a., 24 hrs/day) outcome.

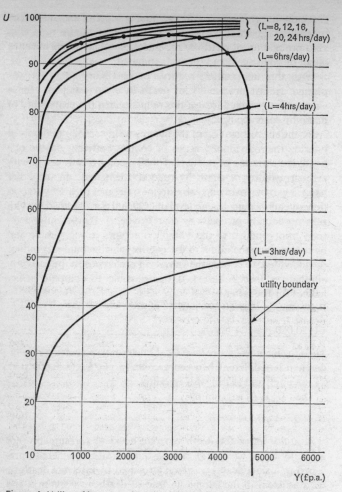

Figure 4 Utility of income schedules (plotted from *N-M* experiment data)

index $U(Y, L)$ determine $p$ such that the individual is indifferent between gamble $[p : (DR), (£20,000 \text{ p.a.}, 24 \text{ hrs/day})]$ and $(Y, L)$ with certainty. Then $U(DR)$ is given by:

$$U(Y, L) = p\, U(DR) + (1-p)\, \varphi$$

The individual concerned believed that subsistence income was of the order of £50 p.a. and subsistence leisure about 3 hrs/day.

The medical profession could, no doubt, supply more definitive information on this subject.

Values of $U[p : (DR), (Y^*L^*)]$ were then computed for various values of $p$ (Table 2) and these, in conjunction with the utility of income schedules plotted from the data in Table 1, were used to estimate maximum $(Y_n - \bar{Y}_n)$ for each value of $p$ (Table 3).

Suppose we wish to know the value, to this individual, of reduction in probability of death by road accident from 0·2 to 0·1. From the 'max. $(Y_n - \bar{Y}_n)$ vs. $p$' curve we have:

$p = 0·1$, maximum $(Y_n - \bar{Y}_n) = £2900$

$p = 0·2$, maximum $(Y_n - \bar{Y}_n) = £3500$

Hence value of reduction in probability from 0·2 to 0·1 is given by:

$$V = £(3500 - 2900) \left( \frac{1 - (1·05)^{-45}}{0·05} \right)$$

$$= £10,600.$$

Table 1 **Probabilities attaching to death by starvation outcome in gamble for indifference between gamble and various income–leisure levels with certainty***

| $Y(£\,p.a.)$ 50 $L(hrs/day)$ | 100 | 200 | 400 | 700 | 1,500 | 3,000 |
|---|---|---|---|---|---|---|
| 24 | 0·105 | 0·095 | 0·091 | 0·063 | 0·053 | 0·032 | 0·012 |
| 20 | 0·111 | 0·100 | 0·095 | 0·077 | 0·059 | 0·035 | 0·013 |
| 16 | 0·133 | 0·111 | 0·105 | 1·100 | 0·083 | 0·040 | 0·016 |
| 12 | 0·167 | 0·133 | 0·125 | 0·111 | 0·091 | 0·063 | 0·032 |
| 8 | 0·250 | 0·200 | 0·182 | 0·125 | 0·100 | 0·091 | 0·048 |
| 6 | 0·455 | 0·333 | 0·286 | 0·222 | 0·200 | 0·154 | 0·091 |
| 4 | 0·590 | 0·555 | 0·525 | 0·455 | 0·400 | 0·286 | 0·222 |
| 3 | 0·835 | 0·770 | 0·715 | 0·667 | 0·625 | 0·590 | 0·525 |

When death by road accident was substituted in the gamble for slow death, the individual required probability of death outcome = 0·060 for indifference between gamble and income – leisure level (£700 p.a., 24 hours/day) with certinty. Hence $U(DR)$ given by:

$$U(£700 \text{ p.a., } 24 \text{ hrs/day}) = (0·060) U(DR) + (0·940) 100$$

but  $\quad U(£700 \text{ p.a., } 24 \text{ hrs/day}) = 95$ (from income utility schedules)

Hence  $\quad\quad\quad\quad\quad U(DR) = 17.$

* Setting $U(DS) = 0$ and $U(£20,000 \text{ p.a., } 24 \text{ hrs/day}) = 100$, utility indices for various income–leisure levels are obtained from probability figures according to:

Utility index $= 100 \, (1 - \text{probability}).$

### Table 2 $U[p:(DR), (Y^*L^*)]^*$ for various values of probability of death by road accident

| Probability of death by road accident | 0·1 | 0·2 | 0·3 | 0·4 | 0·5 | 0·6 | 0·7 |
|---|---|---|---|---|---|---|---|
| $U[p:(DR),(Y^*L^*)]$ | 89 | 81 | 73 | 65 | 57 | 49 | 41 |

* Utility boundary gives $U(Y^*L^*) = 97$. $(Y^*L^*)$ does, in fact, correspond quite closely to the individual's current work–leisure position in this case.

### Table 3 Maximum $(Y_n - \bar{Y}_n)$ for various values of probability of death by road accident*

| Probability of death by road accident | 0·1 | 0·2 | 0·3 | 0·4 | 0·5 | 0·6 | 0·7 |
|---|---|---|---|---|---|---|---|
| Maximum† $(Y_n - \bar{Y}_n)$ (£ p.a.) | 2900 | 3500 | 3800 | 4000 | 4100 | 4400 | 4500 |

* While the first order condition for a maximum was some help in determining these figures from the utility of income schedules, it was clear that schedules for values of leisure time not considered in this exercise would have greatly improved the accuracy of the estimates.

† This individual is apparently prepared to pay as much as £2900 p.a. to effect a permanent reduction in the probability of his own death by road accident from 10 per cent to zero (by reducing leisure time from 18 hrs/day to 8 hrs/day, increasing income from £1370 p.a. to £3660 p.a. and then forfeiting (£2900 p.a.). This figure may seem excessive until it is appreciated that a permanent 10 per cent probability of death by road accident is extremely high compared with the normal risk.

## Conclusions

The analysis relies upon a number of rather strong assumptions: that the individual possesses a consistent set of preferences in income and leisure, that he is perfectly free to choose the porportion of total time to be devoted to earning income, that the opportunity cost of leisure time is a constant for each individual and that each is capable of evaluating his preferences in income, leisure and death in a sufficiently coherent manner for his reaction to the Von Neumann–Morgenstern experiments to be an acceptable basis for any estimation procedure.

The extent to which these assumptions invalidate the estimation procedure is a matter of judgement. Certainly it would seem that continuity of the leisure time choice and constancy of the wage rate are by no means necessary to the basic analysis: these assumptions were made largely to simplify the methodological exposition. The philosophical objections to the use of Von Neumann–Morgenstern utility indices and experiments are far more pertinent and have roots deep in the methodological problems of experiment in the social sciences.

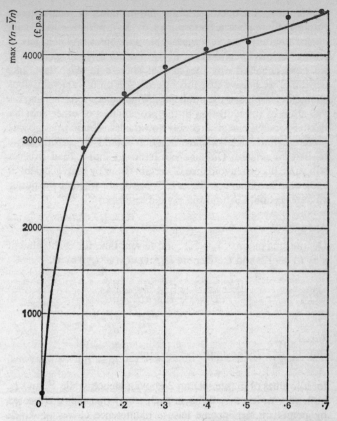

Figure 5 Maximum $(Y_n - \bar{Y}_n)$ vs. probability of death by road accident

It might be argued that if the individual can provide coherent answers to the N.M experiment he ought to be able to give direct valuations of probability reductions. We doubt whether this is so: direct valuation may be much more difficult than the decisions about indifference inherent in the N.M experiment. Furthermore, an individual's direct valuation would be a single once-for-all answer. By performing the N.M experiments we seek to establish the whole pattern of the individual's preferences, so that aberrations are less likely to have a marked effect upon the final result.

However, our primary purpose was to demonstrate that given a set of (more or less) plausible assumptions there is in fact a relationship, albeit perhaps somewhat tortuous, between a man's future income stream (determined by his optimal work-leisure choice and his probable wage rate) and the sums he would pay to reduce various likelihoods of his own death by road accident. If we have achieved any measure of success in this, then, like Schelling, we believe that this information on private valuations should at least assist the public decision-maker in formalizing his valuation of the reduction in the probabilities of other people's death by road accident. Precisely how the translation from private preferences to social welfare function should be performed we hesitate to suggest. Our analysis indicates that a road sweeper will value his own avoidance of certain death by road accident at somewhat less than a millionaire[8] – we doubt whether the public valuation should exhibit the same discrepancy.

### Appendix

Denote 'maximum $(Y_n - \bar{Y}_n)$' and leisure time for each value of $p$ by $(Y_p - \bar{Y}_p)$ and $L_p$. Denote $U[p:(DR)(Y^*L^*)]$ by $U$.

Now
$$\frac{d(Y_p - \bar{Y}_p)}{dU} = \frac{dY_p}{dL_p}\frac{dL_p}{dU} - \frac{d\bar{Y}_p}{dU}$$

$$= -r\frac{dLp}{dU} - \frac{d\bar{Y}_p}{dU}.$$

But $\left(\dfrac{d\bar{Y}_n}{dL_n}\right) U$ constant $= -r_0$ for $\begin{array}{l}\bar{Y}_n = \bar{Y}_p \\ L_n = L_p\end{array}$

for all values of $p'$ (see section 2 above). Hence, while $\bar{Y}_p$ and $L_p$ both vary with $p$ they do so in such a way that they are located by points on the income–leisure indifference curves at which the rate of substitution of income for leisure is $-r$. This, in conjunction with diminishing marginal utility of income and leisure, implies

$$\frac{d\bar{Y}_p}{dU} > 0,$$

and
$$\frac{dL_p}{dU} > 0.$$

Hence
$$\frac{d(Y_p - \bar{Y}_p)}{dU} < 0,$$

8. It is perhaps an encouraging feature of the analysis that the same cannot be said, *a priori*, of the comparative private valuation of a given probability reduction.

but $\quad \dfrac{dU}{dp} \cdot \quad < 0.$

Thus $\quad \dfrac{d(Y_p - \bar{Y}_p)}{dp} > 0.$

That is, the 'maximum $(Y_n - \bar{Y}_n)$ vs $p$' relationship is upward sloping. Predictions concerning $\dfrac{d^2(Y_p - \bar{Y}_p)}{dp^2}$ presumably require assumptions concerning the second partial derivatives of the utility function.

*References*

MUSGRAVE, R. A. (1959), *The Theory of Public Finance*, p. 80, McGraw-Hill.

SCHELLING, T. C. (1968), 'The life you save may be your own', *Problems in Public Expenditure Analysis*, Brookings Institution.

VON NEUMANN, O., and MORGENSTERN, J. (1943), *The Theory of Games and Economic Behavior*, Princeton University Press.

# 14  R. F. F. Dawson

## A Practitioner's Estimate of the Value of Life

Excerpts from R. F. F. Dawson, *Cost of Road Accidents in Great Britain*, Road Research Laboratory, 1967, Ministry of Transport.

[. . .] Road accidents cause a large amount of personal suffering and bereavement which cannot be valued directly but they also cause considerable direct losses on which a monetary value can be placed. An estimate of the total monetary cost of accidents helps to put the problem of road accidents in proper perspective. An average cost of accidents is required for use in the economic assessment of road improvement schemes: this, however, should include an allowance for suffering and bereavement.

The measurement of accident costs is sometimes criticized on the grounds that it is wrong, or impossible, to place a value upon a human life. Unless, however, the community is prepared to say that all lives are beyond value and to act accordingly, then at least an implicit value has to be put on life under many different circumstances. . . .

This study is on the same lines as that carried out by Reynolds (1956) but differs in some respects in the treatment of the loss of output and uses different sources of information. The aim is to measure the present value of the economic consequence of road accidents that occurred in Great Britain in 1963. The figure required is the cost that could be saved as a result of a reduction in accidents. For this purpose it is the marginal cost that is required and the costs of running a system of motor insurance and the costs of accident prevention are excluded. . . .

Road accidents may lead to a loss of output in the current year and in future years. The loss of a person's future output may be complete as in the case of death or a few serious injuries, or for a limited period possibly followed by a period of reduced output – a period which might be the remainder of his or her working life. Depending on the circumstances, this loss may be incurred by the casualty himself, or by his family, or by the taxpayer.

Costs in future years have to be discounted to give present day values. There is no unique discount rate which can be considered the 'correct one'. The rate chosen implies a value judgement on the relative importance of different generations, and must therefore be somewhat arbitrary. Six per cent has been used in this paper; this is lower than the rate currently used in economic assessments but seems reasonable in view of the long period over which some of the discounting takes place.

For fatalities, the number concerned and the extent of the loss of output (i.e. total) are known and by making certain simplifying assumptions the loss in man years can be estimated. In the case of injuries the total numbers are known but there are no direct statistics regarding the extent of the disablement either as regards its effect on output or the length of time for which it will last.

Most output is paid for but some services are provided free. The principal unpaid services are those of housewives. For some comparative purposes the required value of output would be that which enters into the calculation of the National Income; in such cases no value would be placed on the loss of unpaid services. (There might be some underestimate of the loss of paid output as some unpaid services might be undertaken by those which were previously in paid service.)

For most purposes the interest is in the effect of accidents on the nation and it is really immaterial whether or not the items being considered enter into the published estimates of the National Income. It would be quite possible to have a system where husbands paid their wives a wage – such systems have in fact been proposed. If such a system were instituted then the National Income would appear to increase considerably; this however would be a purely book keeping increase and the real wealth of the nation would be unaffected. The services rendered by housewives are an important part of the real income of the country and the loss of these services is a loss to the country. A value should therefore be placed on housewives' services that are lost as a result of road accidents. (Other unpaid services should also in theory be included but these are difficult to measure and the total value is probably relatively small.)

Calculations have been made both including and excluding a value for housewives' services, but they are included in all the figures quoted below, unless it is stated otherwise.

Having decided to include a value for the loss of housewives' services a number of questions then arise:

1. What is the average annual value of such services?

2. Should the same value be used for all housewives irrespective of whether they go out to work or not?

3. Should wives for the point of view of this exercise cease to be considered housewives at any particular age?

The answers to these questions must be largely arbitrary; the following decisions have been made:

1. To value the output of housewives who do not go out to work at the average wage of employed women,

2. For housewives who go out to work, to value their output as housewives at half the average wage rate of employed women. (The reasons for valuing their services at less than those of full time housewives is that some will pay others to undertake part of their household duties and that many will have less than average household responsibilities.)

3. To consider married women as housewives as long as their husbands are working. In practice to avoid complicated calculations, involving the retirement ages of men and the difference in ages between husbands and wives, which would not be justified by the arbitrariness of some of the assumptions it has been assumed that all wives are aged sixty when their husbands retire.

The following sections deal with loss due to fatalities, to serious injuries which may result in permanent or temporary disability, and to slight injuries.

### Loss of output due to death

*Basis of calculation*

When a worker (paid or unpaid) is prevented from working as a result of an injury, then in a time of full employment the community loses his production for the period of his incapacity. In the case of death the position is more complicated, for whilst the community loses his future output it also saves his future consumption. The loss to the community is thus the difference between what would have been his future production and consumption, after both have been discounted to give present day values. The resulting figure is usually referred to as the net loss of production.

It is sometimes argued that if a cross section of the population, as regards age and sex, were killed, the net loss would be zero. Some go even further and argue that the country is overpopulated, is suffering from a balance of payments deficit and therefore the loss of a cross section of the population would lead to a net gain. In a very primitive community this might be so, as the loss of a complete family would not impose an economic loss on the community. If the community were living in an area that was over-populated, because it was being over-hunted or over-cultivated, then the community would gain from the death of a family. The economy of this country however is an extremely complex one. The effect on the economy of a reduction in the population will depend on a number of factors, including the amount of unemployment or shortage of labour, the division between saving and consumption, economies of scale in production, the extent of the division of labour and the available amount of capital per head. It is not clear whether this country is over or under populated; there is a shortage of housing and a shortage of labour. If some of the population are killed then the stock of capital per head will increase, at any rate in the short run, but it does not necessarily follow that there is an economic gain. For example if a cross section of the population of Great Britain were killed, the number of buses per head would increase but as there would be fewer bus drivers the standard of service to the remaining bus passengers would probably be lower. More roads per head would be a gain in some ways which would be offset to some extent by an increase in the fixed costs of maintenance per head.

In the case of child casualties the estimate of the cost of their death to the community could be based on the amount of money that had already been spent on them instead of the discounted value of their future net output. Some young children who are killed in accidents may be replaced by their parents; in these cases the only direct monetary loss to the community might be considered to be the amount that has been spent on them. No estimates have, however, been made of the proportion of child casualties who would be replaced. A disadvantage of basing the calculation of the cost of child fatalities on the amount invested in them is that the estimate of the total cost of fatalities would in different cases be based on opposite premises – past expenditure or future output and the dividing line between the two would be very arbitrary. Taking the loss of output as the basis in all cases and ignoring replacements tends to overestimate the total cost; the overestimate is likely to be small as replacement will mainly apply to the very young for whom the discounted net loss of output is small or even negative.

When a person is killed in a road accident it is difficult to assess what the net effects on the population and the national income will be. In many cases there will be a considerable readjustment: in order to replace fatalities children might be born who otherwise would not have been, widows might go to work who otherwise would have remained at home, a worker being killed might result in a large number of people changing their jobs, future children will not be born because their parents have been killed, etc., etc. The calculations in this paper are based on the rather extreme assumption that a road fatality leads to the removal of a member of the community and that no adjustment takes place. An opposite but even more extreme assumption would be that a death resulting from a road accident had no long term effect but that the community quickly adjusted to a position where the national income per head was the same as before the accident. Such a complete adjustment is unlikely, particularly as road fatalities do not form a cross section of the population as regards age and sex. The truth will be somewhere between these two extremes but it is not possible to make any reasoned estimate of what adjustments will take place. The maximum figure has therefore been used in the present calculations.

In this paper no account is taken of any hypothetical value that a person may place on his own life. Losses due to a death are measured in terms of losses to those remaining alive: his relatives and the community in general. In other words the costs are considered *ex poste*, that is based on the costs to the population after the accident.

## Sources of information and methods of calculation

In order to make an estimate of the net loss, calculations have to be based on a number of averages (average wage, average consumption, average duration of working life etc.) and the values of consumption and production in the future have to be discounted to give present day values. The final answer therefore can only be a very approximate one.

Separate estimates have been made for men and women and for accidents in urban and in rural areas. The age and sex of those killed in road accidents is known but there is no direct information about their income. It has therefore been assumed that incomes of employed persons killed, of whatever age, are and would have been equal to the average earnings of employed people. Average costs are different in urban and in rural areas for although the same average income is assumed, the age distribution of the fatalities is different.

The annual value of the loss of output is measured by the average earned income; separate averages are used for men and for women. Annual consumption per head, for both men and women, is taken as 'the total consumer expenditure and of public authorities' current expenditure on goods and services' divided by the total population (Central Statistical Office, 1964). Production and consumption will vary with age but as the estimates are necessarily very approximate it was not considered that making allowances for age differences would increase the accuracy of the result (Weisbrod, 1961).

Expectations of life and working life of males have been published by the Ministry of Labour; as these relate to 1955 the percentages employed in each age group in 1962 have been used to adjust the expectations of working life to those applicable in 1963. In each male age group the loss of output is calculated as the number of workers killed (number of fatalities in the group times percentage working) times the expectation of working life times the average annual earnings. The saving of consumption is calculated as the number of fatalities times the average expectation of life times the average annual consumption. Loss of production and saving of consumption are discounted at a rate of 6 per cent. Loss of production and saving of consumption occur over different periods of time and have therefore to be calculated separately; the net loss is the difference between the two discounted values.

Whereas the working life of males normally begins when they finish their education and continues until retirement the working life of females is less straightforward. Some women's working life follows the same pattern as that of men but the majority cease work after a few years and an increasingly large proportion of them return to work after a number of years. The average value of lost production per head was estimated from the expectation of life of women (General Register Office, 1964). The average value of lost production per head was calculated from the proportion of women in each age group who are married (Central Statistical Office, 1964) and from the estimates of the proportion of married and single women in each age group who were working in 1962 and the proportions which are expected to be working in 1972 (Beckerman and Sutherland, 1963).

*Results.* The total loss of output due to fatal accidents in 1963 is summarized in Table 1 together with the average cost per fatality in urban, rural and all areas.

A negative loss implies that from a strictly material point of view the community gains from a person's death: however, when the subjective factors are taken into account the losses became positive in all cases.

## Loss of output due to serious injuries
### Loss of output in first year after accident

In order to calculate the value of the loss of output which results from serious injuries, which may be anything from minor fractures to those causing incapacity for life, it is necessary to know the average length of time away from work; for long term incapacities, it is also necessary to know the amount by which the ability to work is reduced and the length of time that this disability continues. This information is not directly obtainable but has been estimated from several sources. The principal source used is the Digest of Statistics Analysing Certificates of Incapacity published by the Ministry of Pensions and National Insurance. The digest is concerned with claims received by the Ministry for Sickness Benefit and for Industrial Injuries Benefit; it gives information on the number of claims, the cause of injury and the length of time benefit is payable. Neither type of claim is payable for absences from work for less than four days. Industrial injury benefits are not paid after six months when, if still incapacitated, the claimant transfers to sickness benefit. Injuries can be classified according to causes of incapacity (e.g. broken leg) and according to external cause of injury (e.g. road accident). (See the International Statistical Classification of Diseases, Injuries and Causes of Death issued by the World Health Organization.) The only analysis in the Digest by external cause of injury is of industrial injury claims. It is not known if 'industrial injuries' caused by road accidents are a biased sample of all injuries caused by road accidents but some check can be made by comparing the durations of incapacity due to road accidents which give rise to industrial injury claims with the duration due to all accidents which give rise to claims for industrial injury or sickness benefit (assuming that sickness benefit also finishes at 6 months). This comparison is given in Table 2.

Table 2 shows that for men the duration of incapacity for general accident cases is very similar for both classes of benefit and that

## Table 1 Total cost of loss of output due to fatalities and average cost per fatality

| | Urban areas | | | Rural areas | | | All areas | | |
|---|---|---|---|---|---|---|---|---|---|
| | Number of net loss of output | | | Number of net loss of output | | | Number of net loss of output | | |
| | fatalities | Total | Average per head | fatalities | Total | Average per head | fatalities | Total | Average per head |
| | | (£000) | (£) | | (£000) | (£) | | (£000) | (£) |
| Males | 2870 | 10,670 | 3720 | 2177 | 11,360 | 5220 | 5047 | 22,030 | 4360 |
| Females | 1332 | −2040 | −1530 | 543 | −60 | −110 | 1875 | −2100 | −1120 |
| Total | 4202 | 8630 | 2040 | 2720 | 11,300 | 4150 | 6922 | 19,930 | 2880 |

road accident cases cause longer incapacity than other accidents. For women the picture is less clear but the differences are small. Women's incapacity as a result of general accidents is longer than that for men, but incapacities due to road accidents are shorter. It seems reasonable therefore to assume that, ignoring incapacities which last longer than six months, 32·5 working days is the average length of incapacity.

Some check on these estimates is given in the Report of the Commissioner of Metropolitan Police. The report contains information on the length and cause of absence from duty of policemen. The average absence due to road accidents, on or off duty, is 23·6 days; averages for different classes of road user vary from 21·9 days for both pedal cyclists and car occupants to 24·8 days for motor cyclists. These figures are lower than those derived from the insurance data but are of the same order of magnitude. There is no reason to think that accidents to the police would be typical of all accidents and policemen are probably of above average fitness which might account for shorter than average absences from duty.

Table 2 **Average duration of incapacity for incapacities of over 4 days and ignoring periods after six months**

| Class of benefit | Classification of injury and WHO reference numbers | Average duration of incapacity (working days) | | |
|---|---|---|---|---|
| | | Men | Women | All cases |
| Industrial injury | Motor vehicle accidents (E810–E835) | 32·6 | 30·2 | 32·4 |
| Industrial injury | Accidents, poisoning and violence (Detailed list numbers 800–856 (except 849) 870–908 (except 889, 899) 920–929) | 25·1 | 32·3 | 25·8 |
| Sickness | – ditto – | 26·6 | 28·1 | 26·9 |

Over 3 per cent of the road accident cases were still incapacitated at the end of six months. If it is assumed that incapacities due to road accidents which last longer than 6 months are of similar duration to accident cases which receive sickness benefit then the average number of working days lost during a year is 41 and about 1 per cent are still incapacitated at the end of the year. The number of working years plus 'housewife years' lost during a year is given in Table 3.

## Table 3 Loss of output in first year as a result of serious casualties

| Age | Males | | | Females | | | |
|---|---|---|---|---|---|---|---|
| | Percentage working | Number of serious casualties Urban | Rural | Percentage working | Percentage housewives | Number of serious casualties Urban | Rural |
| 0–14 | 0 | 7276 | 1249 | 0 | 0 | 3399 | 730 |
| 15–19 | 75 | 9595 | 5012 | 65 | 5 | 2160 | 1467 |
| 20–24 | 96 | 5633 | 4514 | 63 | 46 | 1340 | 1154 |
| 25–29 | 99·5 | 3035 | 2362 | 41 | 74 | 758 | 642 |
| 30–39 | 99·5 | 4043 | 3220 | 43 | 72 | 1239 | 965 |
| 40–49 | 98 | 3634 | 2561 | 49 | 70 | 1664 | 1110 |
| 50–59 | 95 | 3509 | 2103 | 44 | 62 | 1946 | 1045 |
| 60–64 | 90 | 1168 | 457 } | 15 | 0 | 1953 | 618 |
| 65–69 | 44 | 1168 | 456 | | | | |
| 70–79 | 20 | 1267 | 341 | 6 | 0 | 1550 | 267 |
| 80–89 | 5 | 433 | 59 | 0 | 0 | 556 | 64 |
| 90 & over | — | 22 | 3 | 0 | 0 | 27 | 2 |
| Total | | 40,783 | 22,337 | | | 16,592 | 8064 |

* Working housewives counted as one half.

If 41 working days are lost per casualty and the value of a year's work is taken as £960 for men and £530 for women then the working and housewife years lost and the value of lost output are:

|  |  | Years lost | Value |
|---|---|---|---|
| Urban areas: | Men | 3736 | £3,587,000 |
|  | Women | 1280 | £ 678,000 |
| Rural areas: | Men | 2479 | £2,380,000 |
|  | Women | 876 | £ 465,000 |
|  |  |  | £7,110,000 |

*Loss of output in cases of long term incapacity*

The loss of output due to permanent and long term injuries depends on the number of cases, the length of absence from work, and the percentage disability when work is resumed. Because of the lack of data on these subjects several calculations have been made.

1. The most extreme assumption is that the one per cent of serious casualties, who are still incapacitated a year after their accident, are incapacitated for the whole of their working life, so that the whole of their future production is lost without any compensating gain in consumption saved. If this was the case then the present value of the cost of longer term incapacities would be £8·5 million.

2. The Digest for 1954–5 gives the length of incapacities for sickness benefit cases by cause of incapacity and by length of incapacity for periods up to 7 years. If it is assumed that long term road accident cases have similar durations, and if the mid point of the over 7 years group is taken as the average expectation of working life, then the average present value per serious casualty for which incapacity lasts more than a year is £4200. The present value of the cost of all such incapacities is £3·7 million.

3. Persons suffering from the long term effects of industrial injuries may receive a permanent disability pension, a provisional disability pension or a gratuity, which may be on the termination of a provisional pension. In addition there are a number of special allowances of which the most important is special hardship allowance. Some information is available about disability pensions but none that applies directly to road accident casualties. Pensions and gratuities are awarded for a certain percentage of

disability (under 20 per cent and then by tens to 100 per cent) but this does not reflect the extent to which a person's working capability is reduced: it may exaggerate it considerably. 'The assessment of disablement takes no account of the claimant's occupation or any loss of earnings.'

'Disability benefit is payable if ... a person suffers a loss of physical or mental faculty i.e. some impairment of the power to enjoy a normal life which persists beyond the injury benefit period. In assessing disablement no account is taken specifically of any loss of earning power'. Special hardship allowance and in a few special cases unemployability supplements are payable if the injury makes the claimant 'unfit to follow his regular occupation or to perform work of an equivalent standard' (Interdepartmental Committee on Social and Economic Research, 1961).

The majority of pensions are operative only for a limited period. The Government Actuary reports that after five years only 20 per cent of pensions are still operative and thereafter the only cause of cessation will be the death of the pensioner. His estimates of the proportions continuing at different periods of time are given in Table 4.

Table 4 **Disability pensions: percentage disability according to length of time pension has been continuing**

| Period pension has been operative (years) | Percentage of disability pensions continuing |
| --- | --- |
| $\frac{1}{2}$ | 68 |
| $1\frac{1}{2}$ | 32 |
| $2\frac{1}{2}$ | 23 |
| $3\frac{1}{2}$ | 21 |
| $4\frac{1}{2}$ | 20 |
| 5 | 20 |

Thus only one fifth of the pensions granted are or become permanent (at an unknown or unpublished percentage of disability) and the average duration of the others is slightly less than a year. The average percentage of assessment of pensions still in payment at any time is approximately 30 per cent. The average percentage disabilities for special hardship allowances is also 30 per cent.

About 5 per cent of those who receive industrial injury benefits later receive disablement benefits. If it is assumed that:

1. this overall percentage applies to road accident cases,

2. in 80 per cent of the cases the average duration is one year and disability is at 30 per cent (an over-estimate of the impairment to work) and

3. for the other 20 per cent disability is 30 per cent for life, then the cost of loss of output is £2·5 million.

As well as those receiving pensions a further eighth of those who receive industrial injury benefits receive a gratuity. If these are assumed to represent 20 per cent disability for a year the cost is £1·4 million giving a total cost of long term effect of serious injuries at £3·9 million.

*Overall cost of loss of output as a result of serious injuries.* Taking £7·1 million as the cost due to absence from work in the first year after the accident the following estimates of the value of total loss of output due to serious injuries are obtained.

1. £15·6 million. This assumes complete incapacity for all those who have not returned to work within a year after the accident but makes no allowance for loss of capacity by those returning within that period.

2. £10·0 million. Makes no allowance for reduced capacity of those returning to work in less than 1 year.

3. £11·0 million. Based on average disabilities given in Industrial Injury and Sickness Benefit data.

The second and third estimates of long term disability cover slightly different ground but there is a considerable overlap between them and to include them separately giving a total of £13·9 million (7·1+2·9+3·9) would be an over-estimate.

The best estimate appears to lie between £10 million and £16 million and lacking any more precise data it is taken as £13 million.

Persons who die more than thirty days after an accident are classified as serious injuries. An allowance for the loss of output due to death of those dying after thirty days should in theory be included in the costs of serious injuries. The data collected by Jeffcoate (1960) show that deaths after 30 days are about 5 per cent of the number of 'fatalities'. Thus in 1963 there would have been about 350 persons who died as the result of a road accident but were classified as serious injuries. Those who die after 30 days are mainly old people: ninety per cent are over 50 years old, compared with only forty per cent of all fatalities. The average value of loss of output of those dying after 30 days, calculated as above, is £90 per fatality. This amount is so small that there is no need in practice to make any allowance for the measurable cost of those who die more than 30 days after the accident.

£8·1 million of the total cost of loss of output due to serious injuries is attributable to accidents in urban areas and £4·9 million to accidents in rural areas. The average cost per casualty is £141 in urban areas, £161 in rural areas, £174 for men and £81 for women and £148 overall.

## Loss of output due to slight injuries

Slight injuries, '(those) of a minor character such as sprains and bruises', will lead to loss of output by causing some people to be absent from work for short periods. There is no evidence of how long such absences will be. In many cases there will be no absence and in the great majority of cases when there is an absence it will be under four days and therefore will not be recorded in the National Insurance Statistics.

As a third of accidents take place at weekends, and because of the insignificant nature of many slight casualties, it has been assumed that on average one working day is lost by slight injuries to those who go to work. The ages of most slight casualties are not now recorded so it has been assumed that the age distribution is the same as in 1958 (the last year for which the information is available). Table 5 gives the total number of slight casualties and the number who are workers. If it is assumed that the average loss of output is one day per casualty then the number of working days lost is equal to the number of slight casualties who are workers and dividing this figure by 260[1] gives the number of man years lost. The total loss of output due to slight casualties is £546,000 giving an average cost of £2·1 per casualty. The total can be divided into £399,000 in urban areas and £147,000 in rural areas with average costs per slight casualty of £2·0 and £2·3 respectively. The difference between the urban and the rural average is due to the much higher proportion of children in the urban casualties.

1. 312 days are used in the estimates for serious casualties as this is the basis used by the Ministry of Pensions.

**Table 5 Loss of output as a result of slight casualities**

| Age | Men | | | Women | | |
|---|---|---|---|---|---|---|
| | Number of slight casualties | Per-centage working | Number of slight casualties who are workers | Number of slight casualties | Per-centage working | Number of slight casualties who are workers |
| 0–14 | 29,750 | 0 | — | 15,952 | 0 | — |
| 15–19 | 26,762 | 76 | 20,340 | 9664 | 57 | 4678 |
| 20–24 | 27,313 | 96 | 26,221 | 8961 | 62 | 4718 |
| 25–29 | 18,655 | 99·5 | 18,563 | 5802 | 40 | 1971 |
| 30–39 | 27,501 | 99·5 | 27,364 | 10,571 | 44 | 3950 |
| 40–49 | 21,353 | 98 | 20,927 | 11,074 | 52 | 4891 |
| 50–59 | 15,806 | 95 | 15,016 | 9153 | 46 | 3576 |
| 60–69 | 7601 | 67 | 5097 | 6101 | 16 | 829 |
| 70–79 | 3722 | 20 | 744 | 3622 | 7 | 215 |
| 80 and over | 1089 | 0 | — | 1029 | 0 | — |
| All ages | 179,552 | | 134,272 | 81,929 | | 24,828 |
| Man years lost | | | 516 | | | 95 |
| Value of lost output | | | £495,000 | | | £51,000 |

The total is very small compared with other items so any error in the assumption about the average number of days lost will have little effect on the total cost of accidents. No allowance has been made for any loss of housewives' services as a result of slight injuries.

### Summary of cost of loss of output

The cost of the loss of output from all classes of injury is given in Table 6 and the average costs per casualty are given in Table 7.

**Table 6 Value of loss of output as a result of road accidents (£ millions)**

| | Urban areas | | Rural areas | | All areas |
|---|---|---|---|---|---|
| Fatalities | 8·5 | | 11·3 | | 19·8 |
| Serious injuries | | | | | |
| Short term effects | 4·3 | | 2·8 | | 7·1 |
| Long term effects | 3·8 | | 2·1 | | 5·9 |
| (over 1 year) | — | 8·1 | — | 4·9 | — 13·0 |
| Slight injuries | | 0·4 | | 0·1 | 0·5 |
| | | 17·0 | | 16·3 | 33·3 |

The average cost of loss of output per accident is calculated by multiplying the average costs per casualty given above by the average number of casualties per accident. The results are given in Table 8.

**Table 7  Average costs of the loss of output per casualty of different severities (£)**

| Class of casualty | Urban areas | Rural areas | All areas |
|---|---|---|---|
| Fatality | 2040 | 4150 | 2880 |
| Serious injury | 140 | 160 | 150 |
| Slight injury | 2 | 2 | 2 |

**Table 8  Average costs of loss of output per accident (£)**

| Class of accident | Urban areas | Rural areas | All areas |
|---|---|---|---|
| Fatal | 2220 | 4760 | 3160 |
| Serious | 160 | 210 | 170 |
| Slight | 2 | 3 | 2 |

A number of implicit assumptions are made in the above calculations and these may affect the accuracy of the answers, particularly the comparisons between urban and rural costs.

1. That workers who are involved in accidents are a cross section of the working population as regards income,

2. That in each age group the average expectation of working life of those killed was equal to the average expectation of all in the group,

3. That there are no differences in average income between those killed or injured in urban and in rural areas, other than those due to the different age and sex distributions,

4. That those who are working are as likely to be killed as those in the same age group who are not working,

5. That there is no difference in each age group in the proportion working in urban and in rural areas,

6. That the average value of consumption is the same for men and for women.

## Measurable costs per accident

... The average costs per casualty have been multiplied by the
average number of casualties per accident to give the average
cost of loss of output and medical treatment per accident; these,
plus the average cost per accident of damage to property and
administration are given in Table 9.[2]

Table 9 **Average measurable costs per accident (£)**

| Class of accident | Area | Costs | | | | |
|---|---|---|---|---|---|---|
| | | Loss of output | Medical treatment | Damage to property | Administrative costs | Total |
| Fatal | Urban | 2220 | 50 | 110 | 40 | 2420 |
| | Rural | 4760 | 60 | 290 | 40 | 5150 |
| | All areas | 3160 | 60 | 170 | 40 | 3430 |
| Serious | Urban | 160 | 100 | 110 | 30 | 400 |
| | Rural | 201 | 130 | 290 | 30 | 660 |
| | All areas | 170 | 110 | 170 | 30 | 480 |
| Slight | Urban | 2 | 7 | 90 | 26 | 125 |
| | Rural | 3 | 9 | 212 | 26 | 250 |
| | All areas | 2 | 7 | 115 | 26 | 150 |
| Average personal injury | Urban | 80 | 30 | 100 | 30 | 240 |
| | Rural | 260 | 50 | 250 | 30 | 590 |
| | All areas | 120 | 30 | 130 | 30 | 310 |
| Damage | Urban | | | 50 | 10 | 60 |
| | Rural | | | 80 | 10 | 90 |
| | All areas | | | 60 | 10 | 70 |

## Subjective costs

... If the costs given in this paper are to be used in the economic
assessments of road improvements then it is important that they
should reflect the value that the community places on the saving
of life and suffering. From a cold and strictly financial point of
view the community gains from the death of a pensioner, but of
course, humanitarian actions and policies of society frequently

2. The author has, in the omitted sections, presented detailed discussions
and estimates of these additional costs. To save space, only the results of
these calculations are presented here, in Table 9. The interested reader is
referred to the original for fuller discussion (editors' note).

override the strictly financial considerations. An average cost per accident would not generally be accepted as valid if its use in an economic assessment led to the conclusion that particular road improvement should not be carried out as the improvement might save the lives of some old people. It is necessary therefore to try to estimate the value that the community places on the loss of human life, or more precisely what it is prepared to pay to save life.

It has been suggested that the use of awards made by the courts as a measure of the value of loss of life would bring the estimate in line with popular valuation. In fact court awards for fatalities as distinct from injuries are calculated on a similar basis to the estimates made in this paper. To quote Hunkman 'action is based upon financial loss or loss of support . . . it gives no *solatium* for mental distresses, or for the loss or society of a husband or parent' (Hunkman, 1960). Awards for loss of expectation of life are assessed at about £400 for an adult and £200 for a child. There is no indication that these sums bear any relation to the value that is placed on life.

Turning now to injuries there are various heads of damage under which awards may be made; Kemp and Kemp (1961) subdivide them into pecuniary losses and non-pecuniary losses. The pecuniary losses are those that have been estimated in this paper, although some minor items such as the cost of paid help for some who remain seriously injured have not been included here. The non-pecuniary losses consist of:

1. Pain, suffering and shock;
2. Loss of amenities of life;
3. Loss of expectation of life;
4. Inconvenience and discomfort;
5. Exemplary damages.

These are the items for which a value is required.

Legal reference books quote lists of awards and ranges of damages for various classes of injury. There are two drawbacks in trying to use these figures, apart from lack of detailed knowledge about the accidents that occur. Firstly the majority of court cases will be the severer cases and the costs will therefore be above average. Secondly it is usually impossible to separate the payments for non-pecuniary items from many or all of the pecuniary items. 'Judges do not usually break up their global award of general damages into various heads'. This latter point applies equally to settled cases.

The value to be placed on subjective factors is discussed by Thédié and Abraham. They subdivide the subjective losses due to death into

1. Affective injury to family
2. Affective injury to nation
3. *Pretium doloris* (price of suffering)
4. *Pretium vivendi* (price of living).

They arrived at an estimate for 1957 of £2150 (at the official rate of exchange) per person killed; nearly half of this being for the *pretium vivendi*. Their estimates are based to some extent on court awards but they do not discuss the way in which they arrive at their results.

A possible way of arriving at an estimate of the amount that the community is prepared to pay to save life is to examine what, in effect, is paid in a number of different circumstances. Costs, direct and indirect, are incurred in making trains, ships and aircraft safer, in providing fire fighting and lifeboat facilities, and in a number of ways in the field of medicine.

It is possible that, by examining a number of such cases, a value could be arrived at which provides a concensus of opinion. It is, however, possible that the scatter of values would be so wide that no useful result will emerge.

In the meantime it is suggested that the following rather arbitrary, average values should be used for the subjective cost of casualties:

| | |
|---|---|
| fatality | £5000 |
| serious casualty | £200 |
| slight casualty | 0 |

The use of a subjective value £5000 for a death means that when only paid output is valued the total average cost of a death is positive in all age and sex groups. £5000 is thus a minimum value; for if the community wishes to save the lives of persons although it would gain from their death, then the amount of gain which it forgoes is a minimum estimate of the value that is placed on keeping them alive. The figure is somewhat higher than that which Thédié and Abraham calculated for France. A qualitative case could clearly be made for varying these costs according to the age of the victim, but it is not possible at present to do more than take average values.

There are subjective costs in the case of slight injuries and in the case of damage accidents. (The majority of people would be willing to pay something over and above the cost of damage in order to avoid an accident, even if no one was hurt.) The amounts, however, would be small and have little effect on the total – they have therefore been ignored.

The subjective costs per accident based on these costs per casualty are given in Table 10.

**Average costs of an accident including subjective losses**

The amounts which it is assessed that the community would be willing to pay to avoid road accidents are obtained by adding the financial costs and the subjective costs. These amounts are given in Table 11.

Table 10 **Average subjective cost per accident (£)**

|  | Urban areas | Rural areas | All areas |
| --- | --- | --- | --- |
| Fatal accident | 5330 | 5740 | 5490 |
| Serious accident | 220 | 270 | 230 |
| All personal injury accidents | 150 | 330 | 190 |

Table 11 **Average cost per accident including subjective losses (£)**

|  | Urban areas | Rural areas | All areas |
| --- | --- | --- | --- |
| Fatal accidents | 7750 | 10,890 | 8920 |
| Serious accidents | 630 | 930 | 710 |
| Slight accidents | 125 | 250 | 150 |
| Average personal injury accident | 390 | 920 | 500 |
| Average personal inuury with associated damage accidents | 790 | 1330 | 900 |

... A new basis of calculating the cost of road accidents is suggested and the values have been calculated for the total cost of accidents in Great Britain and for the average costs of different classes of accident. These estimates include an arbitrary financial equivalent to the subjective or social costs due to bereavement and human suffering. ...

R. F. F. Dawson 355

For 1965 it was estimated that the total measurable cost was £246 million and the total including subjective costs was £305 million. . . . It was found that over a half of the total cost of all accidents arises from damage to vehicles, and that the subjective costs (assumed to be £5000 per fatality and £250 per serious accident) contribute just under 20 per cent of the total cost. Including subjective costs, just over 20 per cent is accounted for by fatal accidents.

*References*

BECKERMAN, W., and SUTHERLAND, J. (1963), 'Married women at work in 1972', *Nat. Inst. Econ. Rev.*, no. 23.

CENTRAL STATISTICAL OFFICE (1962), 'Estimates of the future working population', *Economic Trends*, no. 107.

CENTRAL STATISTICAL OFFICE (1964), *National Income and Expenditure 1964*, HMSO.

CENTRAL STATISTICAL OFFICE (1964), *Annual Abstract of Statistics*, HMSO, no. 101.

GENERAL REGISTER OFFICE (1964), *The Registrar General's Quarterly Return for England and Wales*, quarter ending 30 June, HMSO.

HOME OFFICE (1965), *Report of the Commissioner of Police of the Metropolis for the Year 1964*, HMSO.

HUNKMAN J. (1960), *Damages for Personal Injuries and Death*, 2nd edn, Butterworth.

INTERDEPARTMENTAL COMMITTEE ON SOCIAL AND ECONOMIC RESEARCH (1961), *Guides to Official Sources No. 5: Social Security Statistics*, HMSO.

JEFFCOATE, G. O. (1960), *The Time That Elapses Between A Fatal Road Accident and Death Resulting Therefrom* (2nd report), Road Research Lab. Note no. RN/3814/GOJ, unpublished.

KEMP, D. A. and M. S. (1961), *The Question of Damages, vol. 1: Personal Injury Claims*, 2nd edn, Sweet and Maxwell.

MINISTRY OF LABOUR AND NATIONAL SERVICE (1959), *The Length of Working Life of Males in Great Britain*, HMSO.

MINISTRY OF PENSIONS AND NATIONAL INSURANCE, *Digest of Statistics Analysing Certificates of Incapacity, 1954–5 and Following Years*, unpublished.

MINISTRY OF TRANSPORT AND SCOTTISH DEVELOPMENT DEPARTMENT (1959), *Road Accidents 1958*, HMSO.

REYNOLDS, D. J. (1956), 'The cost of road accidents', *Journal of the Royal Statistical Society*, Series A (General), vol. 119, pp. 393–408.

THE GOVERNMENT ACTUARY (1960), *Report by the Government Actuary on the Quinquennial Review*, HMSO.

THÉDIÉ, J., and ABRAHAM, C. (1961), 'Economic aspects of road accidents', *Traff. Engn and Control*, vol. 2, pp. 589–95.

WEISBROD, B. A. (1961), *Economics of Public Health*, University of Pennsylvania Press.

WORLD HEALTH ORGANIZATION (1955), *Manual of the International Statistical Classification of Disease, Injuries and Causes of Death*, WHO.

# 15 S. Enke

## Estimating the Benefits of Birth Control

S. Enke, 'The economic aspects of slowing population growth', *Economic Journal*, March 1966, pp. 44–56.

## Introduction

The past decade of planned economic development has been a disappointing experience for many aspiring peoples and their governments. National domestic production in most Less Developed Countries (LDCs) has grown faster than population by only one or two percentage points annually. It is no wonder the United States will now grant technical assistance to reduce births on request,[1] that half a dozen countries have incorporated contraception in their development programme[2] and that the Catholic Church is reconsidering its position on certain birth-control methods other than 'rhythm'.[3]

## Why high birth-rates matter

Reasoned economic concern over high birth-rates in LDCs – usually ten per thousand a year and higher – has little to do with the theories of optimum and static population size. First, high birth-rates cause a natural rate of population increase that is almost too fast to maintain *per capita* output in some countries. Second, high birth-rates mean a higher ratio of dependent children, unable to produce but always consuming.

1. With crude birth-rates continuing at 40 plus per thousand a year, and crude death-rates continuing to fall, many nations' population at present rates of natural increase will double every

1. The Agency for International Development, following President Johnson's 1963 State of the Union pledge to 'seek new ways to use our knowledge to help deal with the explosion in world population' instructed its United States AID missions abroad to henceforth consider requests for assistance in family planning (with two practically unimportant exceptions).

2. India, Pakistan, Taiwan, Korea, Ceylon and Turkey.

3. Involving a consistent reinterpretation of natural law in the light of changed circumstances and new methods having novel or uncertain mechanism of contraception.

25 to 35 years. Perhaps the employed labour force can double as fast. But natural resources cannot increase by definition. And many poor countries cannot save and invest enough yearly to double their stock of capital in, say, 30 years. Therefore unless innovations increase final output to factor input rates rather more rapidly than now seems the case, aggregate output *per capita* may barely increase. Most of these countries cannot have both natural increases in population of from 2 to 3 per cent annually and increases in *per capita* income of 3 per cent a year or better. Even in the most advanced nation, there is an inverse relation between annual rate of increase in population and in output per head.[4]

2. The fraction of population under 15 years of age is highly dependent on age-specific birth-rates, and increases with it. Very approximately indeed, and the interactions are complicated, a country with crude birth-rates of 40 per thousand a year could have as high as 40 per cent of its population under 15 years of age. This percentage might be as low as twenty for a country with an annual crude birth-rate of twenty per thousand. Children under 15 are not significant producers, but only consumers. Lower birth-rates, reducing the relative burden of infant dependency, would 'release' consumption to others. Additionally, depending on private saving propensities and government fiscal policies, perhaps a third of such released consumption could be diverted into useful investment.

Both these ideas are expanded below. Thus, the present discounted value of released consumption – several times the *per capita* income in many countries – provides the bases for several estimates of the economic worth of preventing a birth. And examination of the relative growth rates of output and population leads to the startling conclusion that resources used to retard

4. Consider a modified Cobb–Douglas approach to this problem. Assume $\% \Delta V = (l \cdot \% \Delta L) + (k \cdot \% \Delta K) + \varphi$, where $V$ is national gross value added, $L$ is number of persons in the labour force, $K$ is the value of the aggregate capital stock, $\varphi$ is increase in productivity due to innovations, $l$ is the share of national output paid to labour and $k$ that to capitalists. Suppose $l$ is $0 \cdot 5$ and $k$ is $0 \cdot 2$, these summing to less than unity, indicating diminishing returns due to scarce natural resources. Over 5 years population ($P$) increases, say, 12%, and also $L$, the $P/L$ ratio being constant. Perhaps $K$ increases 30% during these same 5 years. Then there is a $0 \cdot 5$ times $0 \cdot 12$ (i.e. 6%) increase in output attributable to extra labour force. And there is a $0 \cdot 2$ times $0 \cdot 30$ increase in output (i.e. 6%) attributable to capital stock increase. Summing, unless $\varphi$ contributes, there is 12% more output for 12% more people.

population growth can contribute perhaps a hundred times more to higher incomes per head than resources used to accelerate output growth.

## Superior effectiveness of investment in reducing births

Output per head ($V/P$) can be increased by investing resources in making the output numerator larger or the population denominator smaller than they would otherwise be in, say, 1975.

Suppose $0.5 million worth of resources are invested every year in industrial plants to raise national output. The rate of return on these investments is 15 per cent a year. After 10 years $5.0 million has been invested, and the annual output increase ($\Delta V$) attributable to it is $0.75 million a year. Perhaps national output ($V$) at the start in 1965 was $500 million. Then the proportionate change in yearly national output ($\Delta V/V$) due to this $5.0 million investment is 0.0015.

Now suppose $0.5 million of resources – but medical and contraceptive resources this time – are invested each year in a birth-reduction programme that stresses the use of intra-uterine devices (IUDs). The cost per participant each year is about $1, so there are 500,000 participants on an average each year during the 1965–75 time period. And perhaps the live births fertility of a typical woman participant is 0.15 infants a year. Thus, the reduction in births ($\Delta P$) over 10 years is 0.75 million infants. Perhaps national population at the start in 1965 was 5.0 millions.[5] Then the proportionate change in national population ($\Delta P/P$) due to this investment is 0.15.

If $5.0 million over 10 years gives a $\Delta P/P$ of 0.15 when used to retard population growth, and a $\Delta V/V$ of 0.0015 when invested to accelerate output growth, the superior effectiveness ratio of birth reduction over output expansion ($V\Delta P/P\Delta V$) is 100 times.[6]

This ratio of superiority varies proportionately with assumed rates of fertility of women practising contraception ($f$), and inversely both with returns to capital ($r$) and with cost of programme per participant. Table 1 gives examples. It is staggering to encounter such ratios when comparing different economic policies.

5. $V/P$ in this example is accordingly $100/year.

6. A rather similar estimate was expressed by President Johnson in his speech before the commemorative meeting of the U.N. General Assembly in San Francisco in 1965, where he stated: 'Let us act on the fact that less than $5 invested in birth control is worth $100 invested in economic development.'

It does not follow, though, that conventional development investments (*e.g.* power dams and cement plants) should be terminated in favour of birth-reduction programmes. At most, these latter programmes could never usefully cost more than perhaps one twenty-fifth of the formers' budgets. And, in free societies, the State can only use resources to slow population growth to the extent that adults want fewer children, and so voluntarily participate in birth-reduction programmes.[7]

Table 1 **Superior effectiveness ratio** $(V \triangle P / P \triangle V)$
(sensitivity to $f$ and $r$)

| $f$ / $r$ | 0·10 | 0·15 | 0·20 | 0·25 |
|---|---|---|---|---|
| 0·20 | 50 | 75 | 100 | 125 |
| 0·15 | 67 | 100 | 133 | 167 |
| 0·10 | 100 | 150 | 200 | 250 |

## Value of preventing a birth

What is the 'worth' of preventing a birth from the viewpoint of a government that is seeking to increase outputs disposable in future to those alive today? What does a typical infant ultimately cost its society, in this sense, measured at time of birth? What does it mean to 'prevent a birth'?

### Fifteen-year estimates

Not many Heads of Government look beyond 15 years. Any birth prevented between 1965 and 1980 affects *consumption* immediately, but cannot affect *output* significantly during that time. Everyone who can become 15 years old during this period is born already.

The present discounted value of the consumption 'released' if a country does not have 1000 infants born this year, representative as regards sex and other attributes, can be estimated after a fashion. It is necessary to assume survival expectancies through each year. Typical consumption values by age are needed. And there must be agreement on a discount rate that reflects time preferences and capital productivity in the country.

For a country with a *per capita* income, $V/P$, of $100 yearly,

7. This paper does *not* consider the relative worth of improving population *quality* through expenditures on health and education.

from which 10 per cent is saved, the present value of preventing a birth in the sense of released consumption over 15 years is $280 at an interest rate of 15 per cent. At 10 per cent it is $384. And at 20 per cent it is $212.

Such estimates scale approximately with $V/P$, from $100 up to $500 perhaps, so in a country with an output per head of $250 annually these 'worths' for 10 per cent, 15 per cent and 20 per cent would roughly be $960, $700 and $530, respectively.

## Total life estimates

Theoretically, the present discounted value of typical infants' consumption (negative) *and* production (positive) *after* 15 years should be included. Roughly, in a '$V/P$ equals 100' country a typical undiscounted net surplus during 15–55 years of age is perhaps no more than $840. Practically, at 15 per cent return, the present value of this $840 is an insignificant $17 at date of birth. This gives a net $263 at 15 per cent for a country with a $V/P$ of $100. Accordingly, very generally stated, the 'worth' of preventing a birth in a typical LDC is about 2·6 times the output per head.[8]

## Meaning of prevention and postponement

What does it mean to 'prevent a birth'?

The above 'worths' are the values to society of 'permanently' preventing a birth some woman would definitely have otherwise had this year. The probability of the birth this year must be 1·0 without contraception and 0·0 with birth control. Moreover, whatever the probabilities had been of her giving birth next year and in future years, these must remain unchanged. This is an extreme case, admittedly rather unrealistic, and estimates of the 'worth of prevention' made on this basis are not directly relevant to birth-reduction programmes. However, this case needs to be calculated initially, because other important 'estimates of worth' are derived from it.

Most realistic probably is the case of birth *postponement*. This

8. As a standard, per 1000 population, 400 are under and 600 are over fifteen years. If output per head is $100 yearly, and consumption $90, the under-15s may be consuming $70 on an average or $28,000 worth. The over-fifteens are then consuming $62,000 worth or $104 each. Output per head for the over-fifteens is then $167. But perhaps 0·25 of this is attributable to capital and land. Thus, over-fifteens each add $125 to output each year as workers and consume $104. Their net contribution is then $21 a year as workers. Discounted at 0·15, by years from birth, this is about $17.

calculation depends on the fertility rate of exposed and fertile women considering only 'pregnable' women, and excluding those who are already pregnant or have not resumed *menses* following childbirth. Perhaps this rate $(f)$ is 0·25 for such women in their twenties. Effective contraceptive practice during a year, assuming the value of $f$ in immediately following years is not altered, then 'prevents' 0·25 of an infant during the current year. Thus, if the value of 'permanently' preventing a birth is $260 the value of postponing it one year is 0·25 of $260, or $65. This value declines as women age and $f$ falls. Such a calculation of the yearly postponement worth of contraception is especially significant in primitive societies, where women take no precaution against conception at any time.

Sterilization is the only birth-control method where, assuming 'faithful' wives, 'probable' births are completely prevented. If a married man has a vasectomy the present discounted value of the probable future children his wife would otherwise have can be estimated. This in turn should be multiplied by the value of 'permanently' preventing a birth. As estimated above, for a country where $V/P$ is $100, this may be about $260. Then, taking some typical fertility rates, the present discounted value of a vasectomy is roughly $275 when the wife is 25 years old, $193 when she is 30 and $148 at 35 years.

The practical importance of these 'worths' is that they form a basis for determining the maximum cost in resources a government can incur to postpone or 'prevent' a birth. Thus, if three-fifths of all pregnancies result in live births the value of postponing a conception is three fifths the value of postponing a birth.[9] Specifically, if the value of postponing a birth one year is $65, Government should then use less than $39 worth of resources to prevent a pregnancy through birth-control measures.[10]

### Economic cost of reducing births

The resource cost of reducing births is extraordinarily low relative to the apparent economic worth. Estimates of this cost vary, of course, depending on the mix of methods used. For a major

9. The biological distinction between conception and pregnancy is ignored here.

10. This assumed pregnancy wastage of two-fifths does not distinguish between involuntary and induced abortions. Wastage rates in LDCs seem to be much higher than in advanced countries, and certainly higher than reported. Better health measures would reduce mortality at birth, and so raise the worth of preventing or postponing a pregnancy.

national programme stressing a reasonable mix of methods, but with emphasis upon intra-uterine devices (IUDs), over 5 years the annual cost per participant is under $1 and the cost per birth prevented during this half decade is probably $5.

## Costs of methods

Certain methods have a fixed 'starting' cost for initial training, devices, etc., with very low or zero recurrent 'operating' costs thereafter: examples are withdrawal, rhythm, diaphragm, IUD and vasectomy. Other methods have low or zero 'starting' costs but relatively high recurrent costs: examples are condoms, foam tablets and especially pills. Recurrent costs vary with frequency of coitus in the case of condoms and tablets, but not for contraceptive pills.

Table 2, column 1, estimates crudely the cost for each participant over five years, depending upon method. It is assumed that both withdrawal and rhythm require some initial instruction (as noted above). The cost of pills is extremely high compared to other methods. The IUD cost estimate assumes a single insertion and one recheck by a paramedic. The vasectomy cost per year varies inversely with the length of the period considered.

These estimates are of resource cost, assume that participants volunteer without expensive propaganda campaigns, and are independent of whether Government or acceptor pays varying fractions of these costs.

## Cost effectiveness comparisons

Within broad limits it is possible to make cost-effectiveness comparisons of alternative birth-control methods. Rough cost estimates (column 1) must be compared with estimates of effectiveness (column 2). Different methods can be ranked accordingly when the constraint is defined.

A distinction must be made between the *idealised* effectiveness and the *operational* effectiveness of different methods. Some methods that are effective if a couple practises them faithfully as instructed, and notably rhythm, are relatively ineffective where sustained motivation, dependable supply sources or household utilities are lacking. Failure rates for any of the *traditional* methods seem to be higher with poor Asian villagers than with educated and prosperous Westerners. This is not at all true of IUDs and vasectomies, however. Otherwise, lacking good data from primitive cultures, the estimates of column 2 can be little more than intelligent guesses for these methods.[11]

The 5-year costs of column 1, divided by the 5-year effectiveness (pregnancies prevented) estimates of column 2, give the 5-year costs per pregnancy prevented of column 3. These are multiplied by 1·67, allowing for miscarriages, abortions, stillbirths and fatalities shortly after birth, to give the 5-year costs per birth prevented of column 4.

Withdrawal, one of the least effective methods biologically, has supposedly the highest effectiveness per unit cost, because it can be readily explained and involves no purchases or medical treatment. The contraceptive pill, among the most effective methods physiologically, is the worst from an economic viewpoint. As these cost-effectiveness ratios tentatively vary by a factor of 250 times between the most and least costly, and perhaps by a factor of twenty even between rhythm and condom, the choice of a method to stress is important.

Table 2 **Hypothetical costs and effectiveness of alternative contraception measures during a five-year programme**

| | (1) Cost/user (5 years) | (2) Pregnancies prevented (5 years) | (3) Cost each pregnancy prevented | (4) Cost each birth prevented | (5) Births prevented per $1 million, 000 | (6) 'Acceptors' per $1 million, 000 |
|---|---|---|---|---|---|---|
| 0. Zero control | 0 | 0 | 0 | — | — | — |
| 1. Withdrawal | 0·25 | 1·25 | 0·20 | 0·33 | 3000 | 4000 |
| 2. Rhythm | 0·50 | 1·0 | 0·50 | 0·83 | 1200 | 2000 |
| 3. Condom | 12·00 | 1·2 | 10·00 | 16·7 | 60 | 83 |
| 4. Foam tablet | 12·00 | 1·0 | 12·00 | 20·00 | 50 | 83 |
| 5. Diaphragm | 4·50 | 1·5 | 3·00 | 5·00 | 200 | 222 |
| 6. Pills | 90·00 | 1·7 | 52·90 | 88·60 | 11 | 11 |
| 7. IUDs | 2·00 | 1·8 | 1·11 | 1·85 | 540 | 500 |
| 8. Vasectomy | 3·00 | 1·9 | 1·57 | 2·62 | 381 | 333 |

N.B. These magnitudes are good at best to one significant digit. The variable costs assume about 50 exposures a year. No account is taken of possible deaths or reconsorting during the year. Two fifths of all conceptions are assumed to result in early miscarriages, abortions or neo-natal deaths. No allowance is made for drop-outs.

11. The absolute values of col. 2, but not the ranking of methods, are based on the assumption that participants, exposed, pregnable and of representative ages, will have an average fertility of 0·24 a year, allowing for a 0·4 pregnancy and peri-natal wastage.

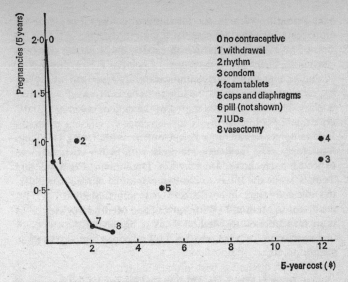

Figure 1 Hypothetical pregnancy reductions and costs associated with different contraceptive methods per acceptor (5-year programme)
Source : Table 2

## What is the best method?

What is the best method depends upon whether the effective constraint of a birth-reduction programme is *budget* or *participants*. Suppose, for example, that the costs and effectiveness of the various methods are again as set out in Table 2. Also assume that the maximum *potential* 'acceptors' in a country is ten million cohabiting women or men.

If acceptors are not the constraint, *i.e.* the budget is the limitation, the 'best' method is that which prevents the most pregnancies per unit cost. Suppose only $1 million is available over 5 years. According to Table 2, column 5, withdrawal is then preferable to all other methods, because 3 million births (5 million pregnancies) are prevented. And the 4 million actual participants shown in column 6 are less than the potential of 10 million.

However, if the budget exceeds $2·5 million over 5 years in this instance the effective constraint will be participants and not funds. Given 10 million actual rather than potential acceptors regardless of method, for each alternative budget over $2·5 million there is a 'best' method that maximizes births prevented. However, at successively higher budgets above $2·5 million the best method in

S. Enke  365

each case will have a lower effectiveness-to-cost ratio. Hence the truly best method is that associated with the best budget. And the best of all budgets is that which equates the cost and worth of preventing births at the margin.

Figure 1 explains this optimization. The vertical axis gives expected pregnancies and the horizontal axis expected costs over 5 years. The scatter points represent the data of columns 1 and 2 of Table 2.[12] Noteworthy is the envelope of efficient methods, linking points representing Zero Control, Withdrawal, IUD and Vasectomy. The inefficient methods, with higher costs or more expected pregnancies, are Rhythm, Diaphragm, Condoms and Tablets, while the Pill is so costly it cannot be plotted. Considering efficient points, in cost-effectiveness terms, Method 7 (IUD) is inferior to Method 1 (Withdrawal), and Method 8 (Vasectomy) is in turn inferior to Method 7, as indicated by the slopes of imaginary rays from the zero point (of no contraceptives) to these scatter points.

But which method is best in marginal terms?

A shift to IUDs from Withdrawal means an extra cost of \$1·75 per acceptor, and an extra pregnancy prevention of 0·55 over 5 years, for a *marginal* cost per pregnancy prevented of \$3·17. Adoption of vasectomy, instead of IUD, means an extra cost of \$1 per participant and an extra 0·1 pregnancy prevented, for a marginal cost of \$10. The question is whether \$3·17 or \$10 best reflects the economic worth of preventing a pregnancy, in the sense of at least postponing it for an average period of 5 years?

Considering even a low-income country with a $V/P$ of \$100 a year, where the value of preventing a birth permanently is around \$250 to \$300, the worth of postponing a pregnancy among participants for 5 years on an average is worth almost \$200.[13] Accordingly, Government would be justified in using \$30 million worth of resources on vasectomies for 10 million men over 5 years, reducing pregnancies by 19 millions during this period. This would be better than spending \$20 million on IUDs, reducing pregnancies by 18 millions, given the assumption of 10 million 'acceptors' regardless of method.

12. Except that column 2 gives expected pregnancies *prevented*, so this value must be substracted from 2·0 (the number of pregnancies expected with *no* birth-control practices) to obtain the ordinate value.

13. Assuming \$263 as the worth of permanent prevention, a fertility rate of 0·24 a year for participants, a 0·6 birth-to-pregnancy ratio and an average postponement of 5 years, then \$263 × 0·24 × 0·6 × 5 gives \$189.

## Preferences of public

Of course, fecund and exposed couples who want to postpone or prevent children are not really indifferent as regards method. Catholics at present are prohibited from any method other than rhythm. Otherwise, often not realising how much contraceptive effectiveness varies among methods, couples who want fewer children will usually prefer the method that 'costs' them least in money, inconvenience and embarrassment.[14]

Thus, Government may have one preference ranking of methods while couples wanting fewer children have differing ranking systems of their own. Politically, Government must usually offer all methods, but this need not preclude it from subsidising one method as against another. Were Government to insert IUDs free, but charge the full price for contraceptive pills, for instance, few participants would use the latter.

The art for Government is only to discourage inefficient methods for which practitioners do not have a strong preference, while encouraging efficient methods for which those who want fewer children do not have a strong revulsion.

## Costs of different mixes of methods

The sensitivity of programme costs to different mixes of methods used is indicated by Table 3. The increasing use of IUDs instead of foams by women, and of vasectomies instead of condoms by men, increases contraceptive effectiveness and reduces cost. There will hopefully be a gradual substitution of 'once-for-all' methods, although requiring individual medical attention, in the place of devices that must be repeatedly supplied and depend for effective use on sustained motivation.

## Magnitude and cost of programmes

The magnitude and cost of a birth-reduction programme will depend, of course, upon goals established by Government. Japan halved its birthrate in 10 years after the Second World War, from 34 to 17 per thousand annually, abortion being widely and openly used; but that nation cannot be considered typical of under-developed countries in Asia or elsewhere. A more probable contraceptive goal might be a one third reduction in crude birth-rates during a decade.

14. Some primitive women do not like to see a male doctor; some couples living with parents do not want them to know contraception is being prac-tised; and poor families may not buy enough birth-control materials in advance.

Achievement of such a goal requires that about half the couples in the procreative age groups, couples over 25 years old being represented somewhat disproportionately, must be effectively practising one or other method of control at any one time.

A typical LDC comprises about 16 men and 16 women per 100 population who are fecund and exposed. Some of these 16 women will not be pregnable in any month, because of pregnancy, or post-partem amenorrhoea. Another substantial fraction will be young couples who want their first boy or girl. If these women who *cannot* conceive or *want* to conceive are deducted, perhaps 8 women (or their partners) per 100 population are 'eligible' in any one month to practise birth control.

Realistically, there will be some rotation of participants among this group, so that perhaps 10 per cent of the population are involved in any year. The cost per 'acceptor' a year varies with the mix of contraceptive methods used, but with Mix B (see Table 3) this is $1. It follows arithmetically that the cost of the national programme per head of population is 10 cents a year.

An annual cost of 10 cents per head means government budgets, assuming all the programme is financed through the State, that are typically about 1 per cent of the economic development programmes in many LDCs. Table 4 gives selected examples. It is astounding to realise that resources having a value of 1 per cent of all those used for development, assuming sufficient participants, could be as effective in raising *per capita* income as the other 99 per cent.[15]

### Using resources and bonuses to increase participation

None of the LDCs currently have 8 women (or their partners) per 100 population practising effective birth control. The number is often not a tenth as large. Sooner or later, as government planners realise how great are the economic advantages to the nation of reducing births, there will be a greater willingness, however, to use resources for public education on contraception. The granting of bonuses to families that practise contraception effectively, or to men who volunteer for a vasectomy, will also become more widespread. It is important also to recognise, in making this choice between education and bonuses, that the latter are transfer payments and have no opportunity production cost.

15. This excludes possible transfer payment bonuses (see p. 370).

Table 3 **Effect of method mix on pregnancies reduced and costs**

| Method mix | A | B | C |
|---|---|---|---|
| *Number of acceptors*, % | | | |
| Condoms – Foams | 70 | 28 | 10 |
| IUDs | 20 | 50 | 60 |
| Vasectomies | 10 | 22 | 30 |
| Reduced pregnancies, 5 years | 132 | 163 | 176 |
| Cost, 5 years per 100 | $910 | $502 | $330 |
| Cost/acceptor/year | $1·82 | $1·0 | $0·66 |
| Cost/reduced pregnancy | $6·90 | $3·08 | $1·88 |

Source: Costs and effectiveness are based on Table 2.

Table 4 **Estimated annual costs of birth-reduction programmes relative to national development budgets for ten selected countries**

| Country | *(1)* Population, 000,000 | *(2)* Estimated cost family planning programme, 000,000 year, $ | *(3)* Total cost development programme 000,000 year, $ | *(4)* Relative cost of programme to reduce births, % |
|---|---|---|---|---|
| Brazil | 80 | 8·0 | 2043 | 0·4 |
| Colombia | 16 | 1·6 | 334 | 0·5 |
| India | 470 | 47·0 | 3921 | 1·2 |
| Korea | 28 | 2·8 | 105 | 2·7 |
| Mexico | 40 | 4·0 | 412 | 1·0 |
| Nigeria | 42 | 4·2 | 227 | 1·9 |
| Pakistan | 107 | 10·7 | 1064 | 1·0 |
| Taiwan | 13 | 1·3 | 149 | 0·9 |
| Tunisia | 5 | 0·5 | 200 | 0·2 |
| Turkey | 30 | 3·0 | 538 | 0·4 |

Col. 1. 1964 estimates.

Col. 2. Population × 10 cents.

Col. 3. Includes United States assistance, country's own contribution and expenditures from other external aid sources expected in financial year 1965.

Col. 4. Col. 2 divided by Col. 3.

*Resources for education*

Various surveys indicate that many simple peoples understand very little about why reproduction occurs and how it can be prevented. The most effective and recent methods of birth control – notably the IUD but also vasectomy – are known but vaguely to a few. Some of this ignorance can be remedied by direct education in secondary schools, to men and women in the civil and military services, and indirectly through radio and movies. However, even if the cost per acceptor a year was thereby *tripled* the annual programme cost would typically be only 3 per cent of all resources used for economic development in a country, and the superior effectiveness ratio could be around 33.

*Bonuses to participants*

It is really much cheaper in terms of resources for Government to encourage participation through offering bonuses that are transfer payments. There is then a transfer of purchasing power from tax-payers to acceptors. Couples who limit births are rewarded by Government in the name of society for behaving more than others in conformity with the public interest.

Such bonuses can be large enough to be influential.

Thus, if the worth of postponing a pregnancy one year is about $39 in a country where $V/P$ is $100 (see p. 362) and the resource cost of a reasonable method mix is $1 per acceptor a year (see Table 3), Government could afford to pay over $30 a year bonus to women who remain non-pregnant. Practically, each participating woman would have to register with a clinic and be superficially examined there each 17 weeks, receiving $10 on each visit if she did not miss her last examination and is again found to be not pregnant (Enke, 1963, p. 377 ff.). How this woman remains non-pregnant is her own affair, but she might well ask for an IUD at the clinic when registering there. And the $30 a year is to her the equivalent of 4 months' *per capita* consumption in her country.

Considerably higher bonuses could be granted to vasectomy volunteers, varying from $260 to $148 (see page 362) in a country where *per capita* income is $100. This could be analogous to a bonus approaching $10,000 in the United States. While the fraction of eligible men who would volunteer as a result might not be high, so large a sum ensures that its availability will be publicised.[16]

16. The bonus-vasectomy programmes in Madras and other Indian States ordinarily require consent of spouse, two surviving children and a waiting period for reconsideration. Vasectomy should not be confused with castration. It affects fertility but not virility, and the operation can be per-

Government, representing all tax-payers, has an interest in making these bonuses less than the full reservation price to the economy. As acceptance of birth reductions became more widespread, these bonus rates could presumably be reduced, sharing more of the gain with society at large. If this shifting 'supply' schedule of participants is relatively elastic, so that the ratio of marginal cost to average cost does not greatly exceed unity, a given budget for these payments will be more effective.[17]

### Other financial incentives

There are other ways in which Government can use funds to extend a birth-reduction programme that partly involve extra resources but also provide generous suppliers' surpluses.

It can offer private doctors generous fees for vasectomies and the insertion of IUDs. It can offer generous fees to midwives and others who 'introduce' new acceptors to the clinics. And it can distribute condoms etc. free to stores and midwives to retail at a generous profit margin.

All such arrangements increase the cost per acceptor, but they also increase the number of participants, and each extra couple reducing births means an extra net product for the economy.

### Conclusion

The main conclusions are important for policy-makers.

1. If economic resources of given value were devoted to retarding population growth, the former resources could be 100 or so times more effective in raising *per capita* incomes in many LDCs.

2. An adequate birth-control programme in these countries might cost as little as ten cents *per capita* yearly, equivalent to about 1 per cent of the cost of current development programmes.

3. The possible use of bonuses to encourage family planning, whether paid in cash or in kind, is obvious in countries where the 'worth' of permanently preventing a birth is roughly twice the income per head. Economists can make a major contribution to

---

formed without hospitalisation and with a local anaesthetic. (See Enke, *Economics for Development*, pp. 379 *et seq.*)

17. It is in the best Pigovian and libertarian tradition that Government should induce individuals to behave socially, whether in the matter of abating smoke nuisances or having fewer children, through the use of special taxes or subsidies.

economic development by refining and explaining such estimates for particular nations.[18]

18. A fair question is whether these same arguments, applied above to LDCs, do not apply equally to More Developed Countries. It is almost certain that *per capita* income would rise faster in the United States if the rate of population increase were lower. But otherwise there are many dissimilarities. First, the burdensome child-dependency ratio is very much a function of the birth-rate, which is much lower in the United States than in LDCs. Second, proportionately more infants survive to productive adulthood in the United States. Third, if interest rates are lower in the United States the productive contributions of adults are discounted less dramatically to time and birth. Fourth, additional natural resources are available in the United States at relatively slight increases in cost of use. Fifth, the United States population is doubling more slowly than in LDCs, giving more time for capital stocks to double and innovations to be made. Sixth, innovations that increase output-to-input ratios seem to be made more rapidly in More Developed Countries. Seventh, and often overlooked, it is mostly the poor and ignorant who have large families and contribute to birth-rates in the US; but they comprise a *minority* of the population instead of the majority (as in LDCs). *They* may need assistance of the kind described in this paper.

## References

BERELSON, B. (1964), 'National family planning programs: a guide', *Studies in Family Planning*, no. 5.

CALDERONE, M.S. (1964), *Manual of Contraceptive Practice*, Williams and Wilkins.

COX, P. R. (1950), *Demography*, Cambridge University Press.

ENKE, S. (1963), *Economics for Development*, Prentice Hall, Part 4.

International Planned Parenthood Federation (1964), *Medical Handbook*.

PERRIN, E. B. and SHEPS, M. C. (1963), 'Human reproduction: a stochastic process', *International Statistical Institute*, August.

TAEUBER, I. B. (1964), 'Asian Populations: the critical decades', *World Academy of Arts and Sciences*.

TIETZE, C. (1962) 'Pregnancy rates and birth rates', *Population Studies*, July.

# Further Reading

These readings are grouped under a number of convenient headings according to the main emphasis of each monograph or paper, but many of these works cover a much wider area of analysis than is suggested by the particular heading they are to be found under.

*General*

S. J. Axelrod (ed.), *The Economics of Health and Medical Care*, University of Michigan Press, 1964.

M. Hauser (ed.), *The Economics of Medical Care*, Allen & Unwin, for the University of York, 1972.

H. E. Klarman, *The Economics of Health*, Columbia University Press, 1964.

H. E. Klarman (ed.), *Empirical Studies in Health Economics*, Johns Hopkins Press, 1970.

G. Myrdal, 'Economic aspects of health', *Chronicles of the World Health Organization*, August, 1952.

R. Stevens, *Medical Practice in Modern England*, University of Yale, 1966.

B. Weisbrod, *Economics of Public Health*, University of Pennsylvania, 1961.

*The nature of the product 'health care'*

M. H. Cooper and A. J. Culyer, *The Price of Blood – An Economic Study of the Charitable and Commercial Principle*, Institute of Economic Affairs, 1968.

A. J. Culyer, 'On the relative efficiency of the National Health Service', *Kyklos*, vol. 25, 1972, no. 2.

S. J. Mushkin, 'Towards a definition of health economics', *Pub. Health Reports*, vol. 73, 1958, no. 9.

R. M. Titmuss, 'Ethics and the economics of medical care', *Medical Care*, vol. 1, 1963, no. 1.

R. M. Titmuss, *The Gift Relationship*, Allen & Unwin, 1971.

*The value of life*

J. A. Dowie, 'Valueing the benefits of health improvement', *Australian Economic Papers*, June 1970.

L. J. Dublin and A. J. Lotka, *The Money Value of a Man*, Ronald Press, 1946.

G. Fromm, 'Comment on Schelling's Paper', in S. B. Chase (ed.), *Problems in Public Expenditure Analysis*, Brookings Institution, 1968.

E. J. Mishan, 'Evaluation of life and limb: a theoretical approach', *J. of Pol. Econ.*, vol. 79, 1971, no. 4.

D. J. Reynold, 'The cost of road accidents', *J. of the Royal Stat. Soc.*, vol. 119, 1956, series A, pp. 393–408.

J. Thédié and C. Abraham, 'Economic aspects of road accidents' *Traffic Engineering and Control*, vol. 2, 1961, pp. 589–95.

## Welfare economics of medical care

K. J. Arrow, 'Uncertainty and the welfare economics of medical care: reply – the implications of transactions, costs and adjustment lags', *Amer. Econ. Rev.*, vol. 55, 1965, no. 1.

K. J. Arrow, 'Economics of moral hazard: further comment', *Amer. Econ. Rev.*, vol. 58, 1968, no. 3.

M. Crew, 'Coinsurance and the welfare economics of medical care', *Amer. Econ. Rev.*, vol. 59, 1969, no. 4.

A. J. Culyer, 'Medical care and the economics of giving', *Economica*, vol. 38, 1971, no. 151.

M. Grossman, 'On the concept of health capital and the demand for wealth', *J. of Pol. Econ.*, vol. 80, 1972, no. 2.

D. S. Lees and R. G. Rice, 'Uncertainty and the welfare economics of medical care', *Amer. Econ. Rev.*, vol. 55, 1965, no. 1.

C. M. Lindsay, 'Medical care and the economics of sharing', *Economica*, vol. 36, 1969, no. 144.

M. V. Pauly, *Medical Care at Public Expense – A Study in Applied Welfare Economics*, Praeger, 1971.

M. V. Pauly, 'The economics of moral hazard: comment', *Amer. Econ. Rev.*, vol. 58, 1968, no. 3.

J. Rothenberg, 'Welfare implications of alternative methods of financing medical care', *Amer. Econ. Rev.*, vol. 41, 1951, no. 2, proceedings (May).

## Need and demand for health care

K. E. Boulding, 'The concept of need for health services', *Millbank Memorial Fund Quarterly*, vol. 44, 1966, no. 4.

M. H. Cooper, 'Rationing and financing health care resources', in N. Hunt and W. D. Reekie (eds.), *Management and the Social Services*, Tavistock Press for the University of Edinburgh, 1972.

A. J. Culyer, 'Assessing government expenditure on health: the problems of need and demand', *Pub. Finance*, vol. 27, 1972, no. 3.

P. Feldstein, 'The demand for medical care' in *Report of the Commission on the Cost of Medical Care*, American Medical Association, 1964.

G. Forsyth and R. F. L. Logan, *The Demand for Medical Care*, Oxford University, 1960.

I. R. Gough, 'Poverty and health – a review article', *Soc. and Econ. Admin.*, vol. 4, 1970, no. 3.

T. Kelly and G. Schieber, *Factors Affecting Health Services Utilization: A Behavioural Approach*, Urban Institute, 1971.

Office of Health Economics, *Without Prescription*, Office of Health Economics, 1970.

Office of Health Economics, *Building for Health*, Office of Health Economics, 1970.

Office of Health Economics, *Prospects for Health*, Office of Health Economics, 1971.

D. Paige and K. Jones, *Health and Welfare Services in Britain in 1975*, Cambridge University for the National Institute of Economic and Social Research, 1966.

M. Rein, 'Social class and the utilization of medical care services', *Hospitals*, vol. 43, 1969, pp. 43–54.

G. D. Rosenthal, *The Demand for General Hospital Facilities*, American Hospital Association, 1964.

G. Teeling-Smith, 'Health, wealth and happiness', *Soc. and Econ. Admin.*, vol. 6, 1972, no. 2.

G. C. Wirick, 'A multiple-equation model of the demand for health care', *Health Services Research*, Winter, 1966.

G. C. Wirick and R. Barlow, 'The economic and social determinants of the demand for health services', in Axelrod (ed)., *op. cit.*, 1964.

*The costs of health*

American Medical Association, *Report of the Commission on the Cost of Medical Care*, American Medical Association, 1964.

M. H. Cooper, 'How to pay for the health service', *Journal of the Royal Society of Health*, vol. 91, 1971, no. 5.

J. T. Dunlop, 'The capacity of the United States to provide and finance expanding health services', *Bull. of the New York Academy of Medicine*, December, 1965

F. R. L. Logan, 'Paying for medical care', *Lancet*, September, 1970.

S. J. Mushkin and F. d'A. Collings, 'Economic costs of disease and injury', *Pub. Health Reports*, September, 1959.

Office of Health Economics, *The Costs of Medical Care*, Office of Health Economics, 1964.

Office of Health Economics, *Work Lost through Sickness*, Office of Health Economics, 1965.

Ff. Roberts, *The Cost of Health*, Turnstile Press, 1952.

C. E. A. Winslow, *The Cost of Sickness and the Price of Health*, World Health Organization, 1951.

US Public Health Service, *Medical Care Financing and Utilization*, US Government.

*Shortage and medical manpower*

B. Abel-Smith and K. Gales, *British Doctors at Home and Abroad*, Codicote Press, 1964.

R. Fein, *The Doctor Shortage, An Economic Diagnosis*, Brookings Institution, 1967.

M. S. Feldstein, 'The rising price of physicians' services', *Rev. of Econ. and Stat.*, vol. 52, 1970, no. 2.

W. L. Hanson, 'Shortages and investment in health manpower', in Axelrod (ed.), *op. cit.*, 1964.

R. A. Kessel, 'Price Discrimination in Medicine', *J. of Law and Econ.*, vol. 1, October, 1958.

H. E. Klarman, 'Economic aspects of projecting requirements for health manpower', *J. of Hum. Res.*, vol. 4, 1969, no. 3.

Office of Health Economics, *Medical Manpower*, Office of Health Economics, 1966.

A. T. Peacock and J. R. Shannon, 'The new doctors' dilemma', *Lloyds Bank Rev.*, January, 1968.

*Organization of health care*

B. Abel-Smith and R. M. Titmuss, *The Cost of the National Health Service in England and Wales*, Cambridge University, 1956.

American Medical Association, 'National health care – the gathering storm', *Medical News*, October, 1969.

R. and O. W. Anderson, *A Decade of Health Services*, University of Chicago, 1967.

British Medical Association, *Health Service Financing*, British Medical Association, 1970.

J. M. Buchanan, *Inconsistencies of the National Health Service*, Institute of Economic Affairs, 1964.

R. and W. Campbell, 'Compulsory health insurance: the economic issues', *Q. J. of Econ.*, vol. 66, 1952, no. 1.

M. H. Cooper and A. J. Culyer, 'An economic assessment of some aspects of the operation of the National Health Service', in British Medical Association, *Health Services Financing*, British Medical Association, 1970.

M. H. Cooper and A. J. Culyer, 'An economic survey of the nature and intent of the National Health Service', *Social Science and Medicine*, vol. 5, 1971, no. 1.

T. E. Chester, 'How healthy is the National Health Service?', *Lloyds Bank Rev.*, September, 1966.

A. J. Culyer, 'The "market" versus the "state" in medical care – a minority report on an empty academic box', in G. McLachlan (ed.), *Problems and Progress in Medical Care*, Oxford University Press, 1972.

Feldstein, M. S. 'An economic model of the medicare system', *Q. J. of Econ.*, Feb. 1971, no. 1.

S. Harris, *The Economics of American Medicine*, Macmillan, 1964.

J. and S. Jewkes, *The Genesis of the British National Health Service*, Blackwell, 1961.

J. and S. Jewkes, *Value for Money in Medicine*, Blackwell, 1963.

D. S. Lees, 'The economics of health services', *Lloyds Bank Review*, April, 1960.

D. S. Lees, 'The logic of the British National Health Service', *J. of Law and Econ.*, vol. 5, October, 1962.

D. S. Lees, 'Health through choice', reprinted with postscript in R. Harris (ed.), *Freedom or Free-for-all*, Institute of Economic Affairs, 1965.

D. S. Lees, 'Health services financing report: review', *British Medical J.*, 31st October, 1970.

R. J. Myers, *Medicare*, Irwin for the McCahan Foundation, 1970.

A. Seldon, *After the National Health Service*, Institute of Economic Affairs, 1968.

H. M. and A. R. Somers, *Doctors, Patients and Health Insurance*, Brookings Institution, 1961.

H. M. and A. R. Somers, *Medicare and the Hospitals*, Brookings Institution, 1968.

*Hospital economics*

R. E. Berry, 'Returns to scale in the production of hospital services', *Hospital Services Research*, Summer, 1969.

W. J. Carr and P. J. Feldstein, 'The relationship of cost to hospital size', *Inquiry*, June, 1967.

H. A. Cohen, 'Variations in cost among hospitals of different sizes', *Southern Econ. J.*, January, 1967.

K. Davis, 'Economic theories of behavior in non-profit, private hospitals', *Economic and Business Bull.*, vol. 24, 1972, no. 1.

J. S. Deeble, 'Economic analysis of hospital costs', *Medical Care*, vol. 3, 1968, no. 3.

M. S. Feldstein, 'Hospital planning and the demand for care', *Oxford Bull. of Stat.*, vol. 26, 1964, no. 4.

M. S. Feldstein, 'Studying hospital costliness', *Hospital Service Finance*, January, 1965.

M. S. Feldstein, *Economic Analysis for Health Service Efficiency*, North Holland, 1967.

W. J. McNerney (ed.), *Hospital and Medical Economics*, Hospital and Educational Trust, 1962.

C. Montacute, *Costing and Efficiency in Hospitals*, Oxford University, 1962.

Office of Health Economics, *Hospital Costs in Perspective*, Office of Health Economics, 1963.

Office of Health Economics, *Efficiency in the Hospital Service*, Office of Health Economics, 1967.

J. A. Rafferty, 'Patterns of hospital use – an analysis of short-run variations', *J. of Pol. Econ.*, vol. 79, 1971, no. 1.

M. Reder, 'Some problems in the economics of hospitals', *Amer. Econ. Rev.*, vol. 55, 1965, no. 2, proceedings.

M. I. Roemer and M. Shain, *Hospital Utilization under Insurance*, American Medical Association, 1959.

B. A. Weisbrod, 'Some problems of pricing and resource allocation in a non-profit industry – the hospitals', *J. of Bus.*, vol. 38, January, 1965.

B. A. Weisbrod and B. J. Feiser, 'Hospitalization, insurance and hospital utilization', *Amer. Econ. Rev.*, vol. 51, 1961, no. 126.

*Variations in health provision*

B. E. Coates and E. M. Rawstron, *Regional Variations in Britain*, Batsford, 1971.

M. H. Cooper and A. J. Culyer, 'Equality and the National Health Service: intentions, performance and problems in evaluation', in M. Hauser (ed.), *The Economics of Medical Care*, Allen & Unwin, 1972.

M. S. Feldstein, 'Hospital bed scarcity: an analysis of the effects of interregional differences', *Economica*, vol. 32, 1965, no. 128.

A. K. Maynard, 'Inequalities in psychiatric care in England and Wales', *Social Science and Medicine*, vol. 6, 1972, no. 3.

## Effectiveness and efficiency

A. L. Cochrane, *Effectiveness and Efficiency: Random Reflections in the Health Services*, Nuffield Provincial Hospitals Trust, 1972.

A. J. Culyer and A. K. Maynard, 'The costs of dangerous drugs legislation in England and Wales', *Medical Care*, vol. 4, 1970, no. 3.

M. S. Feldstein, *Economic Analysis for Health Service Efficiency*, North Holland, 1967.

D. S. Lees, 'Efficiency in government spending – social services: health', *Pub. Finance*, vol. 22, 1967, no. 1.

S. J. Mushkin and B. A. Weisbrod, 'Investment in health – life-time health expenditures on the 1960 work force', *Kyklos*, vol. 16, 1963, no. 4.

M. V. Pauly, 'Efficiency, incentives and the reimbursement for health care', *Inquiry*, Spring, 1970.

M. Reder, 'Some problems in the measurement of productivity in the medical care industry', in V. Fuchs (ed.), *Production and Productivity in the Service Industries*, Columbia University, 1969.

M. Reinhardt, 'A production function for physicians' services', *Rev. of Econ. and Stat.*, vol. 54, 1972, no. 1.

K. R. Smith, *et al.*, 'An analysis of the optimum use of inputs in the production of medical services', *J. of Hum. Res.*, vol. 7, 1972, no. 3.

J. Wiseman, 'Cost benefit analysis and health service policy', in A. T. Peacock and D. J. Robertson (eds.), *Public Expenditure: Appraisal and Control*, Oliver & Boyd, 1963.

D. E. Yett, 'An evaluation of alternative methods of estimating physicians' expenses relative to output', *Inquiry*, March, 1967.

## Studies of particular disorders

I. S. Blumenthal, *Research and the Ulcer Problem*, Rand McNally, 1959.

R. Fein, *Economics of Mental Illness*, Joint Commission on Mental Illness and Health Monograph, series no. 2, 1958, Basic Books.

A. G. Holtmann, 'Estimating the demand for public health services: the alcoholism case', *Pub. Finance*, vol. 19, 1964, no. 4.

H. E. Klarman, 'Syphilis control programs', in R. Dorfman (ed.) *Measuring Benefits of Government Investments*, Brookings Institution, 1965.

Office of Health Economics, *The Price of Poliomyelitis*, Office of Health Economics, 1963.

Office of Health Economics, *The Cost of Mental Care*, OHE, 1965.

Office of Health Economics, *Progress in Mental Health*, OHE, 1967.

Office of Health Economics, *Old Age*, OHE, 1968.

Office of Health Economics, *Obesity and Disease*, OHE, 1969.

Office of Health Economics, *Alcohol Abuse*, OHE, 1970.

Office of Health Economics, *Epilepsy in Society*, OHE, 1971.

Office of Health Economics, *Migraine*, OHE, 1972.

Office of Health Economics, *Hypertension, a Suitable Case for Treatment?* OHE, 1972.

B. A. Weisbrod, 'Costs and benefits of medical research: a case study of poliomyelitis', *J. of Pol. Econ.*, vol. 79, 1971, no. 3.

*Constructing health indices*

R. A. Bauer (ed.), *Social Indicators*, MIT Press, 1966.

W. J. Cohen, 'Social indicators', *Amer. Statistician*, vol. 22, 1968, no. 4.

A. J. Culyer, 'Indicators of health – an economist's viewpoint', in Office of Health Economics, *Evaluation in the Health Service*, OHE, 1972.

A. J. Culyer, R. J. Lavers, and A. Williams, 'Social indicators: health', *Social Trends*, vol. 1, 1971, no. 2.

A. Donabedian, 'Evaluating the quality of medical care', *Millbank Memorial Fund Quarterly*, July 1966.

M. Magdelaine, A. Mizrahi and E. Roesch, 'Un indicateur de la marbilite', *Consommation*, CREDOC, no. 2, April/June, 1967.

C. A. Moser, 'Measuring the quality of life', *New Society*, 10th December, 1970.

A. H. Packer, 'Applying cost-effectiveness concepts to the community health system', *Operations Research*, vol. 16, 1968, no. 2.

D. F. Sullivan, *Conceptual Problems in Developing an Index of Health*, National Center for Health Statistics, 1966, Series no. 2, no. 17.

World Health Organization, *Measurement of Levels of Health*, WHO, 1957.

### Health planning in developing countries

R. Barlow, 'The economic effects of malaria eradication', *Amer. Econ. Rev.*, vol. 57, 1967, no. 2.

S. Enke, 'Leibenstein on the benefits and costs of birth control programmes', *Population Studies*, vol. 24, 1970, no. 1.

M. S. Feldstein, 'Health sector planning in developing countries', *Economica*, vol. 37, 1970, no. 146.

H. Leibenstein, 'Pitfalls in benefit-cost analysis of birth prevention', *Population Studies*, vol. 23, 1969, no. 2.

H. Leibenstein, 'More on pitfalls: reply:', *Population Studies*, vol. 24, 1970, no. 1.

M. Perlman, 'Some economic aspects of public health programs in underdeveloped areas', in S. J. Axelrod (ed.), *op. cit.*, 1964.

# Acknowledgements

Permission to reproduce the following readings in this volume is acknowledged to the following sources:

1 American Economic Association
2 The Clarendon Press
3 *Economica*
4 University of Chicago Press
5 Milbank Memorial Fund
6 Johns Hopkins Press Inc.
7 J. P. Lippincott Co.
8 J. P. Lippincott Co.
9 American Economic Association
10 J. P. Lippincott Co.
11 University of Chicago Press
12 The Brookings Institution
13 *Journal of Transport Economics and Policy*
14 Her Majesty's Stationery Office
15 *Economic Journal* and Professor S. Enke

# Author Index

Ezdorf, R. H. von, 110

Fabricant, S., 93
Farmer, A. W., 149
Fein, R., 112, 121, 127
Feldstein, M. S., 49, 64, 215, 223, 224, 226, 246, 247, 248, 260, 278, 288, 290
Feldstein, P. J., 194, 199, 276, 277, 284, 285, 287, 290
Field, M. G., 23, 26
Fisher, F. M., 217
Fisher, I., 111, 123, 124
Folk, H., 188
Forshall, I., 151
Friedman, M., 16, 28, 283, 290

Garfinkle, S., 109
Gilbert, M., 248
Goldberg, E. M., 154
Goldberger, A. S., 210, 217
Gottlieb, S. R., 283
Gough, I. R., 66
Government Actuary, 347
Grant, E. S., 161
Griliches, Z., 164
Guillebaud Committee, 260

Haefner, D. P., 163
Hansen, W. L., 179, 180, 181
Hawley, K. S., 205
Head, J. C., 64
Health Information Foundation, 103
Henderson, A., 121
Hettinger, J., 99
Hill, E. S., 130
Hirshleifer, J., 175, 249, 287, 289
Hochman, H. M., 65
Hood, W. C., 217
Hoel, P. G., 269
Home Office Reports, 344
Hoover, E. M., 122
Hunkman, J., 353

Igdravidez, P. G., 124

Ingbar, M. L., 276, 278–89
Interdepartmental Committee on Social and Economic Research, 347
International Planned Parenthood Federation, 372
Israel, S., 52

Johnson, R. H., 145
Johnston, J., 192, 217, 290
Jeffcoate, G. O., 356
Jewkes, J., and S., 49

Kaiser, R. F., 149
Kemp, D. A., and M. S., 353
Kendall, M. G., 267, 269
Kessel, R. A., 13, 30, 40, 70
Kirscht, J. P., 163
Klarman, H. E., 49, 52, 136, 137, 158, 162, 210
Klein, L. R., 217
Kleingartner, A., 205
Klem, M. C., 125
Koopmans, T. C., 16, 217
Koos, E. L., 96
Krementz, E. T., 149
Kruger, D. H., 205
Kurtz, R., 283
Kutner, A. G., 150
Kuznets, S., 28

Laitin, H., 127
Lawley, D. N., 267
Lawrence, R. A., 151
Lear, W. J., 125
Lees, D. S., 49, 54, 62, 63
Lees, F. S., 124
Leftwich, R. H., 283
Leibenstein, H., 76
Lerner, M., 168
Leveson, I., 215, 283
Levine, E., 192
Lewison, E. F., 150
Lindsay, C. M., 49, 63, 66
Lindsay, M. I., 150
Little, I. M. D., 14

# Subject Index

## Analytical Welfare Economics

D. M. Winch

Professor Winch writes on the major issues of welfare economics, ranging from the pure theory of welfare maximization in a Pareto setting to the 'real world' issues of economic policy in a political context. Rigorous theoretical tools are developed to provide a basis for policy recommendation. In Part One, the author develops the formal theory of welfare maximization in geometric terms. Special attention is given to the relationships between commodity space and utility space. A critical assessment of the alleged optimality of perfect competition is offered in Part Two. Here stress is laid on the importance of distinctions between factor, goods, income and utility distributions. Part Three is concerned with the assessment of changes in welfare. The theory of surplus and the compensation principle are rigorously analysed from both theoretical and applied viewpoints. To end his cogent analysis, Professor Winch examines the objectives of full employment, stable prices and economic growth in terms of the Pareto welfare function.

D. M. Winch is Professor of Economics, McMaster University, Ontario, Canada.

## Public Enterprise

Edited by R. Turvey

That the public sector is a consumer of resources and a producer of goods and services is apparent. But the methods of ensuring efficiency in public corporations are not obvious. Public enterprise may aim at social as well as commercial ends in conjunction with a private sector which is all too often imperfect in structure and behaviour. This volume of Readings is deliberately selective and provocative in an area where there is much confusion and disagreement.

'I can start by repeating what I said about another book in this series. This is an excellent collection of articles, marvellous value for money, and indispensable reading for the student and interested layman.'

R. Turvey, recently Deputy-Chairman of the National Board for Prices and Incomes, was formerly economist to the Electricity Council and Reader at the London School of Economics. He is the author of *Interest Rates and Asset Prices* and *The Economics of Real Property*

# Cost Benefit Analysis

Edited by R. Layard

Should India build a new steel mill, or London an urban motorway?
Should higher education expand, or water supplies be improved?
These are typical questions about which cost-benefit analysis has
something to say. It is the main tool that economics provides for
analysing problems of social choice. Its study is also an easy way of
seeing what welfare economics is all about.

This book of Readings covers all the main problems that arise in a
typical cost-benefit exercise. Part One surveys the field while Part
Two deals with the valuation of costs and benefits when they occur.
Part Three discusses social discount rate and the social opportunity
cost of capital. The treatment of risk and income distribution is
analysed in Parts Four and Five. The last Part contains a case study
on the location of the Third London Airport. The editor has written
a long elementary introduction to the subject and the Readings,
showing how they might help one to tackle a specific illustrative
problem.

Richard Layard is Lecturer in Economics at the London School of
Economics.